Evaluating
Treatment
Environments

HEALTH, MEDICINE, AND SOCIETY

A WILEY-INTERSCIENCE SERIES

DAVID MECHANIC, Editor

Rudolf H. Moos *Evaluating Treatment Environments: A Social Ecological Approach*

Rudolf H. Moos

Evaluating
Treatment
Environments

A SOCIAL ECOLOGICAL APPROACH

A Wiley-Interscience Publication

JOHN WILEY & SONS, New York • London • Sydney • Toronto

Library of Congress Cataloging in Publication Data:

Moos, Rudolf H   1934-
     Evaluating treatment environments.

     (Health, medicine, and society: a Wiley-Interscience series)
     "A Wiley-Interscience publication."
     Includes bibliographies.
     1. Psychiatric hospitals—Sociological aspects.
     2. Psychiatric clinics—Sociological aspects.
I. Title. [DNLM: 1. Milieu therapy. WM420 M825e 1973]

RC439.M75 1974   362.2'1   73-17450
ISBN 0-471-61503-X

Printed in the United States of America
10 9 8 7 6 5 4 3 2 1

For my Mother and Father,
Herta and Henry Moos,
who told me I could

PREFACE

This book presents a new approach to the comparison and evaluation of treatment milieus. I call it a social ecological approach with some misgiving, since new terms may lead to confusion as well as to clarification. But I believe that the basic focus and organization of this work are unique. A new way of measuring and changing treatment milieus is offered, and ways of relating the characteristics of these milieus to adaptation and functioning are outlined.

In brief, social ecology is concerned with both human adaptation and human milieus. It deals with both the physical and the social environments. I define social ecology as the multidisciplinary study of the impacts of physical and social environments on human beings. Primarily concerned with the assessment and development of optimum human milieus, social ecology provides a distinctive "point of entry" into relevant clinical and applied problems. As I see it, it combines basic research approaches with a dedication to resolving common human problems. For me, the quality of life for patients and staff in psychiatric treatment settings is as significant as the objective empirical and statistical results.

The social and behavioral sciences are now as ever in a state of rapid development. Certain of these developments have influenced me most. In my clinical work I quickly found that I could not understand, much less predict, the behavior of my patients in settings other than my office. Even a decade ago the research literature and my colleagues had convinced me that this was a common problem. I was dissatisfied then with trait notions of personality, much as others are now. I felt that behavior was influenced by situational and environmental forces to a much greater degree than was commonly recognized, at least by psychologists.

About six years ago I became convinced of the importance of deriving alternative methods by which human environments could be understood. I felt that an understanding of human environments would have to precede the assessment of the impact of these environments on human adaptation.

My overall aim is to identify environments that promote opportunities for personal growth, simultaneously enhancing both physical and psychological well-being.

Two thrusts of this work are most important to me. First, research is utilized in a practical, applied manner. Our work illustrates not only that relatively "hard-nosed" objective research can be made interesting and informative to patients and staff, but that it can be utilized by them to improve their own competence in changing their social milieus in directions they themselves desire. In this sense our work is relevant to the task of bettering the quality of life for patients and staff in treatment programs and, presumably, for individuals participating in a broad range of other environments. Second, the distinctive conceptual and theoretical overviews that grew out of the empirical work should help to stimulate and organize further work in this area. Most important, there are similar underlying patterns in a wide range of social environments, and the various methods by which previous workers have attempted to study human environments can be conveniently categorized into six broad types. My hopes and my fears are one: that this work and these concepts will encourage and stimulate their own replacement.

THE BOOK IN BRIEF

This book discusses the development and utility of new methods for evaluating the social milieus of hospital-based and community-based treatment programs in the context of two new broad conceptual overviews that identify underlying theories and patterns of human environments. Part One introduces our concepts. Parts Two and Three focus on the social milieus of hospital-based programs and community-based programs, respectively. Part four summarizes the empirical work and discusses its implications.

Chapter 1 introduces social ecology as a new approach to the study of human milieus and human adaptation. The overall concepts are presented. Naturalistic and evaluative studies of treatment milieus are summarized, evidence that individual behavior varies significantly across settings is considered, and approaches to the measurement of treatment environments are discussed.

In Chapter 2 we discuss the development of the Ward Atmosphere Scale (WAS), which assesses the treatment environments of hospital-based treatment programs. Chapter 3 describes the samples of hospital-based programs that were utilized in collecting information about the current range and variety of treatment milieus. Cross-cultural comparisons of American and British treatment programs and of American and British values regarding ideal treatment programs are made. Chapter 4 deals with the practical utility of measuring social environments; it presents both detailed clinical WAS profile interpretations and a paradigm for utilizing WAS data for the purposes of teaching and encouraging social change. Chapter 5 outlines several relevant program evaluation and program change studies.

In chapter 6 we consider the relationship between the treatment environment and other dimensions characterizing hospital-based programs— that is, structural characteristics (size and staffing), program policies (the amount of adult status allowed patients), and the behavioral characteristics of the patients (the extent of disturbed behavior). Chapter 7 covers work assessing the differential effects of treatment environments. Treatment environments are studied in relation to patient and staff morale and liking for one another, opportunities for the enhancement of self-esteem and personal development, modes of adaptation and coping, and the utilization of different styles of helping behavior. Chapter 8 discusses work that connects treatment environment to objective indices of treatment outcome as assessed by program dropout, release, and community tenure rates. Three perceived climate indices linking these three outcome measures to treatment environments are derived. Chapter 9 deals with two major issues. The first concerns the accuracy of individual perceptions of an environment and the extent to which individuals who perceive an environment in a deviant manner react differently to it. The second issue involves the discrepancy between an individual's perception of a treatment milieu and his views of an ideal treatment milieu.

Part Three is devoted to the social environments of such community-based treatment programs as halfway houses, community care homes, rehabilitation workshops, and day hospitals. Chapter 10 discusses the Community-Oriented Programs Environment Scale (COPES), which assesses the social milieus of community-based treatment programs on 10 dimensions directly parallel to those utilized in the WAS. An informative comparison between the social environments of programs with and without professional staff is made. In Chapter 11 we attempt to determine the clinical utility of COPES in providing feedback about the treatment milieu to members and staff. A useful paradigm for the facilitation and evaluation of social change in treatment settings is presented. Evidence is given that published descriptions of programs do not accurately portray the characteristics of their treatment environments, and guidelines for compiling more useful and complete program descriptions are supplied.

In Chapter 12 we discuss work in community-based programs that replicates and extends the work in hospital-based programs—for example, data indicating that structural and organizational dimensions of programs (e.g., size, staffing, cost) are highly related to their treatment milieus. The effects of deviant perceptions and expectations are discussed. Chapter 13 brings up issues of homogeneity and congruence in treatment settings. Evidence suggests that the average perception and value congruence both among and between patients and staff in treatment programs is considerably greater than the hypothesis of random selection would lead us to expect. Correlates of the degree of perception and value congruence in different programs are presented.

In Part Four, an overview of the ideas, we discuss the conceptual developments that have arisen from this work. Chapter 14 summarizes the empirical work and presents relevant implications for individual clinical practice, for self-initiated change in treatment settings, and for new types of research designs for more comprehensive comparisons and evaluations of both psychiatric and other "treatment" programs. We briefly discuss our work in the Social Ecology Laboratory in other types of social environments. Our idea that the underlying patterns of different social environments are similar is amplified. The relevance of the underlying concepts for comparing different treatment programs and for studying other social environments along commensurate dimensions is explored.

In summary, the most distinctive features of this book include: (1) the use of similar techniques for assessing the treatment environments of both hospital-based and community-based programs on commensurate dimensions; (2) the explicit emphasis on both subjective (i.e., satisfaction, morale, helping behavior) and objective (i.e., dropout, release, and community tenure rates) effects of treatment programs; (3) the emphasis on the clinical utility of research data about program milieus as an aid to teaching, to planning new and innovative approaches to treatment, to identifying trouble spots, and to successfully helping patients and staff change their own social environments; (4) the preparation of guidelines for the compilation of more useful and more complete program descriptions; (5) an emphasis on program homogeneity and congruence that has implications for the high proportion of patients who prematurely terminate or drop out of treatment programs; (6) an emphasis on cross-cultural applications and comparisons of treatment programs, with particular relevance to British and American treatment milieus; and (7) an integration into the literature on treatment environments of relevant research approaches in other institutions.

RUDOLF H. MOOS

Stanford University School of Medicine
Stanford, California
July 1973

ACKNOWLEDGMENTS

My general intellectual debts are too heavy and too numerous to detail. My bibliographic citations give some limited idea of those who have most strongly influenced my thinking. The research was generously supported in part by NIMH Grant MH 16026 and MH 8304, in part by NIAAA Grant AA 00498, and in part by Palo Alto Veterans Administration Hospital Research funds. The work profited considerably from active collaborations with Marvin Gerst, Peter Houts, Paul Insel, Edison Trickett, and Jack Sidman. These individuals provided a rich, stimulating source of new ideas and ever-present challenges. Gordon Adams facilitated significantly the early phases of the work; Marilyn Cohen, Diane House, Susan Lang, Eleanor Levine, Martha Merk, Chris Newhams, Phyllis Nobel, and Karl Schonborn each engaged in a myriad of important tasks. Jim Stein and Bill Lake coordinated the initial computer analyses.

During the last two years of the project the bulk of the detailed work was carried out by Marguerite Kaufman, Jean Otto, Charles Petty, Paul Sommers, Robert Shelton, and Penny Smail. David Mechanic and Richard Price read and competently criticized an earlier draft of the book. Their comments helped me improve and clarify several chapters. Marion Langenberg typed the initial chapter drafts, Susan Glebus and Marcia Insel typed the second drafts, and Louise Doherty and Susanne Flynn typed and organized the final drafts.

David Hamburg, Chairman of the Psychiatry Department at Stanford University, deserves special recognition. For more than a decade he provided the social milieu in which this work flourished. George Coeblo luckily recognized the potential of the work and was instrumental in helping me obtain initial funding. My wife Bernice contributed greatly to the statistical analysis and compilation of the data. Without Bernice, Karen, and Kevin, I might unhappily have finished this book somewhat sooner. They interrupted me, teased me, annoyed me, infuriated me, gumbled and gamboled—and thereby brought me joy.

R. H. M.

CREDITS

Portions of the text have been adapted from the following sources:

R. H. Moos and P.S. Houts, "Assessment of the Social Atmospheres of Psychiatric Wards," *Journal of Abnormal Psychology*, **73** (6): 595-604, 1968. [Pages 36 through 39 in this book.]

W. D. Pierce, E. J. Trickett, and R. H. Moos, "Changing Ward Atmosphere Through Staff Discussion of the Perceived Ward Environment," *Archives of General Psychiatry*, **26:** 35-41, 1972. Copyright 1972, American Medical Association. [Pages 93 through 96.]

P. S. Houts and R. H. Moos, "The Development of a Ward Initiative Scale for Patients," *Journal of Clinical Psychology*, **25** (3): 319-322, July 1969. [Pages 151 through 152.]

J. Sidman and R. H. Moos, "On the Relation Between Psychiatric Ward Atmosphere and Helping Behavior," *Journal of Clinical Psychology*, **29** (1): 74-78, January 1973. [Pages 164 through 166.]

R. H. Moos, R. Shelton and C. Petty, "Perceived Ward Climate and and Treatment Outcome," *Journal of Abnormal Psychology*, **82** (2): 291-298, 1973. [Pages 180 through 189.]

R. H. Moos, "Assessment of the Psychosocial Environments of Community-Oriented Psychiatric Treatment Programs," *Journal of Abnormal Psychology*, **79** (1): 9-18, 1972. [Pages 228 through 232.]

R. H. Moos, "Changing the Social Milieus of Psychiatric Treatment Settings," *Journal of Applied Behavioral Science*, **9** (5): 575-593, 1973. Reproduced by special permission. [Pages 255 through 261 and 265 through 267.]

CONTENTS

Evaluating
Treatment
Environments

PART ONE

*Conceptual
Overview*

Chapter One

CHARACTERIZING
TREATMENT ENVIRONMENTS

Rudolf H. Moos and Penny Smail

THE IMPACT OF TREATMENT ENVIRONMENTS

That treatment environments have a critical impact on the patients and staff who live and function in them is hardly an original notion. In modern times this idea can be traced to Dr. Philippe Pinel, who in 1792 removed the chains and shackles from the inmates of two Paris insane asylums. Most of the patients stopped being violent once they were free to move around. Pinel pointed out that the normal reactions of men to the situation of being restrained or tied up are fear, anger, and an attempt to escape. Pinel applied "moral treatment," in which it was assumed that the social or treatment environment (tolerant and accepting attitudes, setting examples of appropriate behavior, humanitarianism, and loving care) affects recovery from insanity. He stated:

> I saw a great number of maniacs assembled together and submitted to a regular system of discipline. Their disorders presented an endless variety of character; but their . . . disorders were marshalled into order and harmony. I then discovered that insanity was curable in many instances by mildness of treatment and attention to the mind exclusively. . . . I saw with wonder the resources of nature when left to herself or skillfully assisted in her efforts. . . . Attention to these principles of moral treatment alone will frequently not only lay the foundation of, but complete, a cure; while neglect of them may exasperate each succeeding paroxysm, till, at length, the disease becomes established, continued in its form and incurable. (Pinel, 1806).

In 1806 the Quaker William Tuke established the York Retreat in England, emphasizing an atmosphere of kindness and consideration, meaningful employment of time, regular exercise, a family environment, and the treatment of patients as guests. The Quakers brought moral treatment to America, and Charles Dickens (1842) noted the results in a lively descriptive account of his visit to the Institution of South Boston, now known as the Boston State Hospital.

> The State Hospital for the insane is admirably conducted on . . . enlightened principles of conciliation and kindness. . . . Every patient in this asylum sits down to dinner every day with a knife and fork . . . at every meal moral influence alone restrains the more violent among them from cutting the throats of the rest; but the effect of that influence is reduced to an absolute certainty and is found, even as a means of restraint, to say nothing of it as a means of cure, a hundred times more efficacious than all the straight-waistcoats, fetters and handcuffs, that ignorance, prejudice, and cruelty have manufactured since the creation of the world. . . . Every patient is as freely trusted with the tools of his trade as if he were a sane man. . . . For amusement, they walk, run, fish, paint, read and ride out to take the air in carriages provided for the purpose. . . . The irritability which otherwise would be expended on their own flesh, clothes and furniture is dissipated in these pursuits. They are cheerful, tranquil and healthy. . . . Immense politeness and good breeding are observed throughout, they all take their tone from the doctor. . . . It is obvious that one great feature of this system is the inculcation and encouragement even among such unhappy persons, of a decent self-respect. (pp. 105—111)

This era of the recognition of the importance of moral treatment and the social environment of the patient is well documented in Grob's (1966) history of the Worcester (Mass.) State Hospital. He points out that Samuel Woodward, the first superintendent, believed that insanity resulted from impaired sensory mechanisms: "If the physician could manipulate the environment he could thereby provide the patient with new and different stimuli, thus older and undesirable patterns and associations would be broken or modified and new and more desirable ones substituted in their place" (p. 53). Woodward believed that insanity resulted from social and cultural factors. The hospital attempted to institute moral therapy, which essentially consisted of individualized care, including occupational therapy, along with physical exercise, religious services, amusements, and games; physical violence and restraint were deemphasized. Moral treatment implied that the creation of a healthy psychological environment for the individual patient was itself curative. The assumption was that an appropriate social milieu could eliminate undesirable patient characteristics that had been acquired because of "improper living in an abnormal environment" (Grob, 1966, p. 66). Evidence indicates that the results of moral treatment were surprisingly good.

The late nineteenth and early twentieth centuries witnessed a general retreat from the principles of social treatment just described to a reliance on organic and physical treatments. During the past two decades, however, the psychosocial environment of psychiatric wards has again become of increasing theoretical importance and practical concern. There has been yet another reevaluation of the traditional disease model and its assumption that psychological disturbance resides in the individual alone. The theoretical contributions of Hartmann (1951) and Erikson (1950) demonstrate a heightened concern with ego development and the relation between ego functions and external reality. This concern was applied to the social structure and functions of the psychiatric ward, which constituted the "reality" for hospitalized patients. Detailed observations and naturalistic descriptions showing the importance of ward social structure in facilitating or hindering treatment goals were made by Stanton and Schwartz (1954) and Caudill (1958). Stanton and Schwartz noted the need for "a social norm from which the patient can differentiate himself. If there is no social norm or a chaotic one, as occasionally occurs, the experience is if anything far worse for the patient than simple routine treatment. . . . [A] coherent social environment is necessary for elementary ego integrity. . . ." (pp. 337—338).

The contribution of Stanton and Schwartz was important because it revealed that different patient symptoms could be understood as results of the informal organization of the hospital, that is, that the "environment may cause a symptom" (p. 343). The relation between symptoms and the social environment is clearly illustrated for pathological or manic excitement and for incontinence. Stanton and Schwartz found that patients who showed manic excitement were inevitably the subject of disagreement between two staff members who themselves were seldom aware of this disagreement. The patient's manic excitement often abruptly terminated when the staff members were able to discuss seriously the points of their disagreement. Stanton and Schwartz also state that a patient's dissociation may be quite reasonable in the face of certain social situations on a ward; for example, when two staff members violently disagree about how to manage a patient, that patient may himself be of a "divided" mind. When staff disagreement or the "split in the social field" is resolved, patient dissociation usually subsides. Stanton and Schwartz conclude that "profound and dramatic changes such as observed in shock therapy . . . are no more profound and no more rapid than the changes produced . . . by bringing about a particular change in the patient's social field" (p. 364).

Stanton and Schwartz also present an analysis indicating that incontinence almost always occurs when patients are in conflict, when they feel abandoned or neglected, when they are ignored or isolated, when they suffer loss of self-esteem, and when they are denied opportunities to demonstrate their capabilities. Patients were never incontinent immediately after receiving something they had requested. Also, incontinence hardly ever occurred off the ward and never occurred at social activities, such as teas, dances, and sports events. Finally, these authors show how collective disturbances on a ward can result from low staff morale that is perhaps related to staff conflict and lack of communication, which may itself result from other aspects of the social environment (e.g., financial stress on the institution).

Caudill (1958) independently substantiated many of the conclusions reported by Stanton and Schwartz. In one detailed clinical example, he revealed how the behavior of a patient, Mr. Esposito, was directly related to the physical and social structures of his psychiatric ward. It appears that some of Mr. Esposito's excited and disturbed behavior on the ward was due to his personal relationships with his therapist and with other patients. The therapist's interest in Mr. Esposito was both positively and negatively influenced by the attitudes of other staff, and the therapeutic and administrative routines of the hospital system were closely associated with the course of Mr. Esposito's illness. The patient developed a clowning, joking role on the ward which Caudill suggests was necessary because it helped him relate to other patients and reinforced the staff view of him as a clowning, harmless schizophrenic. Caudill concludes that ". . . A patient's pattern of behavior cannot be sufficiently apprehended within the usual meaning of terms such as 'symptom' or 'defense', but must also be thought of as an adaptation to the relatively circumscribed situation in which he is placed" (p. 63). In a final example, Stotland and Kobler (1965) present cogent evidence that a suicide epidemic that occurrred in a hospital was directly related to changes in the financial and social structure of that hospital and to resultant changes in staff morale, attitudes, and expectations of patient improvement.

Some treatment environments produce extremely negative effects on their inhabitants. For example, Goffman (1961) has described "total institutions," which he sees as assuming absolute control over the life functions of people who reside in them. The all-encompassing character of total institutions is symbolized by the barriers to social interchange with the outside world. Total institutions break down the kinds of barriers that ordinarily separate different spheres of an individual's life (e.g., places of work, residence, and recreation). In total institutions all aspects of the residents' lives are conducted in the same place—that is, in the immediate company of a large group of unselected others who are all required to do the same things on a fixed schedule imposed by a presumably indifferent body of officials. Inmates and staff interact with one another only in restricted, formally prescribed ways. Goffman proposes that two different social and cultural worlds develop, one of inmates and one of staff. There is little effective contact between them.

Wing and Brown (1970) provide a detailed description of Kerry ward, which appears to have many of the characteristics described by Goffman. The ward door was always locked, there was no ready access to the outside, and the patients lived almost entirely within the ward. There was little contact with the rest of the hospital and essentially no contact with the outside world. No patient went home, less than half were visited by relatives, and only five were allowed to leave the ward without supervision. Movement about the ward was restricted. Storerooms were locked, as were dormitories and washrooms. Bathing was subject to close control. There were few if any exceptions to the restrictive ward policies. All clothing was provided by the hospital, and few patients even owned a toothbrush. There were few if any personal possessions in the ward. The lack of privacy was almost total. The lavatory doors did not lock, and baths were taken under direct nursing and patient supervision.

Patients were caught up in a daily routine that was geared to staff requirements. The development of personal skills was not encouraged; for example, the patients' beds were made by the staff. In describing the daily routine on Kerry ward, Wing and Brown particularly emphasize the paucity of social interactions and involving activities. For example, they state that ". . . there were long periods when most patients were simply waiting for the next stage of the cycle to begin; this waiting was mostly spent in apathetic inactivity, in doing absolutely nothing. All but one of the 22 patients in the series spent three hours a day sitting at a meal table and half were totally unoccupied except when eating or at toilet" (p. 137). Certainly this severe social and stimulus deprivation must have detrimental effects on patients. The authors present quite important evidence that the social environment of Kerry ward was successfully improved during 2 and 4-year follow-up intervals.

Some vivid and insightful case studies of the impact of positive and negative treatment environments have been compiled by several better-known authors. Mary Jane Ward (1946) wrote of the horrendous physical and social environment of a mental hospital and gave an account of its shockingly detrimental effects in *The Snake Pit*. In Ken Kesey's (1962) *One Flew Over the Cuckoo's Nest*, patients respond adaptively to a highly rigidly structured ward setting that required them to submit to the authority of "Big Nurse". In sharp contrast, a warm supportive therapist and a constructive, humanitarian hospital setting facilitated the recovery of a young schizophrenic girl in *I Never Promised You a Rose Garden* (Greenberg, 1964). In *The Magic Mountain* Thomas Mann (1952) vividly describes how the social environment of a tuberculosis sanitarium slowly and insidiously affects a patient until that patient submits to its procedures and effectively gives up his outside life and identity. Solzhenitsyn's (1969) *Cancer Ward* presents a similar tale, with a different outcome.

Physicians, anthropologists, social scientists, and novelists, for differing reasons, have written of psychiatric hospitals and their social environments. The various authors have also differed in their feelings about the effectiveness of psychiatric treatment, but they all agree on one point: that the immediate psychosocial environment in which patients function determines their attitudes, behaviors, and symptoms, and that this environment can be the most critical factor in determining the outcome of treatment. The evidence just reviewed indicates that pathological excitement, incontinence, collective disturbances, suicide, and the general course of patient illness are related to treatment environments.

Comparative Program Evaluations

Although naturalistic and descriptive studies of treatment milieus made mental health professionals aware of the importance of the environment, they failed to identify precisely which variables affected patient symptoms, satisfaction, and improvement. A number of investigators attempted to isolate specific influences by constructing treatment programs to achieve specific goals and by carefully evaluating these programs in comparison to matched controls.

For example, Jones (1953) founded the Social Rehabilitation Unit at Belmont Hospital in London in order to treat personality disorders in a therapeutic community setting. The emphasis was on communal life and the sharing of feelings to produce a meaningful total life experience in which individuals could grow and learn effective ways of functioning. The ward program was designed to involve patients in activities paralleling those of the nonhospital environments to which they would return. The unit incorporated group therapy, social activities, and work experience to provide patients with the social and work skills they lacked.

A 4-year study of this unit by Rapaport (1960) considered the program ideology, the organization of patient and staff roles, and both the treatment and rehabilitation goals. Rapaport's study is important because it was the first attempt to evaluate the effectiveness of a therapeutic community program based on a specific rationale. The treatment ideology centered on the working hypothesis that "socio-environmental influences are themselves capable of effectively changing individual patterns of social behavior" (p. 269). Untrained staff were utilized to interact with patients, regular staff roles were far less structured than on customary wards, and punitive custodialism was avoided.

Rapaport's study showed that the program was not as effective as its sponsors originally had believed. A major program purpose was to have been the teaching of effective patterns of work and social behavior that could be generalized to the patients' lives in the outside community. Attempts were made to have patients become aware of the reasons for their behaviors and to take an instrumental role in changing them. In choosing the methods for instituting change, individual members were required to assume responsibility within the operation of the unit. Patients had a voice in this "participatory democracy" and thereby became accustomed to determining their living and working environment. However, the staff had failed to recognize that most of the patients were from lower socioeconomic groups and were qualified only for unskilled or semiskilled positions, where they would be heavily supervised and where they would have few decisions to make. Insight into behavior was not particularly valued. The treatment program had taught patients patterns of behavior that were basically inappropriate outside the hospital and thus could not generalize from the hospital to the community environment.

A different type of milieu program was constructed by Fairweather (1964), who considered chronic mental patients as individuals who were capable of establishing roles and statuses in the hospital setting but were unable to do so in the community. The dependent role assumed in the hospital made it difficult to readjust to the community, where such a role is seldom available. Thus Fairweather formed small problem-oriented task groups to provide chronic patients with experience in more active roles that could be transferred to the community at discharge. He structured a small group ward program characterized by autonomous task group meetings and compared it with a more traditional ward program. Each ward had the same number and the same categories of staff and staff changed wards during the middle of the experiment, with the result that patients on both wards had the same exposure to each group of staff.

Successful completion of the experimental program involved four steps. Progressive steps required increased responsibilities that entitled patients to more income and more liberal pass privileges. Task groups were responsible for orienting new members, evaluating members' performances, and making recommendations for job assignments, money allotments, passes, and step level changes. The task groups met with a staff member once a week and submitted their recommendations for comment and approval. By contrast, patients on the traditional program were related to individually, and they requested help or privileges from the staff member assigned to work with them. Their role was much more passive and submissive. The experimental program emphasized involvement, autonomy, program clarity and low staff control.

Evaluations indicated that more patients in the small group would have preferred to be in a program other than their own—they felt that they had been deprived of leisure time and subjected to too much pressure to participate. The experimental program patients, however, rated their ward more positively than the traditional ward patients rated theirs, and they also believed that the ward had helped them more. They credited other patients for this help more frequently than staff.

A 6-month follow-up showed that small group patients spent less time in the hospital, were more frequently employed, and were more actively involved with people outside the hospital. Nevertheless, 50% had returned to the hospital within the 6-month period, suggesting that progress gained in the program was not necessarily maintained in the community. Why was this so? Fairweather reasoned that patients supported one another in the hospital, but they left the institution as individuals to enter the larger community, in which such support did not generally exist. Following this line of thought, Fairweather et al. (1969) established a community lodge and demonstrated that former mental patients could adjust to the community more effectively as a functioning task group than as individuals. The lodge program significantly increased employment and time in the community and enhanced the self-esteem of its members. In addition, its costs were about half the amount of inpatient costs.

The basic implication of the Fairweather studies is that former mental patients can be more successfully maintained in the community when they enter it fortified by newly created supportive and active social roles and statuses.

In a study on chronic schizophrenic patients, Sanders et al. (1967) organized three comparative socioenvironmental treatment programs structured to vary the demand for social interaction. They hypothesized that social interaction could be produced and enhanced by increasing the opportunity and demand for social functioning, and that the greater the external demand for interaction, the more favorable the outcome. A minimally structured program offered opportunities to develop interaction, but no pressure was exerted. A partially structured program, which required group participation in teams responsible for housekeeping, included an interaction program featuring 10 hours of group activities each week. A maximally structured program had the highest demand for interaction; it involved group therapy, patient government, individual work assignments, cottage meetings, and so on. There was also a control group of patients who met the requirements for inclusion in the study but who remained on their original wards.

Improvement was analyzed in terms of global social behavior and in terms of three specific social responses assumed by the investigators to represent a hierarchy of social initiative: awareness of others, interaction in structured situations, and spontaneous social behavior. Socioenvironmental therapy seemed to produce improved social adjustment and psychiatric status for some patients and exaggeration of symptomatology in others. The older male patients, and those with a longer duration of illness, manifested the most favorable social response and the most positive psychiatric adjustment in the maximally structured treatment condition. The less structured treatment program also tended to benefit these male patients, but the effects were less marked. Traditional ward programs were entirely ineffective with such patients.

On the other hand, younger male patients, and those with a shorter duration of illness, generally responded less favorably to socioenvironmental treatment. Apparently some of these patients were disturbed by the interpersonal intimacy with members of both sexes which was demanded by the treatment program. Similar findings were not noted for female patients. A 36-month follow-up study indicated that the effects of socioenvironmental treatment persisted in posttreatment adjustments regardless of degree of structure, although there was some tendency for patients who experienced the two more structured programs to surpass those who participated in the minimally structured program.

Thus these investigators demonstrated that older patients, traditionally regarded as having the poorest potential for recovery, manifested the best treatment outcome under a maximally structured socioenvironmental therapy program. Moreover, this improvement was sustained in subsequent community adjustment. An interaction between type of patient and type of treatment program is clearly evident here.

In a final example, Coleman (1971) designed a treatment program for disturbed delinquent males who had responded poorly to a regular hospital ward. The men were typically 21 years old, single, and had enlisted in the army following difficulties with the courts, school or their families. They often had histories of school dropout, job failure, and trouble with the police. Many servicemen had gone AWOL and had had recurrent fights and difficulty handling routine army assignments.

The program involved custom-designed behavioral plans implemented by specific rewards for learning behavioral skills. Required behaviors for individual patients were related to their target (community) environments. Staff were responsible for establishing a social environment to facilitate the learning of new behaviors. A token economy was used as the reinforcement system. A relative scale of reward was based on the estimated value of specific privileges (e.g., 3-day passes) to patients.

Interestingly, staff found that nondirective group therapy techniques were inapplicable to this patient population, who conceived of the procedure as irrelevant and who did not understand its purpose. As an alternative, "courses" were offered with the object of improving skills on the individual, group, and community levels. These courses were designed around well-defined terminal behaviors, a planned curriculum, and a highly structured class format. The courses taught basic educational and leadership skills by requiring preparation and presentation of material to staff and peers. Practical experiences served to instruct the men in filling out job applications, for example; practice interview situations were also arranged, and there were discussions of how local facilities could be used for inexpensive dates. Follow-up data indicated that the use of educational skills and interests learned in the program persisted, that antisocial behavior reappeared only infrequently, and that positive shifts occurred in attitudes toward work and peer relationships. We studied a somewhat similar hospital-based ward program—intentional social systems therapy (see Chapter 5).

In summary, each program organized a different type of milieu, but each accepted the basic notion that the treatment milieu has important influences on treatment outcome. Jones's program emphasized involvement, peer support, autonomy and independence, and an insight and expression of feeling orientation. Staff control was played down. Fairweather encouraged involvement, peer support, and autonomy and responsibility; however, his program also strongly stressed a practical task orientation. Again a specific attempt was made to minimize staff control. Sanders et al. based their program on involvement and support and, to a lesser extent, on personal problems and the expression of feelings. Finally, Coleman was interested in the effects of involvement and autonomy to a degree, but the strongest thrust of his program was a practical, task-related orientation. Thus we have four quite different milieu programs; each has claimed some success, and each supports the overall thesis that treatment outcome is related to treatment milieu.

THE VARIABILITY OF BEHAVIOR OVER SETTINGS

Behavior is commonly thought of as a joint function of the individual and his environment; until recently, however, theory and research have focused mainly on the person. As a rule, we deal with persons in terms of personality traits, which assume a reasonable degree of consistency of behavior over different settings. For example, when an individual is described as dominant, the implicit assumption is that he will be relatively dominant in a variety of settings. Recent research indicates that this assumption is considerably less accurate than anyone had supposed.

Hartshorne and May (1928) conducted an early and widely cited series of studies bearing on this problem and came to two conclusions: (1) that the conflict between honest and deceitful behavior was specific to each situation and (2) that one could not necessarily generalize about a person's honesty from a few samples of his behavior. They concluded that consistency of behavior from setting to setting was due to similarities in the settings and not to personality traits. The correlations among the different cheating tests they utilized were simply too low to provide evidence of a unified character trait of honesty or deceitfulness.

This issue has also been explored by several other investigators. For example, Raush and his coworkers (Raush, Dittman, and Taylor, 1959; Raush, Farbman, and Llewellyn, 1960) studied the social interactions of a group of preadolescent boys at two phases of residential treatment, 18 months apart. They also studied the social interactions of a matched group of six normal boys. Each child was observed twice in each phase in each of six ward settings (breakfast, other meals, structured game activities, unstructured game activities, arts and crafts, and snacks at bedtime).

Results indicated that the boys differed from one another across settings; that is, individual behavior could be characterized to some extent as more or less aggressive, more or less dependent, more or less dominant, more or less friendly. On the other hand, the six settings also evoked characteristic patterns of social action—settings were more or less competitive, more or less status-oriented, more or less friendly, more or less evocative of dependency. Thus there was some individual consistency in social behavior across settings and some setting consistency across individuals. However, the interactive effects of the child and the setting together contributed considerably more information about behavior than did either the child or the setting alone. Normal children differentiated among social settings more than did disturbed children, and thus situational factors came to play a more potent role in behavior with treatment and maturation. These results argue strongly for the importance of representative sampling of situations in studies of social behavior.

Following a series of questionnaire studies, Endler and Hunt (1968) concluded that persons, settings, and person-by-setting interactions each contributed significantly to the variance in both anxiety and hostility. They found that consistent individual differences among subjects contributed only about 15 to 20% of the variance in hostility and only about 4 to 5% of the variance in anxiety; consistent differences among situations contributed only about 4 to 8% of the total variance. Nearly 30% of the variance for both hostility and anxiety was attributable to the interactions between settings and subjects, settings and modes of response (e.g., modes of response for hostility included swearing, perspiring, becoming enraged, grinding teeth, and wanting to yell), and subjects by modes of response. Thus people react in substantially different ways to different settings. These investigators concluded that the low proportion of variance attributable to individual differences stringently limits the validity coefficients that can be expected from inventories of anxiety (about .25) and of hostility (about .40

to .45). They argue that specifying the situations can appreciably raise these limits. Hunt (1965) has pointed out elsewhere that these results demand substantial revisions in traditional personality theories. Other literature criticizing the empirical legacy of several decades of work with trait models of personality has been cogently summarized by Mischel (1968).

We were impressed by these findings and carried out some related work in our laboratory. We first used a diary method of data collection with patients and staff and found that psychiatric ward subsettings (e.g., community meeting, small group meeting) evoked a specific hierarchy of reactions regardless of whether patients or staff were responding to them. We then more systematically investigated the reactions of patients and staff to a representative sample of daily ward settings. Our results, in direct support of the work reported earlier, demonstrated that persons, settings, modes of response, and their interactions, each contributed statistically significant and practically important proportions of the total variance in behavior. Thus each of these sources of variation must be sampled in measuring and predicting individual patient and staff behavior (Moos, 1968).

Further work replicated the foregoing results and extended them to observations of actual ward behavior (Moos, 1969). This study also revealed a consistent tendency for the proportion of variance attributable to settings to increase over a 3 month interval as patients improved clinically. According to our evidence, ward subsettings elicit varied amounts of therapeutic change in different patients, indicating that these settings are differentially beneficial to different groups of patients and that conclusions about a patient's therapeutic change drawn from observations in one setting do not necessarily generalize to other settings. We also found that patients and staff reacted differentially to the physical characteristics of various rooms (a day room, a dining room, a bedroom, a bathroom, a meeting room) on a ward.

Our studies on individual psychotherapy (Moos and Clemes, 1967; Moos and MacIntosh, 1970) basically supported these results. In one study, for example, each of six patients saw each of four therapists twice. Each of four variables (total activity, feeling words, action words, reinforcements) was scored separately for patients and therapists for each interview. The extent to which patients openly discussed their problems and the extent to which therapists responded empathically were rated for each interview. Consistent differences among therapists accounted for only about 5% of the total variance in therapists' behavior. The patient-by-therapist-by-session interactions, however, accounted for between 6 and 56% of the variance. The results showed that the therapist behaviors were not the result of a "trait" (i.e., of a given tendency to be empathic) or of a consistently applied therapeutic technique, but rather were substantially situationally or patient-determined.

Finally, in an important study, Ellsworth et al. (1968) obtained data on outcome of psychiatric hospitalization as perceived by staff and by schizophrenic patients and their relatives. Patients were assessed twice while hospitalized and twice after their release from the hospital. No congruence was found between patients' initial hospital adjustment and community behavior before admission. There was also no relation between hospital adjustment at release and posthospital adjustment. Ellsworth (1973) points out that patients' behavior in treatment settings often differs markedly from their behavior in community settings. The basic assumption made by many mental health professionals that adjustment in the treatment milieu is highly related to adjustment in the community milieu is simply not correct. All this work, taken together, firmly convinced us that deriving methods for the systematic assessment of ward milieus would richly repay the effort.

ASSESSING TREATMENT MILIEUS

Although physical and sociopsychological settings were clearly recognized as influential in psychiatric treatment programs, major questions remained unanswered. Which setting characteristics relate to which indices of treatment outcome? Which characteristics are situation-specific and which carry over into community settings? What type of milieu program is best for what type of patient? It was clearly necessary to develop milieu assessment techniques to answer these questions and then to set up programs, duplicate them, and systematically compare different treatment environments. A number of tangentially relevant scales have been constructed and cannot be reviewed in detail here, including the Staff Opinion Scale (Rice et al., 1966), the Philosophy of Treatment Form (Barrell, DeWolfe, and Cummings, 1965), the Opinions about Mental Illness Scale (Cohen and Struening, 1963), and the Ward Evaluation Scale (Rice et al., 1963).

In more directly relevant work, Jackson (1964, 1969) constructed the Characteristics of Treatment Environments (CTE) scale, consisting of 72 statements concerning conditions in the immediate environment of a patient in a mental hospital. Stanton and Schwartz (1954) had originally hypothesized that disagreement, conflict, and lack of clarity in authority relations among staff create disturbances in communication that impinge on patients, upsetting them and retarding their recovery. Jackson constructed the CTE to measure these disturbances in communication and their effects on treatment outcome. The instrument was designed to describe objective events in the treatment milieu, rather than perceptions, feelings, and attitudes of individuals.

The CTE originally measured six characteristics of the treatment environment, namely, the degrees to which it developed patients' initiative and creativity, increased their self-esteem, lessened their anxiety, helped them understand their illness, reduced their distortions of reality, and increased their ability to participate. Jackson assumed that the total score reflected the degree to which the environment approximated a therapeutic milieu. These original subscales were oriented principally toward patients and their pathologies or symptoms (e.g., lack of self-esteem, anxiety, distortion of reality).

In a revision of the scoring scheme, Jackson (1969) described five new factor scales labeled as follows: active treatment, socioemotional activity, patient self-management, behavior modification, and instrumental activity. The new scales were oriented toward the environment and its characteristics, (e.g., its restrictiveness or freedom). Bechtel and Gonzalez (1971) have successfully utilized the CTE in a cross-cultural comparison of treatment environments among Peruvian and North American mental hospitals.

Ellsworth et al. (1969) derived a scale to measure the sociopsychological characteristics of treatment settings in order to examine the relation between these characteristics and treatment outcome. Separate Perception of Ward (POW) scales were constructed for patients and staff. The patient POW measures five dimensions—inaccessible staff, involvement in ward management, satisfaction with ward life, receptive and involved staff, and expectation for patient autonomy. The staff POW scale measures four dimensions—motivated professional staff, nursing team as involved participants, dominant professional staff, and praise for work. These POW scales assess important aspects of treatment milieus and have been related to treatment outcome. They are more extensively discussed in Chapters 3 and 8.

Spiegel and Keith-Spiegel (1971) derived a Ward Climate Inventory (WCI) from the POW scales by taking 33 of the statements and adapting the items for administration to both patients and staff. Each statement is rated on a 7-point scale ranging from strongly agree to strongly disagree. A factor analysis yielded three factors, which were labeled personnel concern for patients, ward morale, and patients' concern for patients. These factors were highly intercorrelated with a global ward climate index obtained by summing them, thus suggesting that the WCI assesses only one aspect of those characteristics which differentiate among ward environments.

All the scales mentioned utilize a subjective perceptual methodology in that the staff and/or patients actually functioning in the environment are asked about the characteristics of that environment. There have also been some attempts to develop more objective scales to differentiate among treatment institutions (Wing and Brown, 1970). King and Raynes (1968) developed a 16-item scale that measures practices adopted in the management of children in residential institutions. They derived this measure from the patterns of staff–inmate interactions noted by Goffman as characterizing "total institutions." Goffman, it will be recalled, hypothesized that individual differences among inmates and unique circumstances are disregarded in favor of an emphasis on the routine running of the institution. These are called institutionally oriented practices, in distinction to inmate-oriented practices, in which individual differences and unique circumstances are given recognition and variations in routine are tolerated.

The 16 items on the Inmate Management Scale (IMS) assess the types of processes identified by Goffman. For example, rigidity of routine is assessed by such criteria as whether all the inmates get up and/or go to bed at the same time. Block treatment of children is assessed by ascertaining whether they must wait together in a group before bathing, before coming in for breakfast, and so on. Depersonalization is evaluated according to whether children are allowed to have toys of their own or to possess certain articles of clothing, books, and so on. King and Raynes demonstrate that the IMS significantly descriminates among certain residential institutions.

In a final example, Kellam et al. (1966) studied the atmospheres of psychiatric wards by grouping certain objective, easily observable items along given dimensions. The dimensions used were disturbed behavior, adult status, patient–staff ratio, and ward census. We used this Ward Information Form (WIF) in some studies (Chapter 6), specifically to relate certain characteristics of ward milieus to treatment outcome (Chapter 8), since it represents an objective way of assessing ward milieus.

Thus we found a variety of different scales attempting to measure patient and staff evaluations, opinions, and ideologies. When we started our work on treatment milieus, there were no scales at all that assessed patient and staff perceptions of these milieus. In terms of the more objective characteristics of ward milieus, only the WIF was available. It is noteworthy that in the last few years several relevant measuring techniques have been derived, indicating that other investigators share our overriding concern with the systematic assessment of treatment environments.

To review, our interest in coping and adaptation led us to study therapeutic environments. Previous work on the variability of individual behavior over settings and of person–environment interaction convinced us that techniques for the systematic characterization of human environments had to be developed. Work on naturalistic and descriptive studies of psychiatric ward programs indicated a belief on the part of all theorists that the treatment milieu was of critical import. This basic hypothesis appeared time after time in psychiatric program evaluation studies. Finally, previous work on the assessment of treatment milieus suggested to us that both a subjective perceptual methodology and a more objective ecological methodology were essential.

There is some important serendipity in this work in that the assessment techniques we developed have practical clinical utility. Patients and staff are generally interested in feedback about the characteristics of their environment. This feedback often enhances program analysis and motivates change. Thus the research has applications which are quite different from those we originally intended. Yet an even more important result is the integrative concepts that grew out of this work. First, we developed a point of view regarding social ecology as a growing field of inquiry. Second, we came to an overall conceptualization of six different methods by which human environments could be described. Third, we found that the types of dimensions characterizing social climates were similar in a wide variety of different environments (e.g., psychiatric wards, military training companies, university student living groups). Although in fact these ideas did not precede the research, they are presented next to give the reader the conceptual context for what follows. The ideas provide an overall framework within which further research on treatment milieus and their impacts should be planned.

SOCIAL ECOLOGY:
THE STUDY OF HUMANS AND HUMAN MILIEUS

Current interest in the physical and social aspects of planning for both large and small environmental systems is remarkable. Jordan (1972) notes that more books treating man and his environment from a wholistic and ecological viewpoint have appeared within the past four years than appeared during the preceding three decades. Within our broader society this interest is largely due to technological advances, whose side effects raise critical issues about the delicate ecological balance existing on "spaceship earth." Major human problems that are being extensively discussed include environmental deterioration (particularly water, air, and noise pollution), the probable effects of increasing population and population density, and issues of resource depletion, specifically in relation to food materials.

Partly by drawing attention to issues related to the quality of life, new developments in the social and behavioral sciences are reflecting present concern with the problems just listed. Consideration of physical environments is inextricably linked to a concern about social environments. Concern about human milieus in turn arises mainly from concern about human adaptation.

Social ecology is defined here as the multidisciplinary study of the impacts on human beings of physical and social environments. In its primary concern with the assessment and optimization of human milieus, it is linked to traditional interests of human ecology, both in its emphasis on the measurement of objective physical characteristics of environments (e.g., temperature, noise levels, the shapes, sizes, and physical arrangements of buildings) and in its emphasis on the short-term evolutionary adaptive consequences of these environments. It is linked to traditional areas of the behavioral sciences, particularly psychology and sociology, both in its emphasis on the importance of the social environment and in its explicit consideration of environmental impacts on psychological variables such as self-esteem and personal development. Finally, it is linked to traditional concerns in psychiatry, medicine, and epidemiology in its explicit focus on the identification of dysfunctional reactions (e.g., illness, accidents, anxiety, depression, anger) and their relation to environmental variables.

For example, social ecology examines the effects of temperature and crowding on human aggression, the effects of structural and social environmental characteristics on individual development, and the effects of structural and social environmental characteristics on psychiatric treatment outcome. Each is an ongoing concern in a different field of inquiry. From the range and interconnection of variables generally studied in isolation, social ecology derives a diverse, robust, and socially relevant focus. The field thus provides a distinctive point of entry by which human milieus and their impact on human adaptation can be conceptualized (Moos and Insel, 1974). Several basic assumptions are central to this area:

1. Human behavior cannot be understood apart from the environmental context in which it occurs. This statement implies, for example, that accurate predictions of behavior or of treatment outcome cannot be made solely from information about individuals; information about their environments is essential.

2. Physical and social environments must be studied together, since neither can be fully understood alone. For example, both architectural design and psychosocial treatment milieu can significantly influence patient and staff behavior.

3. Social ecology has an explicit applied value orientation in that it gathers and utilizes knowledge for promoting maximally effective human functioning. The field utilizes basic research and practical techniques for the application of knowledge derived from this research toward the end of increasing the quality of the human environment.

In a sense, the field combines the dissatisfactions of some professionals with the developing concerns of many others. Psychologists have become increasingly intrigued with the notion that environmental and setting effects on human behavior have far more importance than previously had been accorded to them. Sociologists are finding that structural characteristics of institutions account for less variability in human behavior than they had thought. Human ecologists and demographers are concluding that the overall physical and geographical characteristics of environments are not as closely linked to different indices of human behavior as are cultural and social characteristics. Architects and social planners, who are primarily interested in man-made aspects of the environment, are learning that the characteristics of the psychological and social environment may mediate the effects of building designs on people. Community mental health experts, called on to diagnose and change environments, are realizing that they need methods for the systematic assessment of these environments. Finally, practitioners in each of these professional fields must consider the impact of their own knowledge on the task of enhancing the quality of human life.

Whereas social ecology is as much concerned with human adaptation as with human milieus, we focus somewhat more heavily here on the conceptualization and measurement of environments, since this aspect of the field is currently less well developed. Furthermore, assessments of environments must necessarily precede assessments of the impact of such environments on human functioning.

MAJOR METHODS OF CHARACTERIZING ENVIRONMENTS

Six major methods of relating characteristics of environments to indices of human functioning have recently been identified (Moos, 1973). These are: (1) ecological dimensions, which include both geographical–meteorological and architectural–physical design variables; (2) behavior settings, the only units thus far proposed that possess both ecological and behavioral properties; (3) dimensions of organizational structure; (4) dimensions identifying the collective, personal, and/or behavioral characteristics of the milieu inhabitants; (5) dimensions related to psychosocial characteristics and organizational climates; and (6) variables relevant to the functional or reinforcement analyses of environments. The six categories of dimensions are nonexclusive, overlapping, and interrelated. Their common relevance is that each appears to have an important and sometimes decisive impact on individual and group behavior.

For example, ecological dimensions are implicated in the notion of geographic environmental influence, which has been recurrent in many societies. This is essentially the idea that the culture, character, and activities of societies are significantly shaped by the climate (temperature, rainfall) topography, and other geographical features of the region in which the people live. Environmental determinists have hypothesized specific connections between environmental characteristics such as mountainous terrain, soil conditions, and humidity and personality traits such as strength of character, assertiveness, bravery, and laziness. Phenomena of great importance have been attributed to climate; for example, it was widely believed that the riots in Los Angeles and Chicago during the summer of 1965 stemmed partly from the discomforts of hot weather. Indeed, climate may be one of the major factors in economic development throughout the world. On a more individual level, most people seem to feel that their efficiency is impaired by extremes of heat and cold. Climate has also been associated with general health, intellectual performance, admissions to mental hospitals, and organizational participation and interpersonal relations (e.g., Griffitt and Veitch, 1971; Michelson, 1971).

Additional ecological dimensions are related to the man-made environment (i.e., architectural and physical design variables). Behavior must occur in a specific physical context that may impose major constraints on the range of possible behaviors, thus serving to determine particular patterns of individual action. There is a growing belief within the design profession that the man-made physical environment may profoundly influence psychological states and social behavior. In this connection Craik (1970) discusses the technique of "behavioral mapping" of designed environments. Behavioral maps can show the frequency of various activities in different types of available physical locations. Some relevant work has been done on psychiatric wards, which have been analyzed in terms of such variables as behavior density (the frequency of all types of activities at a particular place), diffuseness (the range of different activities occurring at a place), and activity profile (the frequency of specific types of activities occurring at a place). Treatment environments are undoubtedly affected in important ways by both climatological and physical design factors. We did not systematically assess these variables in researching hospital-based programs, but we did begin to evaluate them in the work on community-based programs by developing a Program Information Form that included questions on the physical environments inside and outside the treatment program (e.g., number of rooms in the center; see Chapter 12).

The work on behavior settings has been mainly conducted by Roger Barker (1968), who has demonstrated that behavior settings have pervasive effects on individuals, not only in terms of the specific behavior "demanded" by the setting (e.g., reading and writing in classrooms) but also on both other behaviors and on effects experienced by individuals (mood, self-esteem). Barker has shown that settings in which there are an optimal number of people produce effects differing from those of settings in which there are too few people. For example, students in small schools who have relatively few associates within behavior settings, when compared with students of larger schools having relatively many associates, report twice as many pressures on them to take part in the settings; moreover, the former actually perform in more than twice as many responsible positions in the settings and report that they are more likely to be challenged to be involved, to feel valued, to gain moral and cultural values, and so on. Thus behavior settings have considerable importance in the determination of individual behavior and experience. Unfortunately there has been relatively little work utilizing this methodology aside from that of Barker and his students. We did not use this technique in our studies. Behavior setting analyses, however, can and should be done in a variety of different types of institutions, including hospital-based and community-based treatment institutions.

Dimensions of Organizational Structure

Many investigators have attempted to assess and discriminate among organizations utilizing relatively objective dimensions such as size, staffing ratios, average salary levels, and organizational control structure (March, 1965). Since organizations vary widely in their structural characteristics, it is important to learn how closely differences in organizational structures are related to behavioral and attitudinal effects on the organization members. For example, Porter and Lawler (1965) found that organizational dimensions such as the size of the overall organization and the number of subordinates a manager is responsible for supervising, were significantly related to one or more attitudinal or behavioral variables (e.g., satisfaction, absenteeism, and turnover rate). In similar work done in colleges and universities, attempts have been made to relate traditional indices of institutional quality (faculty–student ratio, percentage of faculty with Ph.D. degree, number of books in the library, etc.) to various indices of student achievement and personal development (Feldman and Newcomb, 1969). In the work reported here we relate organizational indices such as size, staffing, and adult status (Chapter 6) and turnover rates (Chapter 8) to patient and staff perceptions of hospital-based treatment milieus. We also relate a somewhat broader array of organizational indices to perceptions of community-based program treatment environments (Chapter 12).

Personal and Behavioral Characteristics of the Milieu Inhabitants

Various factors related to the characteristics of the individuals inhabiting a particular environment (e.g., average age, ability level, socioeconomic background, educational attainment) can be considered to be situational variables in that they partially define relevant charcteristics of the environment (e.g., Sells, 1963). This idea, which is based on the suggestion made by Linton (1945) that most of the social and cultural environment is transmitted by other people, implies that the character of an environment is dependent in part of the typical characteristics of its members.

The approach is illustrated by Astin (1968), who developed the Inventory of College Activities (ICA), a technique for characterizing environmental stimuli in colleges and universities. The ICA provides information about the average personal and behavioral characteristics of the college environment by the following kinds of items: (1) questions about activites in college, such as whether the individual flunked a course, became pinned or engaged, got married, participated in a student demonstration, changed his or her major field; (2) the median number of hours per week the student spent in different activities such as attending class, studying for school assignments, reading for pleasure or watching TV, watching athletic events, sleeping, playing games; (3) the kinds of organizations to which the student belonged, such as fraternities, sororities, college athletic teams, marching band, religious clubs, and service organization. Remarkable diversity was found among the environments of 246 colleges and universities. The proportion of students who engaged in any particular activity (e.g., dating, going to church, drinking beer) often varied from no students in some institutions to nearly all students in others. Astin feels that this diversity indicates that the college and university environment has great potential for differentially influencing the experience and behavior of the individual student.

The same logic is clearly relevant to psychiatric treatment programs. Assume that a new patient is admitted to a program that is run like a therapeutic community and that certain kinds of environmental stimuli occur relatively frequently: group therapy, discussions about personal problems, staff sensitivity groups, decision-making forums in which patients and staff discuss program policies. Exposed to these and related stimuli, the new patient might feel anxiety about expressing certain personal feelings (a change in immediate subjective experience), increased fear of or hostility toward fellow patients, or increased feelings of inferiority (perhaps due to inability to engage in open self-expression). Presumably the patient would be affected quite differently if he had been admitted to another treatment program. In terms of short-term behavioral effects, the patient may reduce the time devoted to personal interaction in the program; on the other hand, he may vent his feelings of anger, inadequacy, loneliness, low self-esteem, and so on. In the latter case, he may consequently experience greater feelings of integration, belonging-ness, and cohesion with others. Finally, there may be longer-lasting alterations in his self-concept and/or relatively permanent changes in behavior that may persist beyond his discharge from the treatment program (e.g., openly discussing feelings of inadequacy with his wife or a friend).

We utilized this method of characterizing environments in our studies of both hospital and community treatment programs. In hospital programs we used indices such as the average amount of disturbed behavior and the average number of aggressive behavior incidents occurring on the ward (Chapter 6). Indices employed in community programs included average patient chronicity, the proportion of patients working or going to school, and the proportion of staff with college education (Chapter 12). We also utilized average patient background variables in two initial attempts to study the importance of a good person–environment fit (Chapter 13).

Psychosocial Characteristics and Organizational Climate

We relied most heavily on psychosocial characteristics and organizational climate in defining environments. Until recently most of the research in this area involved rather detailed naturalistic descriptions of the functioning of different types of institutions, such as psychiatric wards, colleges, and universities. This work was valuable because it indicated the importance of the immediate psychosocial environment in the determination of behavior, also suggesting various possible dimensions along which psychosocial environments might be compared (e.g., Katz and Kahn, 1966).

A number of perceived climate scales have been developed in the last few years to more systematically measure the general norms, value orientations, and other psychosocial characteristics of different types of institutions. For example, Stern (1970) follows the Murray Need–Press theory and points out that descriptions of institutional environments are based on inferred continuity and consistency in otherwise discrete events. If students in a university are assigned seats in a classroom, if attendance records are kept, if faculty see students outside class only by appointment, if there is a prescribed form for all term papers, if neatness counts, and so on, it is probable that the press at this school emphasizes the development of orderly responses on the part of the students. These conditions establish the climate or atmosphere of an institution. A substantial amount of work utilizing such logic has been carried out in colleges and universities (Pace, 1969; Peterson et al., 1970), elementary schools (Halpin and Croft, 1963), junior high and high school classrooms (Walberg, 1969), and industries (Likert, 1967).

Our related investigations are more fully described in Chapter 14. In addition to our work in treatment environments, however, we have studied total institutions (correctional institutions and military training companies), educational environments (university student living groups and high school classrooms), and naturally occurring community settings (social and task-oriented groups, work environments, and families). We have established three basic types of dimensions that characterize and discriminate among different subunits within each of these different kinds of environments.

1. *Relationship* dimensions, which are very similar in all the environments we have studied, assess the involvement of individuals in the environment and the extent to which they support and help one another. The basic dimensions are Involvement, Support, and Expressiveness.

2. *Personal Development* dimensions assess the basic directions along which personal growth and self-enhancement tend to occur in the particular environment. The exact nature of these dimensions varies somewhat among the different environments studied, depending on their basic purposes and goals. For example, in psychiatric and correctional programs these dimensions assess the treatment goals—for example, Autonomy (the extent to which people are encouraged to be self-sufficient and independent), Practical Orientation (the extent to which the program prepares an individual for training for new jobs, looking to the future, setting and working toward concrete goals), and Personal Problem Orientation (the extent to which individuals are encouraged to be concerned with their feelings and problems and to seek to understand them). An Autonomy or independence dimension is also identified in military companies and work environments. Other dimensions, which are placed in the Personal Development category, are found in university living groups (e.g., Competition, Academic Achievement, Intellectuality), in high school classrooms (e.g., Task Orientation, Competition), and in families (e.g., Intellectual–Cultural Orientation, Moral–Religious Orientation).

3. *System Maintenance and System Change* dimensions are relatively similar across all the environments studied. The basic dimensions are Order and Organization, Clarity of Expectations, and Control.

The major portion of this book discusses the development of perceived climate scales for hospital-based and community-based treatment programs. We present evidence that the three types of dimensions just listed are salient in treatment programs and that they are related to such important criteria as patient morale and indices of coping behavior (Chapters 7 and 12) and different objective indices of treatment outcome (Chapter 8).

We did not explicitly use a functional or reinforcement approach in characterizing treatment environments, in part because we believe the perceived climate approach identifies the basic behaviors that are positively or negatively rewarded in the program. The methodology of functional analysis of environments is an outgrowth of a social learning perspective. The social learning theorist assumes that people vary their behavior extensively in different social and physical environments. In this view people vary their behavior substantially from one setting to another mainly because the reinforcement consequences for particular behaviors differ. Thus the social learning theorist attempts to analyze and identify those stimuli and stimulus changes which produce and maintain behavior and behavior change. People are expected to behave similarly in different settings insofar as those settings are alike (or perhaps are perceived to be alike) in their potential reinforcing properties. For example, if the expression of angry feelings is rewarded in a treatment program but punished in the family setting, it is likely that a patient will express anger on the ward but not at home.

A relevant example is the work of Wolf (1966), who listed the conditions in the environment which were likely to influence the development of intelligence or academic achievement. Among the types of environmental variables identified were the following: the climate created for achievement motivation, the opportunity for verbal development, the nature and amount of assistance provided in overcoming academic difficulties, the level of intellectuality in the environment, and the kinds of work habits expected of the individual. Wolf developed a technique for assessing these variables and found that the relation between the total rating for the degree of intellectual "press" of the environment and measured intelligence was .69. He believes that environments for the development and maintenance of such characteristics as dependency, aggression, and dogmatism could be delineated and measured. This approach has been extensively utilized to set up and study different kinds of treatment programs (Buehler et al., 1966; Cohen and Filipczak, 1971).

As mentioned earlier, these concepts and ideas did not guide this work;

they emerged from it. However, they will help the reader integrate some of the results to be reported. We based our work on three of the foregoing methods: (1) the subjective perceptual methodology of assessing organizational climate, (2) the more objective method of assessing organizational structural dimensions such as size and staffing, and (3) the methodology of characterizing environments by identifying the average personal and/or behavioral characteristics of their inhabitants.

An overview of the scales we constructed, which is given in Table 1.1, will also be helpful to the reader. Chapter 2 presents the development of the Ward Atmosphere Scale (WAS). Our work with this scale is discussed in Chapters 3 to 9. Chapter 10 describes the development of the Community-Oriented Programs Environment Scale (COPES), and our work with this scale is summarized in Chapters 11 to 13.

TABLE 1.1   SUMMARY OF SCALES

	Hospital-Based Programs	Community-Based Programs
Actual program (long form)	99-item, 10-subscale WAS Form C	102-item, 10-subscale COPES Form C
Actual program (short form)	40-item, 10-subscale WAS Short Form S	40-Item, 10-subscale COPES Short Form S
Ideal program	99-Item, 10-subscale WAS Form I (parallel to Form C)	102-Item, 10-subscale COPES Form I (parallel to Form C)
Program expectations	99-Item, 10-subscale WAS Form E (parallel to Form C)	102-Item, 10-subscale COPES Form E (parallel to Form C)

Our initial idea was to relate both perceptual and objective measures of treatment milieus to various indices of adaptation and treatment outcome in hospital-based psychiatric programs. As the work progressed, however, it became clear that we needed to include a wider range of objective variables characterizing the programs. It also became apparent that the assessment of hospital-based programs would be of considerably greater utility if these programs could be directly compared with community-based programs. These considerations led to the work reported in the second half of this book.

REFERENCES

Astin, A. W. *The college environment.* American Council on Education, Washington, D.C., 1968.

Barker, R. *Ecological psychology.* Stanford University Press, Stanford, 1968.

Barrell, R., deWolfe, A., & Cummings, J. A measure of staff attitudes toward care of physically ill patients. *Journal of Consulting Psychology,* **29:** 218–222, 1965.

Bechtel, R. & Gonzales, A. Comparison of treatment environments among some Peruvian and North American mental hospitals. *Archives of General Psychiatry,* **25:** 64–68, 1971.

Buehler, R., Patterson, G., & Furniss, J. The reinforcement of behavior in institutional settings. *Behavior Research and Therapy,* **4:** 157–167, 1966.

Caudill, W. *The psychiatric hospital as a small society.* Harvard University Press, Cambridge, Mass., 1958.

Cohen, H. & Filipczak, J. *A new learning environment.* Jossey-Bass, San Francisco, 1971.

Cohen, J. & Struening, E. Opinions about mental illness in the personnel of two large mental hospitals. *Journal of Abnormal and Social Psychology,* **64:** 349–360, 1963.

Colman, A. *The planned environment in psychiatric treatment: A manual for ward design.* Charles C. Thomas, Springfield, Ill., 1971.

Craik, K. Environmental psychology. *New directions in psychology,* Vol. 4. Holt, Rinehart & Winston, New York, 1970, pp. 1–121.

Dickens, C. *American notes for general circulation,* Vol. 1. Chapman, London, 1842.

Ellsworth, R. Consumer feedback in measuring the effectiveness of mental health programs. In Guttentag, M. and Sturening, E. (Eds.). *Handbook of evaluation research,* to be published, 1973.

Ellsworth, R., Foster, L., Childers, B., Arthur, G., & Kroeker, D. Hospital and community adjustment as perceived by psychiatric patients, their families, and staff. *Journal of Consulting and Clinical Psychology Monograph,* **32:** No. 5, Part 2, 1968.

Endler, N. & Hunt, J. S–R inventories of hostility and comparisons of the proportions of variance from persons, responses, and situations for hostility and anxiousness. *Journal of Personality and Social Psychology,* **9:** 309–315, 1968.

Erikson, E. *Childhood and society.* Norton, New York, 1950.

Fairweather, G. (Ed.). *Social psychology in treating mental illness: An experimental approach.* Wiley, New York, 1964.

Fairweather, G., Sanders, D., Cressler, D., & Maynard, H. *Community life for the mentally ill: An alternative to institutional care.* Aldine, Chicago, 1969.

Feldman, K. & Newcomb, T. *The impact of college on students.* Vol. 1. Jossey-Bass, Inc., San Francisco, 1970.

Goffman, E. *Asylums: Essays on the social situation of mental patients and other inmates.* Doubleday, Garden City, N.Y., 1961.

Greenberg, J. *I never promised you a rose garden.* Holt, Rinehart & Winston, New York, 1964.

Griffitt, W. & Veitch, R. Hot and crowded: Influences of population density and temperature on interpersonal affective behavior. *Journal of Personality and Social Psychology,* **17:** 92–98, 1971.

Grob, G. *The state and the mentally ill: A history of Worcester State Hospital in Massachusetts, 1830–1920.* University of North Carolina Press, Chapel Hill, 1966.

Halpin, A. & Croft, D. *The organizational climate of schools.* Chicago: Midwest Administration Center, University of Chicago, 1963.

Hartmann, H. Ego psychology and the problems of adaptation. In Rapaport, D. (Ed.). *Organization and pathology of thought.* Columbia University Press, New York, 1951.

Hartshorne, H. & May, M. *Studies in deceit.* Macmillan, New York, 1928.

Hunt, J. Traditional personality theory in the light of recent evidence. *American Scientist,* **53:** 40–96, 1965.

Jackson, J. Toward the comparative study of mental hospitals: Characteristics of the treatment environment. In Wessen, A. (Ed.). *The psychiatric hospital as a social system.* Charles C. Thomas, Springfield, Ill., 1964.

Jackson, J. Factors of the treatment environment. *Archives of General Psychiatry,* **21:** 39–45, 1969.

Jones, M. *The therapeutic community: A new treatment method in psychiatry.* Basic Books, New York, 1953.

Jordan, P. A real predicament. *Science,* **175:** 977–978, 1972.

Katz, D. & Kahn, R. *The social psychology of organizations.* Wiley, New York, 1966.

Kellam, G., Schmelzer, J., & Berman, A. Variations in the atmospheres of psychiatric wards. *Archives of General Psychiatry,* **14:** 561–570, 1966.

Kesey, K. *One flew over the cuckoo's nest.* Viking, New York, 1962.

King, R. & Raynes, N. An operational measure of inmate management in residential institutions. *Social Science and Medicine,* **2:** 41–43, 1968.

Likert, R. *The human organization: Its management and value.* McGraw-Hill, New York, 1967.

Linton, R. *The cultural background of personality.* Century, New York, 1945.

Mann, T. *The magic mountain.* Random House, New York, 1952. (Original edition, in German, 1924.)

March, J. (Ed.) *Handbook of organizations.* Rand-McNally, Chicago, 1965.

Michelson, W. Some like it hot: Social participation and environmental use as functions of the season, *American Journal of Sociology,* **76:** 1072–1083, 1971.

Mischel, W. *Personality and assessment.* Wiley, New York, 1968.

Moos, R. A situational analysis of a therapeutic community milieu. *Journal of Abnormal Psychology,* **73:** 49–61, 1968.

Moos, R. Sources of variance in responses to questionnaires and in behavior. *Journal of Abnormal Psychology,* **74:** 405–412, 1969.

Moos, R. Social ecology: Multidimensional studies of humans and human milieus. In Hamburg, D. & Brodie, K. (Eds.) *Frontiers of psychiatry,* Vol. 6, *American handbook of psychiatry,* Basic Books, New York, 1974.

Moos, R. & Clemes, S. A multivariate analysis of the patient–therapist system. *Journal of Consulting Psychology*, **31**: 119–130, 1967.

Moos, R. & Insel, P. (Eds.). *Issues in social ecology: Human milieus.* National Press Books, Palo Alto, Calif., 1974.

Moos, R. & MacIntosh, S. Multivariate study of the patient—therapist system: A replication and extension. *Journal of Consulting and Clinical Psychology*, **35**: 298–307, 1970.

Pace, R. *College and University Environment Scales.* Technical manual, 2nd ed. Educational Testing Service, Princeton, N.J., 1969.

Peterson, R., Centra, J., Hartnett, R., & Linn, R. *Institutional Functioning Inventory.* Preliminary technical manual. Educational Testing Service, Princeton, N.J., 1969.

Pinel, P. *A treatise on insanity*, London, England, 1806 edition (translated from the French by D. D. Davis, MD.).

Porter, L. & Lawler, E. Properties of organization structure in relation to job attitudes and job behavior. *Psychological Bulletin*, **64**: 23–51, 1965.

Rapaport, R. *Community as doctor.* Tavistock, London, 1960.

Raush, H., Dittman, A., & Taylor, T. Person, setting, and change in social interaction. *Human Relations*, **12**: 361–378, 1959.

Raush, H., Farbman, I., & Llewellyn, L. Person, setting, and change in social interaction: 11. A normal control study. *Human Relations*, **13**: 305–332, 1960.

Rice, C., Berger, D., Klett, S., & Sewall, L. Measuring psychiatric hospital staff opinions about patient care. *Archives of General Psychiatry*, **14**: 428–434, 1966.

Rice, C., Berger, D., Klett, S., Sewall, L., & Lemkau, P. The Ward Evaluation Scale. *Journal of Clinical Psychology*, **19**: 251–258, 1963.

Sanders, R., Smith, R., & Weinman, B. *Chronic psychoses and recovery: An experiment in socio-environmental treatment.* Jossey-Bass, San Francisco, 1967.

Sells, S. Dimensions of stimulus situations which account for behavior variance, In Sells, S. (Ed.), *Stimulus determinants of behavior*, Ronald Press, New York, 1963, pp. 1–15.

Solzhenitsyn, A. *Cancer ward.* Bantam Books, New York, 1969.

Spiegel, D. & Keith-Spiegel, P. Perceptions of ward climate by nursing personnel in a large NP hospital. *Journal of Clinical Psychology*, **27**: 390–393, 1971.

Stanton, A. & Schwartz, M. *The mental hospital: A study of institutional participation in psychiatric illness and treatment.* Basic Books, New York, 1954.

Stern, G. *People in context: Measuring person environment congruence in education and industry.* Wiley, New York, 1970.

Stotland, E. & Kobler, A. *Life and death of a mental hospital.* University of Washington Press, Seattle, 1965.

Walberg, H. Social environment as a mediator of classroom learning. *Journal of Educational Psychology*, **60**: 443–448, 1969.

Ward, M. *The snake pit.* Random House, New York, 1946.

Wing, J. & Brown, G. *Institutionalism and schizophrenia: A comparative study of three mental hospitals, 1960–1968.* Cambridge University Press, London, 1970.

Wolf, R. The measurement of environments. In Anastasi, A. (Ed.). *Testing problems in perspective.* American Council on Education, Washington, D.C., 1966, pp. 491–503.

PART TWO

Hospital-Based Programs

Chapter Two

ASSESSING SOCIAL CLIMATES

Like people, environments have unique personalities. Methods have been developed to describe an individual's "personality"; environments can be similarly portrayed with a great deal of accuracy and detail. For example, some people are supportive; likewise, some environments are supportive. Some men feel the need to control others; similarly, some environments are extremely controlling. Order and structure are important to many people; correspondingly, many environments emphasize regularity, system and order. Miller, Galanter, and Pribram (1960) have pointed out that people make detailed plans that regulate and direct their behavior; likewise, environments have overall programs for regulating and directing the behavior of the people within them.

Henry Murray (1938) first wrote of the dual process of personal needs and environmental press. He suggested that individuals have specific needs and that the strength of such needs characterizes "personality." The environment potentially satisfies or frustrates the needs. Murray's model for studying behavior thus consisted of the interaction between personality needs and environmental press. Although Murray's concept of needs provided impetus for the development of measurement techniques for the study of personality, no parallel development in the objective measurement of environmental press was attempted until much later.

Stern, Stein, and Bloom (1956) expanded Murray's contribution. They demonstrated that behavior could be predicted much better when the setting in which the behavior occurred was clearly defined to include the social demands of the situation. Pace and Stern (1958) developed the concept of environmental press further by applying the logic of "perceived climate" to the study of "atmosphere" at colleges and universities. By asking students to act as reporters about the global college environment, they constructed the College Characteristics Index (CCI) to measure that environment. Specifically, the students were requested to answer true-or-false questions covering a wide range of topics such as student–faculty relationships at their college, rules and regulations, classroom methods, and facilities. The logic of this approach suggests that the consensus of students in characterizing their college environment constitutes a measure of environmental climate and that this environmental climate exerts a directional influence on student behavior.

Stern (1970) remarks that descriptions of environmental press are based on inferred continuity and consistency in otherwise discrete events. For example, if patients in a program are assigned specific duties, if they must follow prearranged schedules, if they are liable to be restricted or transferred for not adhering to program policies, if obeying staff is important, and so on, it is likely that the program emphasizes staff control—thus, probably, the development of submissive responses on the part of the patients. It is these conditions which establish the climate or atmosphere of a program.

Our goal was to develop a scale to measure the social climates of hospital-based psychiatric programs by asking patients and staff individually about the usual patterns of behavior in their program. We had three reasons for choosing this method. First, since behavior is shaped and directed by the environment as subjectively perceived by the people in it, we wanted to give each patient and staff member an opportunity to describe the environment as he or she saw it. Second, we wanted to directly compare patient and staff views of their ward culture. Our clinical experience suggested that these two groups often saw the "same" environment quite differently. Third, we wanted to be able to measure people and their environments on similar or commensurate dimensions, because such common dimensions are relevant to the measurement of person–environment congruence or fit. An individual who needs a high degree of support should function better in a highly supportive environment; an individual who needs little support might find such an environment overcontrolling and stifling.

ASSESSING TREATMENT SETTINGS

The Ward Atmosphere Scale (WAS) was developed to measure the social climates of psychiatric treatment programs as perceived by patients and staff. Several sources were used to obtain an initial item pool. Two trained behavior observers with more than a year's experience on psychiatric wards observed three different wards for several weeks, generating several hundred descriptive items. Several popular and professional books (e.g., Maxwell Jones's *Therapeutic Community*, 1953, and Ken Kesey's *One Flew Over the Cuckoo's Nest*, 1962) were read in an effort to identify characteristics associated with different ward environments. Patients and staff who had been on different wards were intensively interviewed about the differences among the wards. These and other sources gave us a pool of more than 500 items. Three steps, resulting in an initial 206-item WAS, were then taken.

1. A set of press appropriate for describing treatment environments was selected from Murray's (1938) and Stern's (1970) categories. Two categories (Personal Problem Orientation and Practical Orientation) were added. Twelve press categories (Involvement, Affiliation, Support, Spontaneity, Autonomy, Practical Orientation, Personal Problem Orientation, Anger and Aggression, Order and Organization, Clarity, Staff Control, and Variety) were adequate to cover all the content areas identified in the item pool, and the items were sorted into these categories by agreement between two independent judges.

2. The item overlap in each of the 12 press categories was eliminated by by deleting highly similar items. To control for acquiescence response set, the number of positively and negatively worded items was approximately equally balanced within each category.

3. Twenty-three additional items were formulated to identify individuals who showed strong positive and/or negative halo in their perceptions.

Some patients might agree with extremely positive items (e.g., "The food here is the best I've ever tasted"; "I never want to leave this ward"), whereas others might agree with extremely negative items (e.g., "In this ward none of the staff ever talks to any of the patients"). These items also helped identify "crazy" or inconsistent answering, since it was easy to determine how often patients endorsed both extremely positive and extremely negative items.

The choice of items was guided by the overall concept of environmental press (Pace and Stern, 1958); that is, an item had to identify characteristics of an environment which could exert a press toward Involvement, toward

Autonomy, toward Spontaneity, and so on. A press toward Involvement is inferred from the following kinds of items: "Patients put a lot of energy into what they do around here," "This is a lively ward," and "The patients are proud of this ward." A press toward Autonomy is inferred from these items: "Patients are expected to take leadership on the ward," "Patients here are encouraged to be independent," and "Patients can leave the ward without saying where they are going." A press toward insight and self-understanding (Personal Problem Orientation) is inferred from still other items: "Patients tell each other about their personal problems," "Personal problems are openly talked about," and "Staff strongly encourage patients to talk about their pasts." Finally, a press toward Order and Organization is inferred from the following items: "Patients' activities are carefully planned," "This is a very well organized ward," and "The staff make sure that the ward is always neat."

THE WARD ATMOSPHERE SCALE

Form A

The resulting 206-item WAS Form A was administered to patients and staff on 14 psychiatric wards. The instructions given to patients and staff were as follows: There are 206 statements in this booklet. They are statements about wards. You are to decide which statements are true of your ward and which are not. Please be sure to answer every statement." The 14 wards represented a broad range of treatment programs in several different institutions. They included three Veterans Administration (VA) hospital wards of relatively acute patients (two all male and one mixed male and female), two VA hospital wards of chronic male patients, two state hospital wards for criminally insane male patients, two regionalized state hospital wards for female patients, one state hospital ward for chronic schizophrenic female patients, one private inpatient ward for acute male and female patients, two coeducational psychiatric wards in general medical community hospitals, and one acute university service ward. The background characteristics of these wards are more fully described by Moos and Houts (1968).

The total numbers of patients and staff tested on the 14 wards were 365 and 131, respectively. Approximately 75% of the patients approached were both willing and able to adequately take the test. This percentage varied from 93% on ward 7 to 45% on ward 11, which housed very chronic schizophrenic patients.

The first question was whether the items discriminated significantly among the wards. For each of the 206 items, one-way analyses of variance were calculated separately for patients and staff. (Only 13 wards were used here because of delay in obtaining data for the fourteenth ward.) For patient responses, 152 of the 183 (83%) press category items (23 of the 206 items were positive or negative halo items) discriminated significantly among wards at the .05 level; 130 of these items (71% of the 183) discriminated significantly among wards at the .01 level. For staff responses, 114 of the 183 items (62%) discriminated among wards at the .05 level, and 95 of these items (52% of the 183) discriminated among wards at the .01 level.

Form B

Items were selected for Form B by the following criteria: (a) The item should significantly discriminate among wards—more than 90% of the items selected did significantly discriminate among wards for patient responses; the figure for staff responses exceeded 80%. (b) The overall item split should be as close to 50–50 as possible—this criterion served to avoid items that were characteristic only of extreme wards. (c) To control for acquiescence response set, each of the 12 press subscales should have an equal number of items scored true and scored false.

The use of these criteria resulted in a 120-item WAS Form B; that is, 12 press dimension subscales each measured by 10 items. The 12 subscale scores were then obtained for each patient and each staff member, and the results of one-way analyses of variance indicated that all 12 subscales significantly ($p < .05$) differentiated among the 14 wards for staff responses, and all but one (involvement) significantly differentiated among them for patient responses.

Form C

The WAS Form B was administered to patients and staff in an extensive normative sample gathered from 160 psychiatric wards in the United States and Canada. The standardization sample is described in Chapter 3. Form C of the WAS was derived from these data. Four samples, two of patients and two of staff, were identified by randomly sampling patients and staff from each of the 160 wards in proportion to their size. The samples were each selected without replacement. The two patient random samples contained

497 and 495 cases, and the two staff random samples had 437 and 439 individuals, in total.

Item intercorrelations, item–subscale correlations, and subscale inter-correlations were calculated for each of these four random samples. The results, which were essentially identical across the four samples, showed that the 12 a priori subscales generally had excellent psychometric properties, except for the Variety subscale, which had very low item intercorrelations and item–subscale correlations. Thus the Variety subscale was dropped from subsequent analyses. Since the Affiliation and Involvement subscales were highly intercorrelated (.58, .64, .65, and .59 in the four samples), these two subscales were collapsed into one subscale labeled Involvement. Otherwise, only the following very slight changes were made in deriving Form C:

1. Three items that had low item–subscale correlations and/or extreme item splits were dropped.

2. Seven items that correlated more highly with another subscale score than with their own subscale score were shifted to the other subscale.

3. Two items were dropped from one subscale (Order and Organization) to decrease item overlap.

4. Two items from the Variety subscale that had showed high correlations with other subscales were added to these subscales.

Table 2.1 lists the 10 final WAS Form C subscales and gives brief definitions of each. The full scale and its scoring key appear in Appendix A.

TABLE 2.1   WAS SUBSCALE DEFINITIONS

1. *Involvement* measures how active and energetic patients are in the day-to-day social functioning of the ward, both as members of the ward as a unit and as individuals interacting with other patients. Patient attitudes such as pride in the ward, feelings of group spirit, and general enthusiasm are also assessed.

2. *Support* measures how helpful and supportive patients are toward other patients, how well the staff understand patient needs and are willing to help and encourage patients, and how encouraging and considerate doctors are toward patients.

3. *Spontaneity* measures the extent to which the environment encourages patients to act openly and to express freely their feelings toward other patients and the staff.

4. *Autonomy* assesses how self-sufficient and independent patients are encouraged to be in their personal affairs and in their relationships with staff, how much responsibility and self-direction patients are encouraged to exercise,

and the influence on staff of patient suggestions, criticism, and other initiatives.

5. *Practical Orientation* assesses the extent to which the patient's environment orients him toward preparing himself for release from the hospital and for the future. Training for new kinds of jobs, looking to the future, and setting and working toward practical goals are among the matters considered.

6. *Personal Problem Orientation* measures the extent to which patients are encouraged to be concerned with their feelings and problems and to seek to understand them through openly talking to other patients and staff about themseslves and their past.

7. *Anger and Aggression* measures the extent to which a patient is allowed and encouraged to argue with patients and staff, to become openly angry, and to display expressions of anger.

8. *Order and Organization* measures the importance of order on the ward in terms of patients (how they look), staff (what they do to encourage order), and the ward itself (how well it is kept); also measures organization, again in terms of patients (do they follow a regular schedule? do they have carefully planned activities?) and staff (do they keep appointments? do they help patients follow schedules?).

9. *Program Clarity* measures the extent to which the patient knows what to expect in the day-to-day routine of his ward and how explicit the ward rules and procedures are.

10. *Staff Control* measures the necessity for the staff to restrict patients—that is, the strictness of rules and schedules, regulations governing relationships between patient and staff, and measures taken to keep patients under effective controls.

The Involvement, Support, and Spontaneity subscales measure *Relationship* dimensions; they assess, respectively, the involvement of patients in the ward, the extent to which staff support patients and patients support and help one another, and the amount of spontaneity and free and open expression within all these relationships. These variables evaluate the type and intensity of personal relationships existing among patients and between patients and staff.

The next four subscales (Autonomy, Practical Orientation, Personal Problem Orientation, and Anger and Agression) deal with Personal Development or *Treatment Program* dimensions. Each subscale assesses a dimension that is specifically relevant to the type of treatment program the ward has developed, and together they assess the four major dimensions along which psychiatric treatment programs vary. With the Autonomy subscale we evaluate the degree to which patients are encouraged to be self-sufficient and independent and to take responsibility for their own decisions. This is clearly an important treatment program variable, and it reflects a major value orientation by staff. The subscales of Practical

Orientation and Personal Problem Orientation are linked to two of the major current psychotherapeutic treatment orientations. For example, token-economy wards and patient-run employment service wards direct patients toward practical preparation for release from the hospital, as in training for new kinds of jobs. On the other hand, some wards strongly emphasize a personal problem orientation and seek to increase patients' self-understanding and insight. These two broad orientations are generally similar to what London (1964) has called the insight and the action psychotherapies.

The Anger and Aggression subscale also assesses a Treatment Program dimension, since the amount of emphasis on the expression of Anger is related to psychotherapeutic values of staff; that is, many professional staff feel that it is beneficial to openly express angry feelings.

The last three subscales of Order and Organization, Program Clarity, and Staff Control assess *Administrative Structure* or *System Maintenance* dimensions. These dimensions are system oriented in that each is related to keeping the program functioning in an orderly, clear, organized, and coherent manner. This tripartite model of the dimensions differentiating among psychiatric treatment programs has direct relevance for a broad range of other social environments (see Chapter 14).

TABLE 2.2   INTERNAL CONSISTENCIES AND ITEM—SUBSCALE CORRELATIONS FOR WAS FORM C SUBSCALES[a]

Subscales	Internal Consistency		Item–Subscale Correlation	
	Patients	Staff	Patients	Staff
1. Involvement (.79)	.78	.82	.51	.51
2. Support (.78)	.65	.60	.44	.44
3. Spontaneity (.69)	.55	.65	.46	.46
4. Autonomy (.76)	.55	.69	.43	.43
5. Practical Orientation (.68)	.59	.63	.46	.44
6. Personal Problem Orientation (.83)	.76	.78	.53	.53
7. Anger and Aggression (.71)	.76	.74	.53	.54
8. Order and Organization (.75)	.75	.82	.53	.53
9. Program Clarity (.76)	.59	.70	.45	.42
10. Staff Control (.77)	.59	.63	.43	.43
Mean	.66	.71	.48	.47

[a]One week test–retest reliabilities for 42 patients shown in parentheses.

Table 2.2 shows the average internal consistencies (Kuder-Richardson Formula 20) and item–subscale correlations for each of the 10 subscales for patients and staff on two random samples of 23 wards each. As Stern (1970) has pointed out, the internal consistencies of tests that measure environmental characteristics may be arbitrarily lowered if the environmental subscales do what they are intended to do; that is, discriminate among different environments. Suppose, for example, most patients and/or staff on one ward answer an item in the true direction, whereas most patients and/or staff on another ward answer the same item in the false direction; that item thus discriminates among environments but also has almost a 50–50 item split, which tends to reduce the internal consistency of its subscale. For this reason, internal consistencies were calculated using average within-ward variances for the items. The subscale internal consistencies are all in an acceptable range, varying from moderate (e.g., Support and Spontaneity) to substantial (e.g., Involvement and Anger and Aggression).

The test–retest reliability of individual subscale scores was calculated on 42 patients, each of whom took the WAS twice one week apart. The results (see Table 2.2, figures in parentheses next to the subscale title) indicate that the 10 subscales have adequate test–retest reliabilities. The reliabilities for the Spontaneity and Practical Orientation subscales are somewhat low, probably because of the relative lack of variability in these subscales on the two wards used in the reliability analysis. The 10 subscale scores were intercorrelated for each of the four random samples. Very few of the correlations were as high as .40 to .50, accounting for only between 16 and 25% of the subscale variance (see Moos, 1974).

Factor analyses were carried out on two (one patient and one staff) of the four random samples. In the patient analysis there were 8 interpretable factors, reflecting 8 of the 10 rationally derived dimensions. Results of the staff analysis were similar; that is, the factor subscales were not very different from the rationally derived subscales. Thus a decision was made to keep all 10 final subscales. By this time we also knew that these subscales were especially useful in giving feedback to patients and staff, since the scales originally derived partly from intensive discussions and observations on wards. The factor analytic subscales, although similar, did not "hang together" in quite as meaningful a manner.

THE HALO SUBSCALE

A thirteenth subscale was constructed for Form B from a group of extremely positively and extremely negatively worded items, using the following criteria: (a) the item should not discriminate significantly among wards, (b) the item should be accepted by fewer than 10% of the patients and staff in the total sample; (c) the subscale should have 10 items—five positive and five negative in content. The resulting subscale was scored for both halo and inconsistency response tendencies (see Moos and Houts, 1968; p. 598).

This subscale was dropped from the WAS for two reasons: first, the items in the 10 final content subscales were only minimally correlated with the halo and inconsistency scores; thus these two response tendencies were essentially independent of the content subscales. Second, inidviduals who answer the WAS inconsistently and/or who do not understand the items tend either to fail to finish the scale or to omit a substantial number of items. Since stringent criteria are applied before a test is included in the sample from a ward (less than 10 missing items, no obvious "runs" of trues and/or falses or alternations between the two, etc.), these two response set scores have proved to be unnecessary.

Equivalence of Forms B and C

Because many investigators have utilized the WAS Form B subscales in their research projects, it should be noted that the correlations between the Form C and the 10 equivalent Form B subscales were calculated for each of our four random samples. The average Form B—Form C correlations are above .90 for all 10 subscales and above .95 for six subscales. Thus statistical analyses(e.g., correlations) on Form B and on the equivalent 10 Form C subscales are essentially interchangeable and are treated as such in subsequent analyses.

The 40-Item Short Form (Form S)

A 40-item Short Form of the WAS was developed for use by investigators or program staff who wish to obtain a relatively rapid assessment of a program's treatment milieu. Four items were chosen from each of the 10 WAS subscales: the items with the highest item—subscale correlations were chosen, provided there was an equal or 3:1 split between items scored true and items scored false (when two chosen items had similar wording, one item was dropped in favor of another less similar item, to cover the subscale content more adequately). Means and standard deviations were then calculated separately for patients and staff, for the 10 four-item subscales for our normative sample of 160 wards. Standard scores were obtained for each of 28 university hospital wards. Intraclass profile correlations between the 10 Form C and the 10 Form S standard scores were calculated for each ward, separately for patients and staff. These correlations assess the similarity between the WAS profile based on only four representative items from each subscale and the profile based on all the items in each subscale. The intraclass correlations between Form C and Form S were greater than .80 for 25 of the 28 wards for patients (the other three were above .70) and greater than .80 for 27 of the 28 wards for staff. Utilizing Form S, therefore, results in profiles highly similar to those obtained with the regular Form C.

The Short Form should be especially useful in following changes in a program over time. However, there are too few items on each subscale to warrant making comparisons among individuals. The 40 items included in the Short Form are marked with an asterisk on the scoring key in Appendix A. The Short Form means and standard deviations for patients and staff for the American reference group sample of 160 wards are given in Moos (1974).

The Ideal (Form 1) and Expectations (Form E) Forms

The Form C items were reworded to allow patients and staff to answer them in terms of the type of ward they would ideally like. This Form was developed to measure the goals and value orientations of patients and staff. What kind of treatment environments do they consider to be ideal? In what areas are patient and staff goals basically similar? In what areas are their goals basically different? To what extent do staff goals vary from ward to ward and/or from hospital to hospital? To what extent do staff of different role orientations (e.g., psychiatrists, nurses) differ in their views of ideal programs?

Another rationale involved comparing real ward and ideal ward profiles, thereby giving patients and staff an opportunity to identify areas in which change is desired. A final purpose was to obtain information on the correlates of the degree of similarity between real ward and ideal ward perceptions for both patients and staff (e.g., are patients and staff more satisfied on wards that show high real—ideal ward similarity?).

There has been much discussion about the overall goals and value orientations of psychiatric treatment programs. Different scales measure staff's opinions about mental illness or staff's attitudes along such dimensions as authoritarian–restrictive and benevolent–democratic (e.g., Cohen and Struening, 1963; Armor and Klerman, 1968); few techniques, however, assess staff ideology in terms of specific ward practices and behaviors. In addition, the value orientations of patients regarding their treatment environments are seldom considered (see Almond et al., 1968), and no available methods assess the goals of patients and staff along the same dimensions.

The WAS Form I can be used in conjunction with Form C in order to identify specific areas in which patients and staff feel that change should occur. Form I also can be used alone if an investigator simply wants to assess the general value orientations or possible value changes in a program or hospital.

The final version of Form I is directly parallel to Form C; that is, each of the items is parallel to one item in Form C. Form I has been given to patients and staff on a sample of 68 different wards in eight hospitals, all in California. Thus the reference group sample is much more restricted in scope than that for Form C. Item—subscale correlations and internal consistencies were calculated for the 10 Form I subscales for a subsample of 20 wards (425 patients and 224 staff). The average item—subscale correlations varied from a low of .33 for Spontaneity to a high of .51 for both Personal Problem Orientation and Anger and Aggression. The subscale internal consistencies varied from a high of .88 for Spontaneity and Order and Organization to a low of .71 for Autonomy. The internal consistencies for Form I were generally slightly higher than those for Form C. Thus Form I has adequate psychometric characteristics. Form I items and instructions are given in Moos (1974).

The Form C items have also been reworded to allow patients and staff to answer them in terms of their expectations about the program they are about to enter. How accurate are these expectations? Does providing systematic information about psychiatric programs result in more accurate expectations? Evidence from both individual and group psychotherapy, and from our own studies of community-based treatment programs, indicates that inaccurate expectations (particularly overly positive ones) can result in poor functioning in the program, absenteeism, and premature dropout (see Chapters 9 and 12). Form E is also directly parallel to Form C, but no separate psychometric data have been obtained on Form E. Form E items and instructions are given in Moos (1974).

DETAILS OF TEST ADMINISTRATION

The various forms of the WAS can be given as paper-and-pencil questionnaires. They may also be administered utilizing tape-recorded instructions. In the latter version, patients and staff mark their answers on an IBM answer sheet. Experience with the tape-recorded testing has been excellent—patients and staff have no difficulty in following the instructions and adequately completing the forms. In addition, the tape-recorded format makes the WAS applicable when potential subjects are either illiterate or cannot read at a sixth-grade level. It is usually best to have separate testing sessions if both the real and the ideal forms are being given; this procedure serves to decrease subjects' fatigue and to clearly differentiate between their impressions of the current program and their conceptions of an ideal program. Each form takes approximately 20 minutes to complete.

The majority of patients and staff are willing and able to complete the forms, assuming that adequate preparations have been made. This aspect of test administration is of critical importance. The procedures are simple and self-evident, but they are often ignored, usually resulting in passive resistance or rebellion (or both!) on the part of patients and staff and thus in a low rate of completed questionnaires.

We follow several basic steps in introducing the concept of assessing ward treatment environments. Since most staff have worked in different treatment milieus, our general approach is quite consonant with their personal experiences. We initially discuss the idea of assessing the program environment with the ward chief or other responsible staff member, and the issues of feedback or results and anonymity of findings are covered. Since the WAS is usually seen as a technique by which to evaluate a program, staff are either overtly or covertly concerned with the use that might be made of the results. Staff usually raise issues about the anonymity and the confidentiality of individual test results (who will be able to see and/or identify *my* responses?) and about the confidentiality of the results for the entire ward. Junior staff are more interested in individual anonymity, whereas senior staff (particularly those who have responsibility for the ward program) care more about the confidentiality of results for the entire program.

These issues are handled differently depending on the purpose of the investigation, the way in which the program was initially contacted (e.g., has the hospital administration been involved or not?) and various other individualized details. The important point is that the issues must be carefully discussed and their solution agreed upon in preliminary meetings. In our experience the ward chief has almost always been interested in the project, and the next step has consisted of having someone from the research project discuss the work in a general staff meeting. In this second meeting arrangements are made for test administration and for giving feedback. The most likely reason for our high response rate (both in terms of the number of programs that agree to be tested and in terms of the proportion of patients and staff who adequately complete the questionnaire) is that we systematically give feedback to each participating program. We feel that some relatively rapid feedback is essential, and we have provided it, at great cost to our studies in terms of both time and money. The methods by which feedback is given and some of the reactions of patients and staff to it are discussed in Chapter 4. In general, patients and staff are appreciative of and interested in the WAS results.

Often a certain proportion of patients either cannot or will not complete the scale. The proportion varies a good deal on different wards; usually, however, an average of about 75% of patients are willing and able to adequately take the test. Exceptions to this are found on geriatric wards and on chronic "back" wards in state hospitals, where the proportion of patients able to complete the test is usually below 50%. Most mentally retarded patients cannot answer the items adequately. Thus patient perceptions of treatment program environment cannot be properly assessed on these types of wards. Staff and/or observers can of course be utilized.

Random Samples on Programs of Varying Sizes

The proportion of people in a program who need to answer the WAS if an adequate profile is to be obtained was investigated by taking 50% random samples of those patients and staff who actually completed the forms, deriving separate profiles for these samples, and assessing the similarity of the profiles by utilizing the intraclass correlation (Haggard, 1958). The average intraclass correlation for the 67 programs with 30 or more patients was above .80 and there was not a single correlation below .80 on any program on whch 20 or more staff members took Form C. Thus a reasonable guideline is that a 50% sample is adequate in programs that have 30 or more patients and/or 20 or more staff members who are able and willing to take the scale.

The advantage of using 50% samples is evident when both the real and ideal forms are employed, since half of each group can take each form. Results for Form I were very similar to those for Form C. However, this procedure is relevant only if an investigator wishes simply to assess the general social environment or value orientations of patients and/or staff. More complete samples are necessary if it is desired to relate individual patient or staff characteristics to either real or ideal ward perceptions.

The Effects of Item Context

A number of investigators who have wanted to give only a portion of the WAS to patients and/or staff have been concerned with the importance of the exact context in which an item is presented. This issue has not been systematically investigated, but some information is available, since there have been three different forms of the scale.

Patients and staff on one ward initially tested with the 206-item Form A were retested 9 and 14 months later with Form B. In the comparison between these testings, the effects of the specific individuals taking the test, the effects of time, and the effects of specific item context are confounded. (As a rule, different sets of individuals took the test at the three administrations.) However, the profile correlations among the administrations suggest that the influence of these factors, thus the effect of item context, is minimal. The intraclass profile correlations for patients were .72 and .71, and those for staff were .97 and .97 for the 9- and 14-month intervals, respectively. The profile stability for another ward tested with Form A and retested with Form B after an interval of almost 2-1/2 years was .83 for patients and .93 for staff. These profile stabilities are as high as those obtained for wards tested at approximately similar time intervals which were given the same Form at each testing. Thus they indicate that the profile stability of the WAS may be extremely high even when items are given in somewhat different item contexts. However, item context may be important for certain individuals, and this issue thus needs further investigation.

The Effects of Subject Anonymity

Two studies were done in collaboration with Jack Sidman in order to estimate the extent to which patients answer the WAS items differentially depending on whether they put their names on the form.

In the first study, done in a VA hospital, patients on two wards were randomly placed into one of two groups. The groups were taken into separate rooms at the same time and were given theWAS under the following conditions. In the first group the standard WAS instructions were given, and the subjects were told: "Fill in your name in the space provided." The subjects in the second group were given the following instruction: "Don't bother to put your name to this test. It is completely anonymous." There were 49 subjects, in the name group and 45 subjects in the no-name group. The 10 Form C subscale scores were calculated for each subject; means and standard deviations were taken for each of the two groups, and T-tests were computed between conditions. None of the 10 subscales differentiated significantly between the name and the no-name groups. Next, separate WAS profiles were drawn for the name and no-name conditions. The two profiles were essentially identical; the intraclass correlation between them was .80, and none of the standard scores for the two conditions differed from each other by more than 0.5 standard deviations. Under the usual conditions of administration, then, it does not make much difference whether patients are asked to put their names on the form.

The second study investigated the effects of anonymity under what were assumed to be "high threat" conditions, since patients in the state hospital in which the study was performed were legally committed and could be released only by consent of the staff. We expected these conditions to give rise to maximum differences between name and no-name instructions.

Patients on each of four wards were randomly divided into two groups and were tested in the manner just described. Patients in the first condition were asked to put their names on the test, whereas patients in the second were told that the test was completely anonymous. There were 70 patients who answered the form anonymously and 70 others who put their names on it. Again subscale scores were calculated for each individual, scale means and standard deviations were taken for each of the two groups, and T-tests were computed for the 10 subscales. Three of the subscales significantly differentiated between the two groups. Patients who put their names on the form perceived significantly more Involvement ($p < .05$) and Order and Organization ($p < .05$) and significantly less Staff Control ($p < .05$). Patients in the name condition viewed their programs somewhat more positively than did patients in the no-name condition. Differences on other subscales were in the same direction, although not statistically significant. The magnitude of the subscale differences between the two conditions was about 0.5 standard deviations.

Under the usual low threat conditions of administration, therefore, few if any effects are related to whether a patient puts his name on the form. In a potentially "high threat" situation, on the other hand, differences between name and no-name conditions may be as great as 0.5 standard deviations.

The differences between responses of identified and anonymous subjects are consistent with those of previous studies (e.g., Ash and Abramson, 1952; Corey, 1937; Gerberich and Mason, 1948; Hamel and Reif, 1952; and Olson, 1936); all these investigators report no significant response distortion by subjects who put their names on questionnaires. Pelz (1959) compared the effects of full anonymity versus confidentiality. Confidentiality meant that the individual subject was identified only to the survey staff. There were almost no differences between these two conditions.

Rosen (1960), attempting to determine the effects of identification on attitudes expressed by college students toward reading in general and toward a specific English course, found that there were significant differences between identified and anonymous groups in the attitudes they expressed toward the specific English course. On the other hand, the differences between the two group means were very small. Rosen concluded that identification of respondents in attitude questionnaire surveys conducted under less than highly threatening circumstances is not likely to result in serious statistical or practical distortion" (p. 679).

In a recent study, Klein, Maher, and Dunnington (1967) compared attitude survey responses between identified and nonidentified employees under two conditions of identification. One involved a face-to-face designation by the employee's manager of which group the subject was to be in (high threat), whereas the other involved a random allocation as the employee entered the testing room (low threat). All subjects were assured of confidentiality of their responses, and the nonidentified individuals were assured anonymity. A positive distortion in responses took place under both identified conditions, but significantly more distortion occurred under the high threat condition.

King (1970) reviewed the effect of anonymity versus identification in drug usage surveys and obtained contrasting results—namely that neither the percentage of return nor the percentage of respondents admitting to drug use was a simple function of the anonymity of the questionnaire. In one study the identified questionnaires yielded a higher percentage of both returns and admission of the use of drugs. In no instance, however, was the difference between the anonymous and the identifiable questionnaires significant at the .05 level. King concludes that his findings, at the minimum, cast doubt on the validity of the "obvious" notion that a coded identifiable questionnaire necessarily yields a significantly smaller percentage of returns and a significantly smaller percentage of admissions of the use of illegal drugs.

These studies suggest that there may be less response distortion due to questionnaire identification than has previously been thought, although many subtle situational factors seem to affect the degree of distortion that does occur. Klein, Maher, and Dunnington (1967) also propose that items of different content may be differentially susceptible to change under conditions of identification. They found that items dealing with salary and with ratings of top management produced consistent positive distortions, whereas items dealing with the subject's situation (i.e., work pressure and subject's manager) produced little or no distortion even under conditions of high threat. Since the items in the WAS ask about the environment, rather than about either personality or attitudes, they are the kinds of items that should give rise to relatively little distortion.

In summary, lack of anonymity produces little or no distortion in WAS items under conditions of low threat and moderate amounts of positive distortion under conditions of presumed high threat. These conclusions hold only for patients. There may be larger effects for staff. We have not replicated these studies with staff, since we felt that the potential negative effects of not telling staff the truth about our procedures were not worth the additional information that might be produced. However, staff are usually highly ego-involved in the treatment environment they are creating. Staff are more likely to respond under conditions they perceive to be threatening; thus positive response distortion by staff may be more likely than positive response distortion by patients.

Even though patient identification makes relatively little difference, it is probably best for investigators to gather data anonymously unless they wish to relate individual responses to other measures. Appropriate coding procedures to guarantee confidentiality must always be followed if the WAS is given by a staff member. Anonymity is important, otherwise this condition is similar to the high threat condition described by Klein et al. (1967) in that the patient knows that his responses can be identified by a staff member in the program. Different investigators must make these decisions to the best of their ability. The conditions of test administration have important effects on the response rate of completed questionnaires and on the exact results. The care with which these conditions should be arranged cannot be overemphasized.

REFERENCES

Almond, R., Keniston, K., & Boltax, S. The value system of a milieu therapy unit. *Archives of General Psychiatry*, **19**: 545-561, 1968.

Armor, D. & Klerman, G. Psychiatric treatment orientations and professional ideology. *Journal of Health and Social Behavior*, **9**: 243—255, 1968.

Ash, P. & Abramson, E. The effect of anonymity on attitude-questionnaire research. *Journal of Abormal and Social Psychology* **46**: 722—723, 1952.

Cohen, J. & Struening, F. Opinions about mental illness: Mental hospital occupational profiles and profile clusters. *Psychological Reports*, **12**: 111—124, 1963.

Corey, S. Professed attitudes and actual behavior. *Journal of Educational Psychology*, **28**: 271—280, 1937.

Gerberich, J. & Mason, J. Signed versus unsigned questionnaires. *Journal of Educational Research*, **42**: 122—126, 1948.

Haggard, E. *Intraclass correlation and the analysis of variance*. Dryden, New York, 1958.

Hamel, L. & Reif, H. Should attitude questionnaires be signed? *Personnel Psychology*, **5**: 87—91, 1952.

Jones, M. *The therapeutic community*. Basic Books, New York, 1953.

Kesey, K. *One flew over the cuckoo's nest*. Viking, New York, 1962.

King, F. Anonymous versus identifiable questionnaires in drug usage surveys. *American Psychologist*, **25**: 982—985, 1970.

Klein, S., Maher, J., & Dunnington, R. Differences between identified and anonymous subjects in responding to an industrial opinion survey. *Journal of Applied Psychology*, **51**: 152—160, 1967.

London, P. *The modes and morals of psychotherapy*. Holt, Rinehart & Winston, New York, 1964.

Miller, G., Galanter, E., & Pribam, K. *Plans and the structure of behavior*. Henry Holt, New York, 1960.

Moos, R. *Ward Atmosphere Scale Manual*. Consulting Psychologists Press, Palo Alto, Calif., 1974.

Moos, R. & Houts, P. Assessment of the social atmospheres of psychiatric wards. *Journal of Abnormal Psychology*, **73**: 595—604, 1968.

Murray, H. *Explorations in personality*. Oxford University Press, New York, 1938.

Olson, W. The waiver of signature in personal reports. *Journal of Applied Psychology*, **20**: 442—449, 1936.

Pace, C. & Stern, G. An approach to the measurement of psychological characteristics of college environments. *Jornal of Educational Psychology*, **49**: 269—277, 1958.

Pelz, D. The influence of anonymity on expressed attitudes. *Human Organization*, **18**: 88—91, 1959.

Rosen, N. Anonymity and attitude measurement. *Public Opinion Quarterly*, **24**: 675—679, 1960.

Stern, G. *People in context; Measuring person environment congruence in education and industry.* Wiley, New York, 1970.

Stern, G., Stein, M., & Bloom, B. *Methods in personality assessment.* Free Press, New York, 1963.

Chapter Three

THE SOCIAL CLIMATES
OF HOSPITAL—BASED
TREATMENT SETTINGS

AMERICAN TREATMENT PROGRAMS

Great care was exercised in order to obtain an American reference group sample that would be fully representative of the breadth and diversity of current inpatient treatment programs. Our overall goal was to provide a new measurement technique that would be standardized well enough to be applicable to the widest possible range of psychiatric programs. An attempt was made to secure a broad regional representation of wards from different parts of the United States; for example, hospitals in several southern and southwestern states were included. When more than one ward was tested in a hospital, we tried to take a representative sample of wards in that hospital. Wards that had unusual or innovative treatment programs were identified and were usually included because of high staff interest in them.

The final American normative sample included wards located in 16 states: Alabama, California, Colorado, Illinois, Kansas, Massachusetts, Mississippi, New York, North Carolina, Oklahoma, Oregon, Pennsylvania, Texas, Virginia, Washington, and Wisconsin. The summary characteristics of this sample are given in Table 3.1. We assessed 160 wards in 44 hospitals, approximately one-third of the sample being collected from hospitals and wards in California. Included were 55 wards in 10 state hospitals, 55 wards in 14 Veterans Administration Hospitals, 28 wards in 24 university and teaching hospitals, and 22 wards in 6 community and private hospitals. The total numbers of patients and staff tested were 3575 and 1958, respectively.

TABLE 3.1 SUMMARY CHARACTERISTICS OF AMERICAN NORMATIVE SAMPLE

Type of Hospital	Number of Hospitals	Number of Wards	Number of Hospitals in California	Number of Wards in California	Number of States Represented
State	10	55	5	24	4
VA	14	55	4	14	11
University	14	28	4	10	8
Community and private	6	22	3	3	4
	44	160	16	51	16

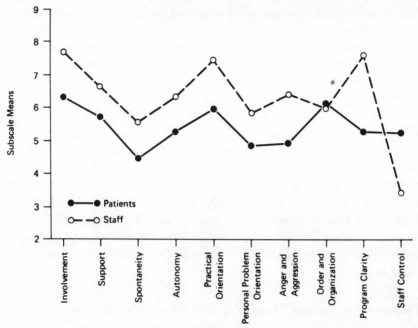

Figure 3.1   WAS Form C means for patients and staff on 160 American programs.

Figure 3.1 plots the means of the Form C subscales over the 160 wards, separately for patients and staff. It should be noted that we did not collect a truly random sample of psychiatric wards, even though the total range and variation of different types of treatment programs are represented. Also, wards having mainly geriatric patients, mentally retarded patients, and/or very chronic patients were not included in the sample because the patients could not adequately complete the form.

The most important finding is that there are significant differences between patients and staff on all subscales but one (Order and Organization). Since patients and staff were answering exactly the same items, this indicates that there are substantial discrepancies in the overall manner in which the two groups perceive psychiatric wards. These results corroborate the importance of conceptualizing two distinctly different patient and staff subcultures, although patients and staff in some programs do show very close agreement.

To identify items on which the two groups showed particularly large disagreements, the average proportion of true responses was calculated separately for patients and staff for the total sample for each of the items.

Patient–staff differences were 20% or greater on 25 items, but only 10% or less on 36 items, indicating that the items are differentially sensitive to such differences. For example, items on which staff answered true at least 20% more often than patients included: "Discussions are pretty interesting on this ward," "Staff are interested in following up patients once they leave the hospital," "New treatment approaches are often tried on this ward," "On this ward staff think it is healthy to argue," and "Staff tell patients when they are getting better." Staff answered false considerably more often than patients on certain other items, including ; "Once a schedule is arranged for a patient the patient must follow it," "Patients will be transferred from this ward if they don't obey the rules," "It's not safe for patients to discuss their personal problems around here," and "If a patient argues with another patient he will get into trouble with the staff." These items give substance to what the overall results indicate—namely, that staff on the whole present a significantly more positive picture of programs than do patients.

Differences Among State, VA, and University Wards

To learn whether there were broad differences in treatment environments in wards at different types of hospitals the total sample of 160 wards was divided into 55 state hospital wards, 55 VA hospital wards, 28 university and teaching hospital wards, and 22 private hospital wards.

The 55 state hospital wards included alcoholic wards, adolescent wards, wards mainly for acute and wards mainly for chronic patients, token-economy wards, and regionalized wards. There were slightly more male than female wards. The number of patients per ward varied from 7 to 90; the number of full-time day staff from 1 to 14, and the patient—staff ratio from 1.75 to 28 patients per staff member. The total number of patients and staff tested was 1231 and 568 respectively. The median length of patient stay varied from less than 3 months to more than 6 years. Thus these wards included the full range of variation usually found in state hospitals. The 10 hospitals were Agnew, Atascadero, DeWitt, Modesto, and Napa State Hospitals in California, Fort Logan Mental Health Center (Colorado), Galesburg State Research Hospital (Illinois), Mendota State Hospital (Wisconsin), Peoria State Hospital (Illinois), and Philadelphia State Hospital.

The 55 VA hospital wards included 52 wards for males, two wards for females, and one ward for males and females. The number of patients per ward varied from 20 to 140, the number of full-time day staff from 1 to 20, and the patient–staff ratio from 3 to more than 20 patients per staff member. The median length of patient stay varied from less than 2 months to more than 5 years; thus the full range of acute and chronic patients was represented. Tested were 1687 patients and 590 staff. The 14 hospitals were located at American Lake (Washington), Bedford (Massachusetts), Biloxi (Mississippi), Los Angeles, Philadelphia, Salem (Virginia), Salisbury (North Carolina), Syracuse (New York), Topeka (Kansas), Tuscaloosa (Alabama), and Waco (Texas).

Almost all the 28 university and teaching hospital wards were coeducational. The number of patients per ward varied from 10 to 40, the number of full-time day staff from 6 to 40, and the patient—staff ratio from less than 1 to slightly more than 3 patients per staff member. These wards usually had acute patients who stayed for only short periods. The numbers of patients and staff tested were 391 and 532, respectively. The number of staff tested was particularly high because trainees (e.g., psychiatric residents psychology trainees, social work and nursing students) and evening and night shift staff were usually included. The wards were affiliated with the following institutions: Hahnemann Medical Center, Michael Reese Institute (technically a private hospital that was classified as a university and teaching hospital because of its long tradition and reputation in this area), Stanford University, University of California at Los Angeles and at San Francisco, University of Colorado, University of Montreal, University of New York at Syracuse, University of Oregon, University of Pennsylvania, Rochester University, and the University of Virginia.

The 22 private wards and community hospital wards inluded male wards, female wards, and mixed wards. The number of patients varied from 10 to 30; the number of full-time day staff from 2 to 26, and the patient—staff ratio from 1 to 6 patients per staff member. Median length of patient stay varied from 1 to 2 weeks to more than 6 months. There were 266 and 268 patients and staff tested, respectively. The number of staff members tested is again particularly high because of the inclusion of trainee and evening and night shift staff on a number of wards. Since only a small number of hospitals is involved in this subsample, anonymity is best preserved by not identifying the institutions.

Figure 3.2 compares patients' perceptions of state, VA, and university hospital programs. The results for private and community hospital wards are not plotted because of the limited sample. The results indicate that

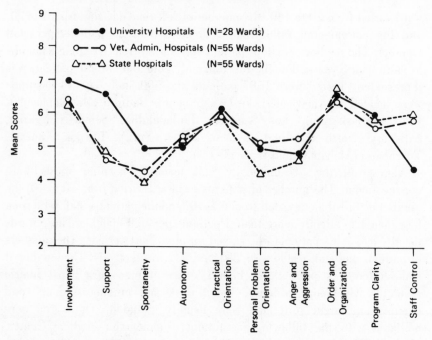

Figure 3.2 Patient WAS Form C means for 55 VA wards, 55 state hospital wards, and 28 university hospital wards.

there are some overall differences among the three types of programs but that these differences are not substantial. University programs reveal somewhat greater emphasis on all three Relationship dimensions and somewhat less emphasis on Staff Control. The differences are in the same direction for staff, but they are much smaller. The VA wards score lowest on Spontaneity, Personal Problem Orientation, and Anger and Aggression, and highest on the System Maintenance dimensions of Order and Organization and Staff Control. This trend fits with the view of VA wards as being somewhat more likely to be well-organized, rule-oriented, and "unexpressive."

Perhaps the major finding, however, is the degree of overlap among the three types of wards. The variation in results *within* state, VA, university, and private and community hospital wards is extremely large. This is directly consistent with the finding that the variation in treatment environments may be as great on different wards within one hospital as on wards in different hospitals. These results support the conclusion that specific characteristics of the ward treatment program, rather than hospital administrative policies per se, are of critical import in determining the actual treatment milieu.

BRITISH TREATMENT PROGRAMS

A sabbatical year at the Institute of Psychiatry and Maudsley and Royal Bethlem Hospitals in London provided the opportunity to collect a cross-cultural sample. The process of becoming familiar with the range of available psychiatric ward settings and conducting interviews with patients and staff oriented toward making the WAS applicable to wards in the United Kingdom went slowly at first. This was because of unanticipated differences in ward organization and difficulties in obtaining the necessary administrative approvals required before the research could be begun. After this relatively mild "culture shock" was overcome, the work proceeded rapidly. Pretest data from selected wards indicated that the American version of the WAS could be utilized in Britsh psychiatric settings with little or no change. Only some relatively minor changes in wording (e.g., "complain" for "gripe", "tidy" for "clean") were necessary.

A total of 36 wards was collected for a British normative sample. The wards were drawn from eight different hospitals and included three psychiatric wards in general medical hospitals, several wards in four different university teaching hospitals, and wards in both small and large psychiatric hospitals in urban and rural areas. There were adolescent wards, a geriatric ward, acute admission wards, wards for chronic patients, a long-stay psychotherapy ward, and so on. Some of the wards were only for male, some only for female, and some for patients of both sexes. Programs with radically different treatment orientations were included—for example, wards in the sample ranged from those in which there was essentially no milieu orientation to those in which patients and staff jointly made almost all important decisions in large community meetings.

The size and staffing of the wards was quite varied, the median size being slightly more than 20 patients (range from 7 to 77) and the median number of full-time day staff about 4 patients per staff member (range from 0.9 to more than 30). The totals of patients and staff tested were 450 and 290 respectively. Further details about this sample, internal consistencies for the 10 subscales, subscale intercorrelations, and sample British WAS profiles are given elsewhere (Moos, 1972).

The differences between British patients and staff were almost identical to those between American patients and staff. Overall, British staff perceived significantly greater emphasis than British patients ($p < .01$) on all the dimensions except for Order and Organization and Staff Control. British patients perceived significantly more emphasis on Staff Control. This was exactly the result obtained in the American sample. Thus the conclusion that staff view psychiatric programs much more positively than patients generalizes cross-culturally to a British sample. The actual means and standard deviations are given in Moos (1974).

COMPARISONS OF AMERICAN AND BRITISH TREATMENT PROGRAMS

In making a cross-cultural comparison of American and British programs, a subsample of 36 wards was chosen from the total American normative sample. These 36 wards were selected to match the range of ward sizes and staffing ratios obtained in the British sample.

From Figures 3.3 and 3.4, which compare the 36 British wards with the 36 matched American wards, we see that the general pattern of results is similar in American and British wards. However, American patients and staff perceive significantly ($p < .01$) greater emphasis on the Relationship dimension of Involvement, the Treatment Program dimensions of Autonomy, Practical Orientation, and Personal Problem Orientation, and the System Maintenance dimension of Staff Control than do British patients and staff. American staff also report significantly ($p < .01$) more emphasis on Anger and Aggression than do British staff.

Some items were much more sensitive to cross-cultural differences than others. For example, 57 items showed differences of 10% or less, whereas 13 items showed differences of 20% or more, in the average proportion of American and British patients who answered them true. Staff displayed similar differences on 11 of the latter 13 items. Examples of items on which both American patients and staff answered true at least 20% more often than both British patients and staff include: "Patients often do things together on the weekends," "Patients are pretty busy all the time," "Patients can leave the ward whenever they want to," "Patients can wear what they want," "The staff act on patients' suggestions," "Patients are expected to take leadership on the ward," "If a patient breaks a rule he knows what will happen to him," and "Patients who break the ward rules are punished for it." These items distinctly suggest the major differences between American and British wards; namely, there is less emphasis on

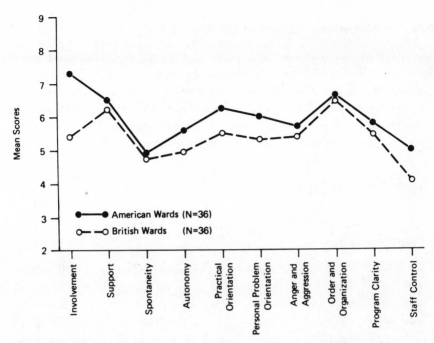

Figure 3.3   Patient WAS Form C means for 36 American and 36 British wards.

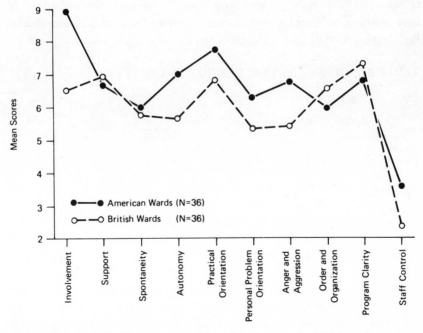

Figure 3.4   Staff WAS Form C means for 36 American and 36 British wards.

Involvement, on Autonomy and Independence, and on Clarity and Control on British than on American wards. On the other hand, there is substantial overlap in the two samples (e.g., some British wards have more emphasis on Involvement and Autonomy than some American wards). Consistent with general cultural stereotypes, however, British staff tend to leave their patients more "to their own devices" than do American staff.

TEST STATISTICS

Profile Stability

We know that the 10 WAS subscales have adequate test–retest reliabilities (see Table 2.2). From the point of view of characterizing treatment programs, a more important question is related to the stability of the overall ward profile. Table 3.2 presents the stability results obtained for WAS profiles derived from patients and staff at different test–retest intervals. These profile stabilities were obtained by calculating intraclass correlations (Haggard, 1958) on the standard scores of the different administrations on each ward. The intraclass correlation was used because it is sensitive to both level and relative position differences.

TABLE 3.2 TEST—RETEST PROFILE STABILITY

Test–Retest Interval	Number of Wards	Average Profile Correlations	
		Patients	Staff
1 week	2	.92	.91
1–2 months	7	.76	.85
4–7 months	4	.77	.89
9 months	2	.70	.78
14–15 months	2	.70	.92
2–2.5 years	7	.76	.83
3 years, 4 months	1	.73	.96

The results indicate that the profile stability of wards that have a consistent treatment philosophy is extremely high over relatively long periods of time. This is true for both patients and staff, although the stabilities for staff are somewhat higher than those for patients, particularly over the longer time intervals. The profile stabilities for test–retest intervals of 9 months or longer may be especially high because the wards involved had stable staff and an ongoing research program and/or were specifically interested in continuing reevaluation of their treatment environments. Even considering these factors, the average profile stabilities over 2- to 3-year time intervals are remarkable. Very few if any of the same patients were tested on both occasions on wards on which the test–retest interval was 6 months or more. Thus we can tentatively conclude that the treatment environment of a program does not necessarily depend on the specific patients in that program.

Differences Among Programs

We were concerned about the proportion of subscale variance accounted for by differences among programs. This is similar to the problem of the relative proportion of variance accounted for by persons, settings, and person-by-setting interactions in responses to questionnaires and in behavior. The proportions accounted for by different sources varies greatly depending on the particular sample of persons, settings, and response modes under study. Thus no single answer can be given to this question. The analysis of variance of WAS subscales among wards is almost always statistically significant for both patients and staff, particularly when the wards under study are sampled from different hospitals.

Estimated Ω^2 (Hays, 1963) was used to calculate the average proportion of the total subscale variance accounted for by differences among programs. Three different sets of analyses were conducted across 8, 28, and 36 wards, respectively. The proportion of variance accounted for by differences among wards varied from a low of less than 2% to a high exceeding 50%. On the average, differences among wards account for about 20 to 25% of the variance for patients and 25 to 30% of the variance for staff. Thus the proportion of variance accounted for by between-ward differences may be quite substantial. In addition, it is very similar to the proportion of variance that is usually accounted for by individual difference measures of personality traits (Mischel, 1968). On the other hand, an important proportion of subscale variance is attributable to individual differences of perception among patients and among staff within wards. Correlates of different types of individual "deviancies" of perception are discussed in Chapter 9.

Ellsworth and Maroney (1972) have dealt with the issue just described in relation to the Perception of Ward (POW) scales, and Centra (1970) has discussed it with respect to the student perception section of the Questionnaire on Student and College Characteristics (QSCC). Ellsworth and Maroney found that only between 2 and 11% of the total variance of the POW subscales was between-ward variance. This finding may be partly attributable to the following circumstances: (1) the POW items were not initially chosen on the basis of their ability to discriminate among wards; (2) the 34 wards used (sampled from only eight different hospitals, five of them being VA hospitals) do not represent a particularly broad range of wards; (3) since the POW data on 19 of the wards were collected over fairly long time intervals, the within ward variance is partly due to changing program characteristics; (4) some of the wards were very large (average number of beds was 140), and evidence indicates that the degree of disagreement among patients and staff about their ward milieu (thus the extent of within ward variance) is significantly positively correlated with ward size (see Chapter 6).

Centra derived 8 student perception factors on data from a broadly representative sample of 116 colleges and universities and used Estimated Ω^2 to calculate the proportions of the total factor variance attributable to differences among institutions. These proportions ranged from 21 to 68% with a mean of 35% for the 8 factor subscales and from 3 to 75% (mean of 21%) for the 77 items. Thus the proportions of variance due to between-college differences were quite substantial, although usually still less than those accounted for by differences among students within colleges. Centra rightly concludes that the proportion of variance due to institution differences is an important criterion in selecting items for scales primarily oriented toward assessing institutional environments.

Relationships Between Subscales and Background Variables

To acquire information on the extent to which perception of ward treatment environment is a function of individual background characteristics, we calculated correlations between the 10 subscales and the background characteristics of sex, age, and length of stay (or time worked) on the ward. Correlations for our initial sample of 365 patients on 14 wards are presented in Moos and Houts (1968, p. 599). Only 5 of the 30 correlations were above .20. Similar correlations were calculated for a second sample of 186 patients on 8 other wards, and only 2 of the resulting 30 correlations were above .20. Correlations were also calculated for staff. Only 3 of 30 correlations for the 131 staff on our initial sample of 14 wards were above .20, and only 5 of 30 were above .20 in a second sample of 63 staff on 8 additional wards.

Thus the relationships between the three background variables named and the WAS subscales are quite low. These results are consistent with our findings on other perceived environment scales—for example, low correlations between the Correctional Institutions Environment Scale (CIES) subscales and age and length of stay of residents in correctional units (Moos, 1968), and close similarity between male and female residents' perceptions of three coed dormitories (Gerst and Moos, 1972). More work remains to be done before precise statements can be made, since other personality and/or background factors may bear closer relation to perceptions of ward atmosphere than the background factors of sex, age, and length of time spent on the ward. However, it is also possible that background and personality factors do not strongly affect environmental perceptions because such perceptions concern relatively objective aspects of the environment rather than the personality, motivations, or attitudes of individuals.

Relationships Between Subscales and Social Desirability

Next we attempted to ascertain how perceptions of milieus are related to the degree to which patients and staff answer items about themselves in socially desirable directions. The two scales utilized were the Crowne-Marlowe Social Desirability Scale and the Social Desirability subscale of the Ward Initiative Scale (WIS), which is composed of items indicative of concrete initiatives that can be taken by patients on psychiatric wards (Houts and Moos, 1969). This subscale consists of nine items that have high correlations with and similar content to the Crowne-Marlowe.

First, the 10 WAS subscales were correlated with the Crowne-Marlowe for 262 patients on eight different wards in one state hospital, and for 186 patients on eight other wards located in four hospitals. These correlations were generally low, although there was a slight tendency for the Crowne-Marlowe to be negatively correlated with the Treatment Program dimensions (average $r = -.18$) and positively correlated with the System Maintenance dimensions (average $r = .11$). The correlations were contrary to expectation, since they indicated that patients who answered Crowne-Marlowe items in less socially desirable ways perceived their wards somewhat more positively. Since these correlations confounded intraward and interward differences, another set of correlations was calculated for patients *within* each of four different state hospital wards. There were slight positive relationships between the Crowne-Marlowe and the WAS Relationship dimensions (average $r = .12$). The Crowne-Marlowe was not correlated with the other WAS dimensions (see Moos, 1974).

Finally, correlations were calculated for 94 staff members on four different wards in one state hospital. These correlations indicated that staff who answer items in socially desirable directions have a slight tendency to also answer the WAS items in somewhat more desirable directions. The correlations were generally low, although four of them were above .20. Overall, patient and staff perceptions of treatment milieus are only minimally if at all related to their tendency to answer items about themselves in socially desirable directions. These results are consistent with those obtained on our other perceived climate scales (Moos, 1968; Gerst and Moos, 1972).

PERSONALITY AND BACKGROUND CORRELATES OF ENVIRONMENTAL PERCEPTIONS

The extent to which individual personality and background characteristics effect or determine perceptions of the environment is important. If these factors are strongly influential, perceived environment scales could be regarded simply as personality scales that happen to have items asking about the social milieu. There is some evidence on this question, most but not all of it consistent with the notion that individual characteristics are only minimally correlated with environmental perceptions.

Some studies have been done with the WAS. Westmaas (1971) found that the only sex difference of any size was on the dimension of Order and Organization. Female staff members perceived less order than males but wanted more order on their ideal ward. Kish, Solberg, and Uecker (1971a) predicted that a patient's perception of his treatment environment would be related to his perception of the locus of control of his reinforcements. They utilized the Rotter Internal–External (I–E) Control Scale (Rotter, 1966). In general, individuals having high internal scores are more striving and persistent in the face of frustration and more self-confident than externals. Externals are more passive, apathetic, and anxious; yet they are less self-confident, feeling that they are not in control of the reinforcements they receive.

Kish et al. took two groups of subjects from the upper and lower extremes of the I–E distribution and found that patients scoring high on the I–E Scale perceived their wards more positively in terms of emotional support, practical orientation, fostering of independence and affiliation, and clarity regarding program goals and procedures. An internally oriented patient tends to perceive his ward as a locus of active treatment, whereas an externally oriented patient is apt to take a more custodial perspective. Kish et al. point out that each alternative may be a realistic appraisal, since the internally oriented patient is seen by staff as having greater potential for improvement and is thus treated in a more therapeutic fashion, whereas the external oriented patient is treated in a more custodial fashion. However, since Kish et al. did not control for differences among wards, their findings may simply indicate that high internal and high external patients are assigned to wards with different treatment environments.

Kish et al. (1971b) also related Ellsworth's (1965) version of the Opinions about Mental Illness Scale (OMIS) to staff perception of treatment environment. The attitude dimensions were (a) Restrictive Control or Conventional Attitude, (b) Protective–Benevolence, and (c) a Nontraditional or Accountability attitude. These three attitude scores were correlated with WAS subscale scores for 54 psychiatric aides. There were only a few significant correlations; for example, the more conventional aides saw their wards as deemphasizing Autonomy and Personal Problem Orientation, and aides who perceived the locus of Accountability as lying with the patient saw their wards as promoting insightful discussion of patients' problems and feelings. However, these relationships might again be based on real between-ward differences in treatment environments.

Ellsworth and Maroney (1972) correlated POW subscale scores with background variables of age, length of time in hospital, and marital status ($N = 1449$ patients), and with psychological test scores such as self-confidence in physical skills, thinking and planning, and work capacity ($N = 57$ admissions). Only 6 of the 45 correlations presented were above .20, indicating that these variables accounted for little of the variance in patient perceptions.

This issue has been extensively pursued in relation to perceived environment scales constructed for other types of environments, particularly in the educational area. For example, McFee (1961) studied the relation between student perception of the college environment as measured by the College Characteristics Index (CCI) and student personality needs as measured by the Activities Index (AI). She failed to find any correlation between scale scores of individuals on the CCI and their parallel scores on the AI. In addition, no strong relationship appeared between personality needs and the student's perception of environmental press as reflected by individual items. The responses to 88% of the 300 CCI items were independent of the parallel personality needs of the respondent. Differences in the objectivity of individual items produced moderate differences in uniformity of response to the items but no discernible differences in the influence of need on the item responses. Items about conditions the student was unlikely to have encountered (i.e., those low in "exposure value") yielded less agreement and were more influenced by need than were items about widely shared experiences.

In a somewhat different approach, Herr (1965) used the High School Characteristics Index (HSCI) to describe the perceptions of students at differing achievement and extracurricular participation levels. He found that students categorized as high or middle achievers perceived more press for affiliation, for intense open emotional display, for detached impersonal problem-solving and analysis, and so on. The low-achieving students perceived more press for such factors as self-depreciation and self-devaluation, for indifference or disregard for the feelings of others, for withholding friendship and support, and for compulsive organization of the immediate physical environment. Herr also noted some minor differences in environmental perceptions related to the degree of extracurricular participation by the student.

Herr concluded that responses to the HSCI items provided descriptions of the different environmental demands faced by students. He argued that these individual differences had implications for counseling and might be used to identify students who did not perceive environmental demands on themselves that were strongly evident to the majority of other students. Relationships between ability levels and the extent of extracurricular participation and environmental perceptions may demonstrate the effect of personality on perception; alternatively, they may be taken to indicate that different types of students function in somewhat different subenvironments within the larger environment.

Several studies have investigated this issue, using the College and University Environment Scales (CUES). Pace (1969, p. 10) reported that responses to CUES items are not influenced by the personal characteristics of the students. He states:

Of 245 correlations between the responses of individuals about their environments and such personal characteristics as are measured by the Allport-Vernon-Lindzey Study of Values, the Omnibus Personality Inventory, the Heston Personality Inventory, the Activities Index, the ACE Psychological Examination, and the College Qualification Test, 86 percent have been between .00 and plus or minus .29.

Both Spradling (1970), utilizing Cattell's 16PF, and Berdie (1967), utilizing high school percentile rank and Minnesota Scholastic Aptitude Test scores, came to essentially similar conclusions. Yonge (1968) had 102 students take the CUES and the Omnibus Personality Inventory (OPI). He intercorrelated the subscale scores and reported 90 correlations; of these, only 11 were above .20 and none above .30.

On the other hand, Jansen (1967) found that social-political action leaders perceived less friendliness, cohesiveness, and emphasis on the search for personal meaning in their campus environment than other types of campus leaders. Liberal social-political action leaders had significantly lower mean scores on the CUES Community, Awareness, and Propriety scales than their more conservative counterparts. Finally, Marks (1968) has performed a sophisticated study in which he systematically assessed item content, item ambiguity, and selected personality and motivational factors as measured by Jackson's (1965) Personality Research Form and two other scales relating to motivational aspects of educational behavior. He found that descriptions of the college environment were not independent of the properties of the subject or of the properties of the items. A fairly high proportion (30%) of the correlations between selected CUES subscales and subject variables were statistically significant; however, the number of subjects was high ($N = 570$), and Marks gave no indication of the magnitude of the correlations. For selected subject and item characteristics, he concluded, a reliable portion of the response to a given environmental characteristic can be attributed to certain properties of the subject, arguing that for some CUES items it is the sample of students and not the environment that is being characterized.

In this connection, Marks noted a lack of association between judgments of CUES item ambiguity and students' reported item–response certitude. He stated that students seem to develop a set of stable perceptions and cognitions about the environment which is independent of the number and clarity of environmental cues available. Like McFee, he believes that some of this response consistency may be attributable to selected personality and need structures of the student, especially when environmental cues are vague or conflicting.

The current status of this line of research suggests that some relations exist between individual personality and/or background characteristics of subjects and their perceptions of the environment but that such connections are seldom very substantial. It is also unclear to what extent they reflect differences in the subenvironments actually experienced by the individual perceivers. On the other hand, as both McFee and Marks indicate, it seems reasonable that an individual who is under high environmental uncertainty and high need will answer an environmental item in a way that conforms to or is congruent with his particular need structure. The role position of an individual in an environment (e.g., patient or staff, political or fraternal campus leader, active or inactive in extracurricular affairs) may have a substantial effect on his perceptions of that environment. Thus personality and background variables might be correlated with environmental perceptions through the mediating effects of role position. Some of these issues are discussed in Chapter 9, which explores the correlates of deviant perceptions of the environment.

CONSTRUCT VALIDITY: CORRELATIONS WITH SIMILAR SCALES

As reviewed in Chapter 1, several other scales have been used in attempts to assess dimensions of ward milieus. Correlations between the WAS and the Ward Information Form (Kellam et al., 1966) are presented in Chapter 6. Correlations have been calculated between the WAS and two similar scales. Ellsworth and Maroney (1972) calculated the correlations between the 10 WAS subscales and the 5 Perception of Ward (POW) subscales for a sample of 111 patients on three psychiatric wards. They found that the POW subscales of Inaccessible Staff and Receptive–Involved Staff correlated ($r = -.65$ and $.64$, respectively) highly with the WAS Support subscale. The POW Involvement in Ward Management subscale assesses the same content dimension as the WAS Autonomy subscale ($r = .41$), whereas the POW Satisfaction with Ward subscale measures the same content dimension as the WAS Involvement subscale ($r = .57$). Finally, the POW Expectation for Patient Autonomy subscale correlated $.23$ with WAS Autonomy. On the whole, the correlations between the WAS and the POW subscales make good sense, contribute to the construct validity of both scales, and indicate the existence of some overlaps in the types of ward milieu dimensions assessed by the two scales. On the other hand, some of the WAS subscales have no parallels in the existing POW subscales; for example, none of the correlations between the POW subscales and the WAS subscales of Spontaneity, Practical Orientation, Personal Problem Orientation, Anger and Aggression, or Staff Control was above .40.

Correlations were also calculated between the WAS subscales and the Ward Climate Inventory (WCI) for 254 patients and 173 staff on eight different wards. Spiegel and Keith-Spiegel (1971) derived the WCI from the POW scales by taking 33 statements reflecting attitudes toward the ward environment and adapting the items for administration to both patients and staff. Since the three separate factor scores and the total Ward Climate Index were very highly intercorrelated, we calculated correlations only for the total WCI. Three of the correlations were above .40 for patients (Involvement, Support, and Program Clarity), whereas only two were above .40 for staff (Involvement and Support). The WCI is highly related to the WAS Relationship dimensions, but it does not assess most of the aspects of either the Treatment Program or the System Maintenance dimensions.

WAS FORM I NORMATIVE SAMPLES

The American Form I reference group sample consists of 2364 patients and 897 staff from 68 wards. This sample is less extensive than that for Form C; however, a reasonably broad range of value orientations is represented. The current British Form I reference group sample is based on 242 patients and 124 staff on 23 wards. The Form I norms are given in Moos (1974).

Figure 3.5 compares the American patients and staff on the 10 Form I subscales. The overall patient and staff views of ideal treatment milieus are relatively similar, although staff think of an ideal program as having more emphasis on all the *Relationship and Treatment Program* dimensions and less emphasis on Staff Control. These patient–staff differences are quite similar to those which exist in their perceptions of actual program environments.

British staff want more emphasis on all three Relationship dimensions, on all four Treatment Program dimensions, and on Program Clarity, although seeking less emphasis on Staff Control than do British patients. Thus the patient–staff differences are almost identical in the British and the American samples. The patient–staff differences are quite important, since they indicate that staff may be trying to develop treatment environments that patients do not want. Thus the "two-subculture" phenomenon is applicable to concepts of ideal programs as well as to perceptions of actual

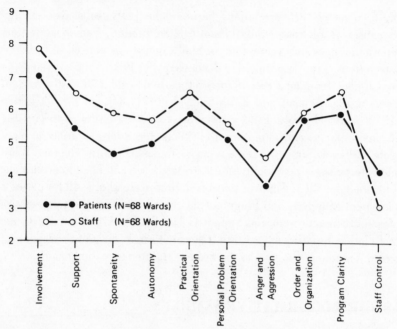

Figure 3.5 WAS Form I means for patients and staff on 68 American wards.

programs. It also holds for both British and American wards.

Although overall notions of ideal treatment environments are quite similar in the two countries, there are some differences. For example, American patients and staff would ideally like more emphasis on Personal Problem Orientation and Staff Control than would British patients and staff. In addition, American patients wish to have more emphasis on Involvement and Practical Orientation than do British patients. There were three items on which both American patients and staff answered true 20% more often than both British patients and staff: namely, "Patients would be expected to take leadership on the ward," "Patients would be expected to share their personal problems with each other," and "Patients who broke the ward rules would be punished for it." These items illustrate how British and American views of ideal treatment programs do differ.

The standard deviations of the 10 Form I subscales are quite substantial for patients and staff alike in both the American and British samples, indicating that there are important differences of opinion about the ideal treatment milieu. This empirically substantiates what many clinicians feel—that is, different patients want and presumably would do better in different treatment milieus. Although less has been written about it, this is just as true for staff. To our knowledge, no systematic attempt has yet been made to place staff on wards that have treatment environments consistent with their orientation and preferences. In this connection it should be noted that individual formulations of ideal programs are highly stable over time; indeed, the average Form I profile stabilities for four wards retested after intervals of 6 to 12 months were .78 for patients and .82 for staff.

The findings described in Chapters 2 and 3 indicate that the WAS has excellent psychometric properties and may be a valuable tool for evaluating the differential effects of various treatment environments. The next two chapters present information on the utility of the scale in describing individual programs, in making longitudinal comparisons of contrasting programs, in helping teach psychiatric residents and other staff about the characteristics of their own programs, and in assisting staff in changing their treatment milieus in directions more consonant with their preferences.

REFERENCES

Berdie, R. F. Some psychometric characteristics of CUES. *Educational and Psychological Measurement*, **27**: 55–66, 1967.

Centra, J. A. The college environment revisited: Current descriptions and a comparison of three methods of assessment. College Entrance Examination Board Research and Development Reports, No. 1, August 1970.

Ellsworth, R. B. A behavioral study of staff attitudes toward mental illness. *Journal of Abnormal Psychology*, **70**: 194–200, 1965.

Ellsworth, R. B. & Maroney, R. Characteristics of psychiatric programs, and their effects on patients' adjustment. *Journal of Consulting and Clinical Psychology*, **39**: 436–447, 1972.

Gerst, M. & Moos, R. The social ecology of university student residences. *Journal of Educational Psychology*, **63**: 513–525, 1972.

Haggard, E. *Intraclass correlation and the analysis of variance*. Dryden, New York, 1958.

Hays, W. *Statistics for psychologists*. Holt, Rinehart & Winston, New York, 1963.

Herr, E. L. Differential perceptions of "environmental press" by high school students. *Personnel and Guidance Journal*, **7**: 678–686, 1965.

Houts, P. & Moos, R. The development of a Ward Initiative Scale for patients. *Journal of Clinical Psychology*, **25**: 319–322, 1969.

Jackson, D. Personality Research Form. Research Psychologists Press, Inc., Goshen, New York, 1965.

Jansen, D. Characteristics of student leaders. Doctoral dissertation, Indiana University. *Dissertation Abstracts*, **28**: 3768A, 1967.

Kellam, S., Shmelzer, J., & Berman, A. Variation in the atmosphere of psychiatric wards. *Archives of General Psychiatry*, **14**: 561–570, 1966.

Kish, G., Solberg, K., & Uecker, A. Locus of control as a factor influencing patients' perceptions of ward atmosphere. *Journal of Clinical Psychology,* **27**: 287–289, 1971a.

Kish, G., Solberg, K., & Uecker, A. The relation of staff opinions about mental illness to ward atmosphere and perceived staff roles. *Journal of Clinical Psychology,* **27**: 284–287, 1971b.

Marks, E. Personality and motivational factors in responses to an environmental description scale. *Journal of Educational Psychology,* **59**: 267–274, 1968.

McFee, A. The relation of students' needs to their perceptions of a college environment. *Journal of Educational Psychology,* **52**: 25–29, 1961.

Mischel, W. *Personality and assessment.* Wiley, New York, 1968.

Moos, R. The assessment of the social climates of correctional institutions. *Journal of Research in Crime and Delinquency,* **5**: 174–188, 1968.

Moos, R. British psychiatric ward treatment environments. *British Journal of Psychiatry,* **120**: 635–643, 1972.

Moos, R. *Ward Atmosphere Scale Manual.* Consulting Psychologists Press, Palo Alto, Calif., 1974.

Pace, R. *College and University Environment Scale,* Technical manual, 2nd ed., Educational Testing Service, Princeton, N.J., 1969.

Rotter, J. Generalized expectancies for internal versus external control of reinforcement. *Psychological Monograph,* **80,** (whole # 609) 1966.

Spiegel, D. & Keith-Spiegel, P. Perceptions of ward climate by nursing personnel in a large NP hospital. *Journal of Clinical Psychology,* **27**: 390–393, 1971.

Spradling, J. An analysis of personality and environmental press in two church-related colleges and a state university. Doctoral dissertation, University of South Dakota, 1970.

Westmaas, R. A study of social atmosphere on Pine Rest Christian Hospital intensive treatment units. Unpublished manuscript, Pine Rest Christian Hospital, Grand Rapids, Mich., 1971.

Yonge, G. Personality correlates of the College and University Environment Scales. *Educational and Psychological Measurement,* **28**: 115–123, 1968.

Chapter Four

PROFILE INTERPRETATION, FEEDBACK, AND PROGRAM CHANGE

PROFILE INTERPRETATIONS

Some primary uses of the WAS are the derivation of detailed descriptions of ward programs to compare patient and staff perceptions, the assessment of program changes over time, and the contrasting of different programs with one another. We routinely provide staff (and sometimes patients) with detailed feedback about their treatment environment. Several illustrative profile interpretations are offered here. In these profile descriptions the ward as a whole is the central object of study, analogous to the individual patient in a clinical case description.

A wide diversity of WAS profiles was included in our normative sample, and only a few examples of the more typical ones are given. Profiles for wards in different types of hospitals are presented. One program is discussed in greater depth to illustrate comparisons between actual and ideal ward profiles.

Wards 205 and 272: University Teaching Hospital Programs

Ward 205 is a heavily staffed, 28-bed, university service, acute treatment unit for male and female patients. The ward functions as a therapeutic community in a general hospital. There are between 18 and 26 full-time patients and between 5 and 15 part-time patients. At the time of testing there were two faculty members—the ward administrator (a psychiatrist) and a psychologist; four psychiatric residents (one third-year resident on a

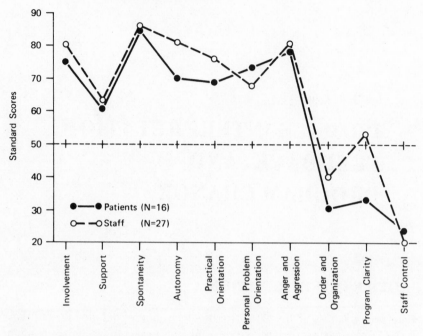

Figure 4.1 WAS Form C profiles for patients and staff on ward 205.

4-month rotation and three first-year residents on 6-month rotations); three vocational rehabilitation counselors; two psychology trainees; and two part-time social workers. In addition, the ward had one public health nurse, a full-time nursing staff of eight registered nurses, five licensed practical nurses, and seven psychiatric aides. There were also student nurses, medical students, a ward clerk, and from two to four housekeepers. The average length of patient stay on the ward was about 2 months.

Figure 4.1 compares the WAS Form C profiles for patients and staff with the average score obtained by patients in our 160-ward American normative sample. The most striking aspect of this profile is the unusually high agreement between patient and staff perceptions. Both patients and staff perceive the ward as substantially (more than 2 standard deviations) above average in its emphasis on the Relationship dimensions of Involvement and Spontaneity and on all four Treatment Program dimensions. The emphasis on Support is seen as moderately (1 standard deviation) above average. Patients and staff agree that the emphasis on Order and Organization is moderately below average, whereas that on Staff Control is substantially below average. The only subscale on which patients and staff disagree is

Program Clarity—staff report about average emphasis, whereas the patients' judgment is moderately below average.

Except for the unusually high degree of patient–staff agreement, this intriguing profile is similar to the profile often found in university teaching settings. Patients are seen as active and involved, as spending time constructively, and as having group spirit and pride in the program. They express their feelings relatively freely and emphasize the discussion and understanding of personal problems and the open expression of anger and aggression. Encouraged to be self-sufficient and independent, they are oriented toward preparing themselves for release from the hospital. The ward is high on Practical Orientation and Personal Problem Orientation, indicating that a program may simultaneously put strong emphasis on both areas.

The foregoing contention is supported by descriptions of the actual treatment program (Grant and Saslow, 1971). A patient initially learns the community's "basic expectations," which must be fulfilled if the patient is to earn necessities such as his meals and a mattress (e.g., lunch is earned by morning attendance at whatever formal treatment activity is part of a patient's individual treatment program). To earn a mattress, a patient must hand in a personal "daily program" each evening. This "behavioral" approach contributes to the high emphasis on Practical Orientation. On the other hand, patients obtain points by fulfilling personally defined treatment goals which are quite diverse—for example, to become more involved with people, to increase self-confidence, to show and express feelings more adequately. One patient was awarded points for discussing an emotionally charged situation, for listing her reactions when dieting, and for venting feelings about her desire to eat. Such individualized goal orientation, which usually includes goals related to the open expression and understanding of feelings, contributes to the emphasis on Personal Problem Orientation.

Patients on this ward feel that they receive little support; they are also quite unclear about what to expect in the day-to-day routine of the program. It seems apparent that patients who need to earn points in order to obtain meals, and so on tend to feel a certain lack of staff support. It is also reasonable to suppose that highly individualized goals and strong emphasis on all four Treatment Program dimensions can lead to lack of clarity about the direction and explicitness of the program.

The treatment environment of this program is further illustrated by some items on which more than 80% of both patients and staff agree. Examples of these items on the Relationship dimensions are "This is a lively ward,"

"Discussions are pretty interesting on this ward," "There is very little group spirit on this ward" (false), and "When patients disagree with each other they keep it to themselves" (false). Examples of relevant items on the Treatment Program dimensions are "Patients can wear what they want," "Patients are expected to take leadership on the ward," "Patients here are encouraged to be independent," "New treatment approaches are often tried on this ward," "Patients are encouraged to learn new ways of doing things," "Patients tell each other about their personal problems" (100% of both patients and staff agreed), and "On this ward staff think it is a healthy thing to argue." Finally, examples of relevant items on the Staff Control subscale are "It's not safe for patients to discuss their personal problems around here" (false), "It's a good idea to let the doctor know that he is boss" (false), and "If a patient argues with another patient he will get into trouble with the staff" (false).

Ward 205 was retested after 4 months because staff wished to assess the temporal stability of their treatment milieu. At the time of the second testing more than half the staff including all the primary therapists, had been on the ward less than 2 months. Nonetheless, the retest results were extremely close to the initial results, with patients perceiving slightly less Involvement and Spontaneity and slightly more Practical Orientation and Program Clarity. There were only small changes in staff perceptions. The profile stabilities (intraclass correlations) were .92 for patients and .96 for staff, indicating extremely high milieu stability over the 4-month interval, even though all but one of the patients and most of the staff had changed. Grant and Saslow (1971) discuss these profiles and the value of obtaining regular outside assessments of treatment milieus.

Figure 4.2 represents a contrasting profile for a different university teaching hospital program—another very small and very heavily staffed ward. There were 13 patients and 11 full-time staff members on ward 272 at the time of testing. The staff included a psychiatrist, a psychiatric resident, a psychologist, and several nurses and nursing assistants. The average length of stay was approximately 6 weeks to 2 months, and often the patients were acutely disturbed when admitted.

Although the structural and patient background characteristics on this ward are strikingly similar to those on ward 205, the WAS profiles are in striking contrast. Patients and staff on ward 272 show moderate to substantial disagreement about the characteristics of their milieu. They agree in perceiving above-average emphasis on Support, Personal Problem Orientation, and Anger and Aggression, as well as average emphasis on

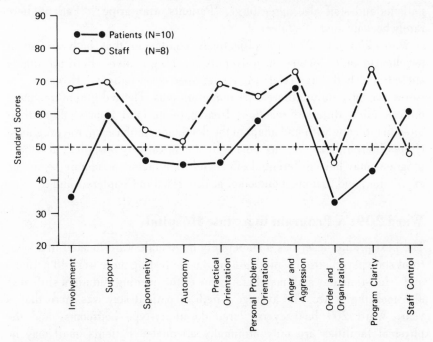

Figure 4.2 WAS Form C profiles for patients and staff on ward 272.

Spontaneity; but they strongly disagree on Involvement, Practical Orientation, and Program Clarity. Staff see substantially more emphasis on each of these areas than do patients. Thus ward 272 has a treatment milieu quite different from that of ward 205. The program on ward 272 encourages patients to be concerned with and to seek to understand their feelings and personal problems and to express openly their angry feelings. According to the patients, the program is moderately helpful and supportive; control is relatively strict.

The differences between these programs are concretely illustrated by the Staff Control items on which over 80% of the patients and staff on ward 272 agree. These items are "Staff don't order the patients around" (false), "Once a schedule is arranged for a patient, the patient must follow it," "The staff very rarely punish patients by restricting them" (false), "Patients can call nursing staff by their first names" (false), "Patients who break the ward rules are punished for it," and "It's not safe for patients to discuss their personal problems around here." The distinctive "feel" of this program's treatment milieu is further illustrated by the nature of some of the items on the Anger and Aggression subscale on which 80% of ward 272 patients and staff also agree (e.g., "Patients often gripe," "Patients here rarely become angry"—false).

Ward 205 and 272 are objectively similar in that both are small psychiatric units located in university teaching centers. Both are highly staffed; and both have relatively acute, short-term patients. However, the two wards have quite different treatment milieus. These different treatment milieus elicit different reactions from patients (and from staff) in their attempts to cope with and adapt to the dominant emphases in the programs. Quite different behaviors are positively and negatively rewarded, and these programs may have differential effects on such factors as morale, symptom expression, and treatment outcome, as discussed in Chapters 7 and 8.

Ward 209: A Program in a State Hospital

The next profile describes a moderately large male ward located in a large rural state psychiatric hospital. At the time of testing there were 48 patients and 7 full-time day staff members. Some of the evening and night shift staff also took the WAS. The average length of patient stay was more than a year. Ward 209 has several large dormitory-type bedrooms, and the physical facilities are only minimally adequate. Patients' mail may be censored, and patients cannot wear their regular street clothes. Even though patients submit to certain relatively strict procedures and to a lack of privacy, the ward has a very active treatment program. The program emphasizes a strong psychotherapeutic orientation, and several therapy groups meet regularly on the ward. There is also a very active elected patient government.

The ward profile (Figure 4.3) indicates that patients see above-average emphasis on the Relationship dimension of Involvement and on the Treatment Program dimensions of Practical Orientation and Personal Problem Orientation. In addition, staff report strong emphasis on Support, Spontaneity, and Anger and Aggression. Patients and staff agree that there is relatively little encouragement for patients to be autonomous and independent; they disagree on the System Maintenance dimensions, with staff perceiving more emphasis than patients on both Order and Organization and Program Clarity, whereas the reverse is true for Staff Control.

Thus patients and staff generally agree on the Relationship and Treatment Program dimensions, although staff see more emphasis on each of the areas and a somewhat more differentiated program than do patients.

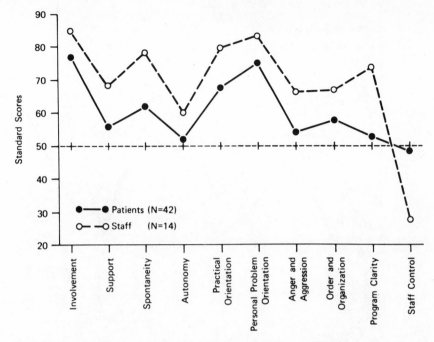

Figure 4.3   WAS Form C profiles for patients and staff on ward 209.

On the other hand, staff and patients are in some disagreement about the degree of emphasis on each of the System Maintenance dimensions. This profile is included to show the type of treatment milieu that can be created with what must objectively be regarded as difficult patients living in a relatively poor physical situation in a hospital with quite restrictive overall policies and regulations. This is not a typical profile for a large ward in a rural state hospital; rather, it illustrates that social milieus may to some extent be independent of physical facilities.

Wards 203 and 462: VA Hospital Programs

Figure 4.4 is the WAS profile for a moderately well-staffed VA hospital ward on which there are between 30 and 35 patients and between 5 and 8 full-time staff members. The patients are all male, tend to be moderately but not acutely disturbed, and stay on ward 203 for an average of 2 to 3 months. The entire range of psychiatric disorders is represented. This profile is included to illustrate the diversity of existing ward treatment environments and to show that a relatively low patient–staff ratio and

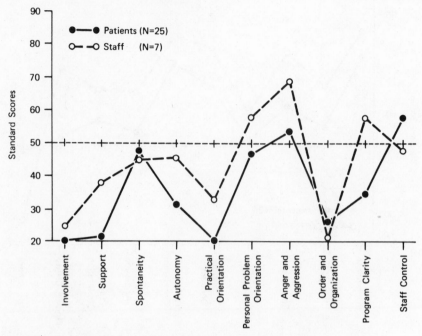

Figure 4.4 WAS Form C profiles for patients and staff on ward 203.

excellent physical facilities in a new remodeled location do not necessarily result in an active, coherent treatment program.

Patients and staff on ward 203 generally agree on the characteristics of their treatment environment, although staff see more emphasis in some areas than do patients (e.g., the Relationship dimension of Support, the Treatment Program dimensions of Autonomy and Anger and Aggression, and the System Maintenance dimension of Program Clarity). Patients are moderately encouraged to express their feelings openly, including their feelings of anger, and to discuss their personal problems with other patients and with staff. However, this emphasis is in a context notably lacking in Involvement, Support, Order and Organization, and Program Clarity (the latter as perceived by patients at least). This is not a particularly unusual WAS profile, but it is somewhat extreme, serving to illustrate a program in which the open expression of feelings and personal problems is empahsized within a context of moderate to high Staff Control and moderate to low Involvement and Support. On such wards the expression of feelings is ritualized and "wooden," lacking real openness, personal commitment, or follow-through. Staff are pursuing a certain psychotherapeutic orientation without a detailed knowledge or understanding of what that orientation implies. The push to openly express angry feelings within a context of bickering and lack of general support is usually detrimental to both patient and staff morale.

The "flavor" of the social environment of this ward is illustrated by items on which more than 90% of the patients and 6 of the 7 staff agreed. On the Relationship dimensions these items include "A lot of patients just seem to be passing time on the ward," "The ward has very few social activities," "The patients are proud of this ward" (false), and "Patients tend to hide their feelings from the staff." Similar items on other subscales include "Patients often gripe," "Patients often criticize or joke about the ward staff," "Things are sometimes very disorganized around here," "The ward sometimes gets very messy," and "The day room is often messy." Surprisingly, there was a high degree of interest in the WAS profile feedback in this program. As might be imagined, the feedback session was a long and difficult one, but the ward staff were genuinely motivated to institute important and far-reaching program changes.

Figure 4.5 shows a quite different profile for a large male ward in another VA hospital. The profile for ward 462 is illustrative of a treatment environment in which all three System Maintenance dimensions are relatively highly emphasized. It also demonstrates that a relatively low staff–patient ratio does not necessarily result in unclear expectations or a disorganized milieu.

We obtained several profiles on which the three System Maintenance dimensions were the only above-average dimensions. The profile for ward 462 is more highly differentiated. Patients and staff agree that there is a high degree of Order and Organization, that ward rules and procedures are explicit, and that patients know what to expect in the day-to-day ward routine. In addition, there is some emphasis on the orderly scheduling of program activities and on patients keeping within clearly defined limits. Patients and staff also agree that there is some stress on Involvement, Autonomy, and Practical Orientation, although staff perceive more emphasis on each of these areas than do patients. Patients and staff agree quite closely, however, that the program does not systematically encourage understanding oneself and discussing personal problems or expressing angry feelings openly.

An idea of the milieu is given by some of the items on the System Maintenance dimensions on which more than 80% of patients and staff agree: "Most patients follow a regular schedule each day," "Patients'

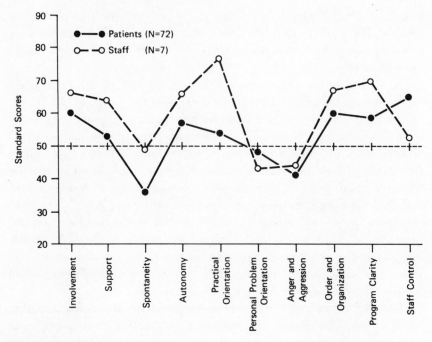

Figure 4.5 WAS Form C profiles for patients and staff on ward 462.

activities are carefully planned," "This is a very well organized ward," "The staff makes sure that the ward is always neat," "On this ward everyone knows who is in charge," "Ward rules are understood by the patients," "Once a schedule is arranged for a patient, the patient must follow it," "Patients who break the ward rules are punished for it," and "Patients will be transferred from this ward if they don't obey the rules." In addition, more than 80% of patients and staff agree on the following items, representing other areas: "The patients are proud of this ward," "The ward staff help new patients get acquainted on the ward," "Patients are encouraged to learn new ways of doing things," and "Patients must make plans before leaving the hospital."

Thus ward 462 is a fairly large, not particularly well-staffed VA hospital ward where all three System Maintenance dimensions are treated as important. The relatively large size and low staffing may make this necessary to keep the ward functioning adequately. On the other hand, staff also stress certain aspects of the Relationship and Treatment Program dimensions, most notably Involvement, Autonomy, and Practical Orientation. Taken together, the WAS profiles for wards 203 (small, relatively

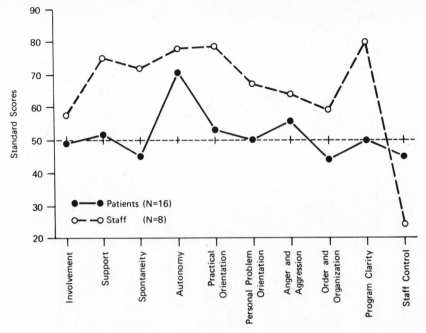

Figure 4.6   WAS Form C profiles for patients and staff on ward 238.

well-staffed and 462 (large, relatively poorly staffed) indicate that size and staffing do not necessarily determine the characteristics of the treatment environment.

Ward 238: Real and Ideal Program Profiles

The last example illustrates in greater detail the information available when both real and ideal ward perceptions are obtained from patients and staff. Ward 238 is a small VA ward with between 20 and 25 male patients. The average length of patient stay was between 4 and 6 months. There were seven full-time day staff members on the ward at the time of testing.

Figure 4.6 presents the usual comparison of WAS Form C profiles. Patients see the program as emphasizing independence and self-sufficiency and as encouraging them to make their own decisions. For example, more than 80% agreed that "The staff act on patients' suggestions," "Patients are expected to take leadership on the ward," and "Patients here are encouraged to be independent." Staff feel that the treatment milieu is much more differentiated and varied than do the patients. Staff see above-average

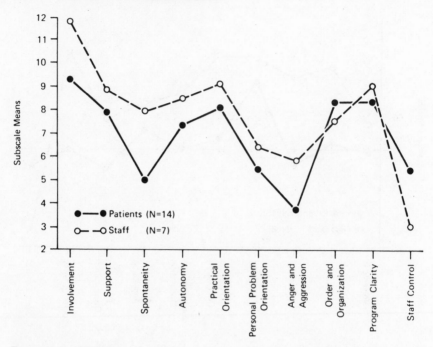

Figure 4.7   WAS Form I profiles for patients and staff on ward 238.

emphasis on the Relationship dimensions of Support and Spontaneity, on all four Treatment Program dimensions (particularly Autonomy and Practical Orientation), and on the System Maintencnce dimension of Program Clarity. Staff also believe the emphasis on Staff Control to be well below average.

The average raw scores of patients and staff on the WAS (Form I) in Figure 4.7 permit comparison of patient and staff ideas about an ideal program. Patients and staff disagree about their actual program environment; they also disagree, although not quite as strongly, on their desired program environment. Staff wish more emphasis on the Relationship dimensions, particularly Involvement and Spontaneity, than do patients. On the other hand, patients and staff agree fairly well on the desired amount of emphasis on the Treatment Program dimensions, particularly Autonomy, Practical Orientation, and Personal Problem Orientation. Patients ideally prefer somewhat less emphasis on Anger and Aggression than do staff. Patients and staff are in accord regarding the emphasis they wish on both Order and Organization and Program Clarity, but staff desire much less emphasis on Staff Control than do patients.

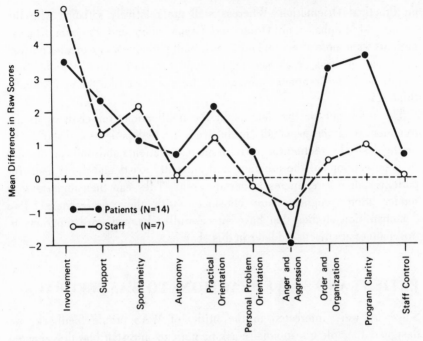

Figure 4.8 Real–ideal discrepancies as perceived by patients and staff on ward 238.

Figure 4.8 compares the degree of change that patients and staff on ward 238 would like in the treatment program. The degree of change desired is calculated by subtracting the mean score for patients for the actual program (Form C subscale means) from their mean score for an ideal program (Form I subscale means). The same is done for staff. For the program to become an ideal program in the eyes of patients and staff, each area would have to increase or decrease as shown in the profile. The line in the center of the profile indicates that no change is desired (i.e., that there is no discrepancy between real and ideal subscale means). For example, staff desire no change in the amount of emphasis on Autonomy or Staff Control. Positive scores designate a desire for increased emphasis in an area; for example, both patients and staff would like more emphasis on all three Relationship dimensions. Negative socres reveal a desire for decreased emphasis; for example, both groups would like less emphasis on the expression of Anger and Aggression than currently exists in the program.

Thus, patients and staff agree that more emphasis on each of the Relationship dimensions is desirable. They would also like more emphasis on Practical Orientation. Whereas staff are relatively satisfied with the amount of emphasis on Order and Organization and Program Clarity, patients want more stress on both areas. Staff perceive much greater current emphasis on these areas (see Figure 4.6) than do patients. Patients may simply wish the treatment program to become more like the staff already think it is.

The relevance of the data is in the implications for changes in the treatment program, especially in the areas in which patients and staff agree on the desired direction for program change. Patients and staff can discuss their perceptions of the program as it currently exists and the reasons for patient–staff discrepancies in certain areas. They can then undertake to render their program more consonant with their preferences. Two demonstration studies that have successfully changed ward programs in this manner are discussed later in this chapter.

PATIENT AND STAFF REACTIONS TO WAS FEEDBACK

Since we were interested in the utility of WAS profile feedback, we designed a simple questionnaire asking patients and staff how they reacted to the feedback. This questionnaire, which contained three questions, was given to a sample of 50 staff members and 28 patients.

Patients and staff were asked how *accurate* they felt the profiles were. They were asked to make separate judgments, on 4-point scales; for both staff and patient results and for both real and ideal profiles. The allowed responses were as follows: not at all accurate, somewhat accurate, fairly accurate, and quite accurate. About 75% of patients and staff felt that both their real and ideal ward profiles were either fairly accurate or quite. accurate.

The next question asked was "How *complete* do you feel your ward profile was in describing staff and patient perceptions of the ward (i.e., how much of the important aspects of ward climate did it seem to capture)?" Judgments were also made on a 4-point scale. Approximately 66% of the staff and 75% of the patients felt that both their real and ideal ward profiles were either fairly complete or quite complete.

Finally, patients and staff were asked to assess the implications of the feedback data for self-evaluation and for specific changes in ward practices or programs. They made judgments on a 5-point scale that varied from "no real implications" to "a number of major implications." More than 80% of the patients and staff felt that the feedback had either minor or major implications for changes in ward practices or policies. The detailed written comments were most informative, for example:

> We have found the WAS a valuable and accurate tool in making objective many of the things which we feel have been happening to the ward in the last year. It's useful because it puts at one remove the discontents, dissatisfactions and hurts which we have been feeling and gets it out where we can discuss them more safely.

> I was sure that staff and patients alike felt that the staff was supportive. Evidently there should be more communication between staff and patients so that we understand one another's feelings. Patients were not relaying the message to us that they felt we were not supportive.

> It was an eye-opener to me that patients and staff both agreed that our ward needs more clarity and personal problem orientation. It will probably motivate me to encourage staff and patients to communicate with each other more closely.

Thus patients and staff generally feel that the WAS profiles are both accurate and complete and that they have some important implications for changes in ward policies and programs.

CHANGING PROGRAM TREATMENT ENVIRONMENTS

The WAS as a Teaching Device

Dr. Peter Hauri, a research psychologist, gave the WAS to patients and staff on a small, heavily staffed university teaching hospital ward on four different occasions: October 1968, December 1969, February 1970, and November 1970. The ward was originally used in our normative sample. The first profile and a detailed feedback letter were sent to Dr. Hauri, who discussed the information with ward staff. A reassessment was made in December 1969. At that time patients perceived the emphasis on all 10 WAS dimensions to be within 1 standard deviation of the overall mean. They perceived the emphasis on Involvement and on all four Treatment Program dimensions to be somewhat below the mean. The staff agreed quite closely with the patients, although they reported more emphasis on Personal Problem Orientation and Anger and Aggression and less emphasis on Staff Control than did the patients.

After Dr. Hauri had given the ward staff feedback on this profile, the staff then began to discuss developing a ward therapeutic community program. When the WAS was readministered in February 1970, however, it was revealed that only slight changes had occurred from the profile obtained 2 months earlier. During the summer of 1970 a therapeutic community came into full swing under the leadership of a psychiatric resident who agreed to stay on the ward for an extra year. Dr. Hauri's utilization of the WAS as a teaching device generally followed a common-sense approach. First he presented the WAS real ward results with a straightforward discussion of the profiles in relation to the overall norms and of agreement and disagreement between patients and staff. When relatively large disagreements occurred (more than 1 standard deviation), the subscales were discussed item by item to isolate the reasons for the discrepancies. Second, the perceptions of different staff groups were compared; for example, nurses saw less emphasis on Spontaneity and more emphasis on Order and Organization and Program Clarity than did residents.

Actual and ideal profiles, particularly for staff, were compared in the third step. Subscales with large real–ideal discrepancies were analyzed and discussed item by item. It sometimes occurred that a characteristic initially thought to be ideal lost this status on exposure to discussion and more explicit consideration. Sometimes Form I subscales had relatively large standard deviations, indicating disagreement among staff about the characteristics of their ideal ward. According to Dr. Hauri, this may suggest the need for further in-depth study, as topics for special seminars, for example. The large standard deviations are often caused by differences among staff members of different roles. For example, the supervisor and the psychiatric residents on this ward surpassed the nurses in their ideal wish for more emphasis on Involvement and Spontaneity and less emphasis on Staff Control.

After intensive discussion of the results, an attempt was made to formulate a relatively modest common goal—for example, that the emphasis on Involvement and Autonomy be increased. The items from these subscales were then put on the staff bulletin board. At first, Dr. Hauri noted, they were followed rather slavishly; however, within a few weeks, the patients and staff began to assimilate the spirit of the subscale.

The results of the November 1970 reassessment indicated that substantial changes had been obtained with the procedure. The ward had developed a much more active, differentiated treatment milieu. Moreover, patients and staff saw significantly greater emphasis on the Relationship dimension of Involvement and on all four Treatment Program dimensions in November 1970 than they had in December 1969. The substantial changes in these five dimensions brought the program much closer to an ideal program as perceived by both patients and staff. The basic thrusts of the program were to emphasize autonomy and independence and to encourage patients to express and to seek to understand their personal problems.

Patients reported no changes in their perceptions of the three System Maintenance dimensions; however, staff saw more emphasis on both Program Clarity and Staff Control. As ward staff actively direct and change a treatment program, both clarity and control usually increase. However, since these changes are often confusing to patients, it is not surprising that their perception of Program Clarity failed to increase. It would probably increase if reassessed when the new program had been stabilized after a period of functioning. The overall change in the social milieu of this ward demonstrates that assessment and intensive staff discussion can act as a stimulus for positive change.

Clinical Change Through Staff Discussion

The second study, which is reported in more detail in Pierce et al. (1972), took place on a psychiatric unit of a general hospital located in an urban area. Ward 60 serves about 25 male and female patients both as full-time inpatients and as day patients. It is an acute, short-term treatment service and has a major commitment to training mental health professionals. The trainees include psychiatric residents, psychology interns, psychiatric social work fellows, recreation therapy trainees, and medical interns. Because of the training commitment, the staff–patient ratio is high (about 1–1.5 on day shift). The treatment orientation is psychoanalytic, and the major modes of treatment include individual and group psychotherapy for each patient. The patients participate in community meetings in which the focus is on such issues as rules, scheduling activities, and the introduction of new staff and patients. The patients also participate in recreation therapy and body-movement sessions.

The staff decided to use the WAS to describe the ward milieu and to identify ways in which it could be used in the continuing effort to create a maximally beneficial treatment program. There were three administrations of the WAS: (1) Form C was given to patients ($N = 17$) and staff ($N = 31$) in May; (2) Form C and Form 1 were given to staff only ($N = 23$ and 17,

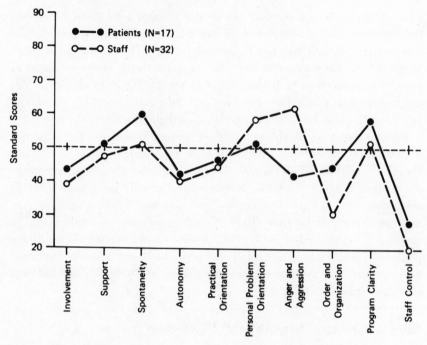

Figure 4.9 May WAS Form C profiles for patients and staff on ward 60.

respectively) during the last part of October and the first part of November; (3) Form C was given again to patients ($N = 14$) and staff ($N = 18$) during mid-December.

Figure 4.9, the May WAS profile, indicates that neither patients nor staff saw substantial emphasis on any of the Relationship or Treatment Program dimensions. Actually, both patients and staff perceived somewhat below-average emphasis on Involvement, Autonomy, and Practical Orientation. Patients and staff also saw the emphasis on both Order and Organization and Staff Control as somewhat below average.

Change Attempts

Between the latter part of September and the end of October, the May data were discussed with the staff in feedback sessions. Staff comments focused on Autonomy and Staff Control, reflecting a concern about lack of patient movement. The program did not foster patient autonomy; staff did not exert sufficient "push" or influence on patients, and patients were thus too dependent and comfortable. Staff felt that this deficiency was especially evident in the lack of progress of a certain number of patients who had been on the ward for a relatively long time. Another issue involved dealing with acting-out behavior that was clearly beyond the ward rules and required limit setting by staff. The Order and Control subscales were applicable here. Who was primarily responsible for limit setting and how could the limit setting be consistently implemented by ward personnel? What role could the community meeting play in this implementation?

From these discussions a committee was formed to generate suggestions and to attempt to make the community meetings function in a more meaningful manner in the total program. Another committee began to review the activity program and to offer suggestions that would increase staff and patient participation in ward activities. The committees were made up of representatives from permanent staff and trainees. The treatment-team and staff meetings centered on patients whose length of stay exceeded the "average" expectation for the ward and on improving the consistency of staff limit setting of acting-out behavior.

At the end of the feedback sessions in October, the WAS was administered again to obtain a current assessment of the ward milieu before any major changes were introduced and to evaluate the stability of the milieu (as perceived by staff) over a 5-month period. Two weeks later the ideal form of the WAS was also administered to staff. Staff felt that it would be too burdensome to patients to have them take the WAS again, especially since still another administration was planned. Thus, unfortunately, we did not obtain data on patient perceptions at the October testing.

Several changes were initiated as a result of the committee reports and the new focus in the staff and treatment-team meetings. Staff agreed that the community meeting should continue to be a forum for general ward issues but decided that it should also be used to define, explain, and reiterate staff expectations of patients and to transmit ward norms and values. It was also agreed that staff would more actively structure the meetings.

It was determined that management of limit-breaking behavior would be the responsibility of the treatment team and that decisions would be followed by all staff. The treatment team was assigned to communicate decisions and changes of decisions. The staff also decided that continuity on treatment issues would be enhanced if outside private therapists were more actively encouraged to attend and participate in discussions and decisions concerning individual patients. In the middle of December the

WAS was again given to patients and staff to obtain a final assessment of the ward milieu and to evaluate changes toward the staff-perceived ideal atmosphere.

Results

Results indicated that staff saw the program as closer to their ideal in December than they had in October. All nine of the WAS subscales that showed change (Staff Control showed essentially no change) changed in the direction of the staff's perception of an ideal ward ($p < .01$, binomial test). Four subscales revealed significant change toward the ideal: Involvement ($p < .01$), Support ($p < .05$), Personal Problem Orientation ($p < .05$), and Program Clarity ($p < .01$). Importantly, staff did not consider the program to be closer to their ideal in October than they had in May. Only three of the nine subscales displaying changes had changed in the direction of the staff ideal between these two testing sessions. Thus staff perceptions moved significantly closer to their views of an ideal program between the October and December testing, whereas this was not true between the May and October testing. This indicates that the changes occurring between October and December were probably due to the staff attempts to change the ward environment.

Figure 4.10, which presents the December profiles for patients and staff, further illustrates the results. A comparison of Figures 4.9 and 4.10 indicates that patients and staff agreed that the emphasis on Support, Practical Orientation, and Personal Problem Orientation had increased and that the emphasis on Order and Organization had decreased. Staff showed significant increases (one-tailed tests, $p < .05$) between the May and December testing on the Support, Practical Orientation, and Clarity subscales; patients showed significant increases on the Support and Autonomy subscales. In addition, the December profile is more differentiated (several scores substantially above the mean; further deemphasis on Order and Control), indicating movement toward a more coherent, defined treatment program. On the other hand, the overall shape of the profile remained relatively stable, reflecting the fact that the ward changes were taking place gradually, within a dominant treatment philosophy that was generally consistent.

Items to which patients and/or staff answered true more often in December than in May illustrate the specific changes that had occurred—"The healthier patients on this ward help take care of the less

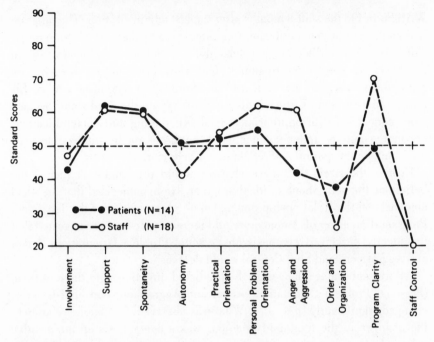

Figure 4.10   December WAS Form C profiles for patients and staff on ward 60.

healthy ones," "Patients set up their own activities without being prodded by the staff," "Patients are expected to take leadership on the ward," "New treatment approaches are often tried on this ward," "Patients must make plans before leaving the hospital," and "Staff don't order the patients around."

Several charts of patients whose progress and movement had become an area of focus during the time of the study were reviewed. The charts revealed increased staff activity and increased patient movement. Notations indicated that the patients were being discharged to private therapists and day care programs; they were being transferred, too, from full-time to day-patient status. A review of overall ward statistics during the period of the study brought out a trend in the direction of more rapid patient turnover—namely, that patients were staying less time in December than in November or October. Although the data are minimal and longer-time comparisons are necessary to draw reliable conclusions, it seems that the ward became more active in terms of patient movement and turnover.

In a follow-up to this study, Lowell Cooper (1970) readministered the

WAS Form I to the staff 8 months after the last administration. The program had continued to change during this interval, and there had been a major shift from an individual psychoanalytic psychotherapy model to an emphasis on short-term treatment for crisis intervention, focusing on resocialization within the context of the therapeutic community. After this change there was no further individual therapy on the ward. Staff became more concerned with appropriate social functioning and communication, encouragement of independence, and emphases on hospitalization as a crisis and on the control and regulation of behavior.

Cooper theorized that these changes would predictably influence the beliefs of the staff about an ideal program. He hypothesized that the ideal emphasis on the Relationship dimension of Spontaneity and the Treatment Program dimension of Autonomy would increase. He further suggested that the ideally perceived emphasis on Personal Problem Orientation, Anger and Aggression, and Staff Control would decrease.

All five subscales changed in the predicted direction, and three of them (Personal Problem Orientation, Anger and Aggression, and Staff Control) changed significantly ($p < .05$). What was observed, in specific relation to the changes in the treatment program, was a deemphasis on the positive value of the expression of feelings and the concern with intrapsychic processes, a deemphasis on patients taking a "good patient" role of submitting and of being cared for by the staff, and greater stress on the control of impulses such as anger and aggression. Two of the predictions were not supported statistically, in that both the Spontaneity and Autonomy subscales changed only slightly. Cooper speculated that the strong emphasis on control of impulses and on patients working together in groups may have made staff overconcerned with group controls and thus less willing to push for Autonomy and Spontaneity. In summary, staff ideals are influenced in predictable ways by the nature of the values in the setting itself. This is highly significant both for the training of ward staff and for the inculcation of a set of values in a patient community.

Change-Oriented Teaching and Research

The demonstration studies cited here are exploratory attempts at facilitating changes in treatment programs using a measurement device that yields systematic information about how the program is perceived by patients and staff. Originally we saw the WAS primarily as a way of clarifying the existing shared perceptions of the ward—both real and ideal—and of assessing changes over time, leaving the implications for specific action up to the initiative and ingenuity of the staff involved. The results of these studies indicate that wards can be altered in a direction more congruent with staff preferences. Several general issues merit consideration in this connection.

First, although no claim is made that the feedback and discussion of WAS data cause changes in treatment environments, the systematic information about program perceptions does aid staff in formulating and articulating their current concerns. The use of the WAS in discussion sessions is an important supplement to the staff's knowledge of the ward, and as such it is a meaningful contributor to the change process as well as an evaluator of change. Second, some staff who infrequently spoke of their concerns were able to discuss ward issues in terms of the WAS information. Thus WAS feedback may have motivating properties that help staff become involved in talking over ward policies and programs.

Third, certain specific findings may have generality. The patients' perception of decreased Program Clarity in the second study indicates that negative effects may occur (temporarily, it is hoped). Apparently the various committees and discussions of ward policies incidental to the WAS feedback increased staff perception of Clarity (this was true in both studies), but this increase was not adequately translated into patient perceptions. Decisions about program changes arrived at by staff committees and in staff discussions, may initially confuse patients. Since patients wonder about impending changes, staff must explain as fully as possible the overall ward plan for modifications in policy. The second study illustrates that this item is particularly important because change may occur very rapidly, as it did in the 6 to 7 weeks between the October and December testings.

Ward program changes may take place within a generally consistent treatment ideology, as in the second study, or they may involve the initiation of a new program as in the first study. A ward can institute a series of carefully thought-out and graduated changes in their program while still retaining the same overall direction and ideology. However, it may be difficult to stop change once it has been initiated; in the second study, for example, change continued beyond the formal research. This continuing change was generally consistent with directions that had been initiated during the project; in the end, however, the overall treatment ideology of the program had changed fairly drastically. This major change coincided with the appointment of a new ward director.

Since treatment environments explicitly emphasize certain directions, Cooper's important finding that values may be changed by the actual practices in such environments indicates that they may have differential effects on value systems, which, by implication, may generalize to ideal notions of other social climates (e.g., families and social or work groups). Thus a patient or staff member who functions in a ward milieu that strongly emphasizes Autonomy and Spontaneity may eventually value these dimensions more highly in hospital milieus and elsewhere, as well.

In interpreting these results it should be noted that treatment environments, as assessed by the WAS, remain highly stable over relatively long periods of time when no change attempts are made. For example, the staff in the second study showed very high stability in their perceptions of their treatment environment on two assessments that were made 5 months apart before change attempts were instituted. Thus it is highly improbable that later changes are due to any simple test–retest phenomenon. It may be that "self-fulfilling prophecies" influence the results (e.g., staff perceive more Support because they have tried to enhance Support), but the existence of specific behavioral and structural changes, as detailed previously, militates against this explanation. Ideally, independent outside observers should be used in future studies, even though there is the risk that they themselves may become involved in the change process.

A last but very important point is that feedback and discussion sessions allow practical applications to be made of ongoing teaching and research. By initially tying teaching or research to current issues for a ward, staff can help design and cooperate in projects that are acceptable and relevant to their felt needs. The issue of the relevance of research to a busy hospital staff has often gone begging. Feedback and discussion sessions can be an important mechanism in the acceptance and use of research, as well as a critical source of information and ideas about future relevant research. In this regard, easily administered assessment instruments such as the WAS may be feasible short-term information-gathering techniques for overburdened staff lacking extensive facilities or personnel for evaluation.

REFERENCES

Cooper, L. "Staff attitudes about ideal wards before and after program change." Unpublished paper, Mount Zion Hospital and Medical Center, San Francisco, 1970.

Grant, R. & Saslow, G. Maximizing responsible decision making, or how do we get out of here? In Abroms, G. & Greenfield, N. (Eds.). *The new hospital psychiatry.* Academic Press, New York, 1971.

Pierce, W., Trickett, E., & Moos, R. Changing ward atmosphere through staff discussion of the perceived ward environment. *Archives of General Psychiatry,* **26**: 35–41, 1972.

Chapter Five

PROFILE
COMPARISONS AND
EVALUATIONS

THE SOCIAL ECOLOGY OF TWO TREATMENT PROGRAMS

An innovative attempt to design a new treatment milieu, conducted at the Palo Alto Veterans Administration Hospital, was compared with a more traditional ward program. The WAS was utilized to specify and contrast the treatment environments of the two programs, which were also involved in a comparative outcome study. Research designed to evaluate the differential outcome of treatment programs should include measures of the psychosocial environment (i.e., of the actual "treatment" by which patients are presumably influenced to change). This use of the WAS demonstrates the utility of having an assessment of the psychosocial environment for several purposes: (*a*) as an aid to the specification of the salient characteristics of a treatment program, (*b*) as a way of systematically comparing two programs, and (*c*) to help ensure that attempts at replicating a particular program are successful.

The programs were on two adjacent 30-bed VA hospital wards which were architecturally mirror images of each other. Male patients were randomly assigned to the two programs and were heterogeneous in terms of such factors as income, skill level, age, education, and diagnosis. The experimental and control group patients were closely comparable. The patients were gradually aging (mean age approximately 40) and most had been in and out of hospitals several times. They had relatively high levels of education (average approximately 12 years), work skill, and previous income, although most had had unstable work records and were alienated from former family relationships. The mean number of previous hospitalizations was approximately 4, and the mean days of prior hospitalization in the past 10 years exceeded 500. About half the patients carried a current diagnosis of psychosis. Detailed descriptions of the patient groups appear elsewhere (Daniels, 1970).

On the experimental ward the basic goal was to design an intentional social system model of treatment through the reorganization of the program into a problem-solving organization of task groups that called for a division of labor and interdependence among patients and staff. Group membership, processes, and tasks were considered to be core treatment elements; that is, the social system and task groups were perceived as curative agents per se, not as mainly supportive of more specific treatments. This experimental reorganization of a treatment program into patient–staff task groups involved the formation of a nonprofit corporation (Dann Services Inc.) for the delivery of psychiatric services; patients participated at all levels, including corporate directorships, management, and therapy.

The task groups included a patient–staff planning and progress team, which made decisions about patients' treatment plans and discharges, an industrial workshop, and, at the end of the research, a community housing planning group. Patients receiving services were simultaneously involved in delivering them. Although staff roles became more indirect and consultative, traditional treatment activities were also utilized. These included (as on the control ward) medications, individual therapy, and group therapy in the form of task groups, community meetings, and recreational outings. The primary difference was in the emphasis on structured program elements provided by the task group orientation. Decision-making power on the experimental ward was distributed equally between staff and patients, and the social system furnished opportunities for the patients to move upward into positions of responsibility and leadership. Practical problem solving and crisis resolution were stressed. Theoretically it was assumed that a change in social behavior would lead to personality change and subsequently to psychological insight. Action and adjustment were stressed. Hence restoration of function and employment often went hand in hand.

The basic attempt of the intentional social system therapy model is to create a treatment system that facilitates ego growth and mutually satisfying social behavior. The model is based on a synthesis of principles drawn from ego psychology, social adaptation theory, role theory, and organizational theory. As the means of repairing ego damage, especially impairments in social role functioning, the intentional social system attempts to develop, facilitate, and utilize a combination of organizational structure and approaches to the individual.

Daniels (1970, pp. 12–14) has summarized the essential elements of the intentional social system as follows:

1.   Meaningful, clearly specified tasks and roles must be established, requiring interdependence and a division of labor among members. The tasks represent various degrees of complexity, challenge, and responsibility. Roles should approximate as nearly as possible those required for general living, and their fulfillment must be essential for the functioning of the intentional social system.

2.   The organizational structure should provide for supportive group membership, participation in decision making by all group members, graded responsibility, accountability, and a series of challenges to the participants ranging from problems of everyday living to naturally occurring crisis situations.

3.   Incentives and group rewards are linked to task performance. Feedback on performance should include all members—staff and patients alike.

4.   Self-government by members is in accord with general standards of the community at large. The power of members to make policies and decisions regulating their own behavior should require living with the consequences of these decisions.

5.   An ideology and value system is necessary that inculcates enthusiasm and positive expectations, particularly warmth, encouragement, and support.

6.   Participants will closely scrutinize and explore actual roles, interpersonal behavior, and their consequences in the here and now. Such scrutiny and exploration help to develop self-awareness, a sense of reality, and more satisfactory interpersonal relationships.

7.   Regularized assessment should be a core treatment component and should include evaluation of outcome on both "hard" and "soft" criteria.

Daniels believes that through the use of these elements a milieu program becomes a problem-solving, supportive, self-maintaining social system, that is, an intentional community.

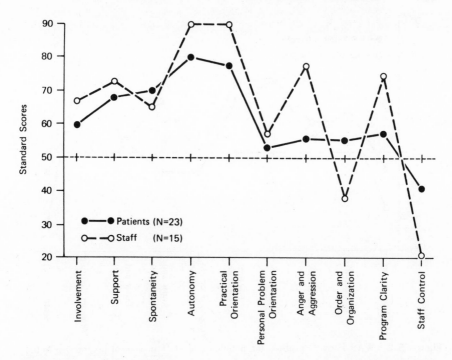

Figure 5.1 WAS Form C profiles for patients and staff in experimental program in initial project phase.

In contrast, a now traditional model of treatment was utilized in the control program. The milieu or social system was viewed essentially as supportive to more specific therapies. Formally these included medications, individual therapy, community meetings, recreational outings, and hospital "industrial" therapy. The control program, which emphasized interpersonal relationships as the core of treatment, highly valued the staff team, the philosophy of participation and sharing, nursing care, and individual therapy. The "people equal program" slant meant that the program relied heavily on the individual effectiveness of staff in their treatment of patients, rather than on structural program elements.

In this program staff had the decision-making power and delivered all treatment services directly. The general focus was on individuals, and individual patient goals were considered to be most important. It was hoped that understanding and conflict resolution would promote personality change and subsequent change in social behavior. Employment placement generally followed discharge (i.e., the restoration of personality function).

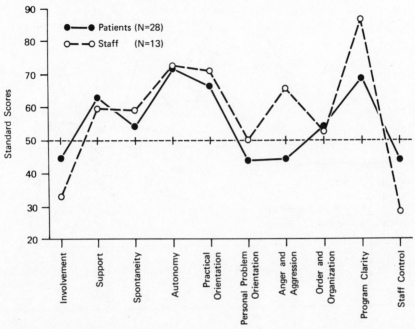

Figure 5.2   WAS Form C profiles for patients and staff in control program in initial project phase.

The Initial Project Phase

The WAS was administered to patients and staff in each program. Figures 5.1 and 5.2 present the WAS profiles of the first administration. Patients in the two programs saw an identical emphasis on Involvement; however, patients in the experimental program noted more emphasis on Support and less on Spontaneity ($p < .05$) than did patients in the control program. The staff in the two programs perceived these three Relationship dimensions almost identically. Patients in the experimental program thought there was greater emphasis on Practical Orientation and Anger and Aggression ($p < .05$) than did patients in the control program. Staff in the experimental program found more emphasis on Autonomy ($p < .01$), Practical Orientation, and Anger and Aggression ($p < .01$) than did control program staff. There were no significant differences between patients' perceptions of the three System Maintenance dimensions, but control staff reported more emphasis ($p < .01$) on all three dimensions than did experimental staff.

The initial profiles indicate that both programs were seen in a positive manner; that is, the emphasis on the Relationship and Treatment Program

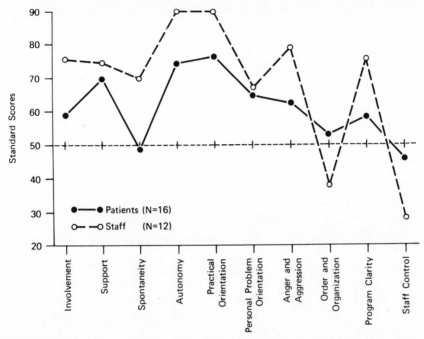

Figure 5.3   WAS Form C profiles for patients and staff in experimental program in active research phase.

dimensions was moderately to substantially above average. Patients and staff in the experimental program perceived more emphasis on Practical Orientation and Anger and Aggression, reflecting this program's emphasis on out-of-hospital work, outside community issues, on confrontation, openness, and the sharing of angry feelings. The control patients noted greater stress on Spontaneity, reflecting a more traditional concern with the expression of feelings per se (although not specifically the expression of angry feelings). Staff in the experimental program saw much more emphasis on the Treatment Program dimensions, whereas control staff saw much more on the System Maintenance dimensions. This is not surprising, since the experimental staff were instituting a new treatment program, whereas the control staff were maintaining a more traditional program.

The Active Research Phase

Figures 5.3 and 5.4 show the profiles for the active phase of the research, by which time the experimental program was fully developed. As expected,

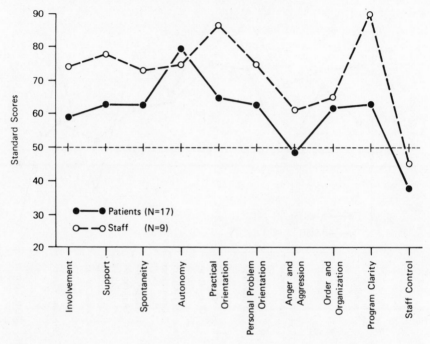

Figure 5.4 WAS Form C profiles for patients and staff in control program in active research phase.

there were greater differences between the two programs during this phase. The results indicate three major conclusions.

1.   Patients in the experimental program believed that there was much more emphasis on the Relationship dimensions of Involvement ($p < .01$) and Spontaneity ($p < .01$) than did control program patients. Staff in the experimental program saw more emphasis on Involvement ($p < .01$) and Support ($p < .10$) than did control staff. An important finding was that the patient and staff groups in each program agreed closely about the amount of emphasis on these three dimensions.

2.   Experimental program patients saw much greater emphasis on the Treatment Program dimensions of Autonomy ($p < .10$), Practical Orientation ($p < .10$) and, to a lesser extent, Personal Problem Orientation and Anger and Aggression ($p < .10$). Experimental program staff generally agreed.

3.   Finally, patients in the experimental program reported less emphasis on Program Clarity than control program patients. Staff in the

experimental program perceived more emphasis on all four Treatment Program dimensions and less emphasis on all three System Maintenance dimensions than did control program staff.

The experimental program was more stable during the 8-month interval than the control program. The intraclass profile correlations for the experimental program were .72 for patients and .97 for staff ($p < .01$), indicating extremely high program stability over time. The patient profile on the control program exhibited decreases in Involvement and Personal Problem Orientation; in the staff profile there were substantial changes in the three Relationship dimensions, in Practical Orientation and Personal Problem Orientation, and to a lesser extent in all three System Maintenance dimensions. The intraclass correlations for the control program were .68 for patients ($p < .01$) and .41 for staff (not statistically significant).

The changes in the control program corresponded to a period of leadership crisis, low staff morale, and low patient discharge rates. Only the emphasis on Program Clarity was higher in the control program, probably reflecting its somewhat simpler and more familiar organization. A senior permanent professional was planning on leaving the program, thus exposing its major weakness—namely, the almost exclusive emphasis on "people as therapy" and the relative lack of concern with structured program elements such as the employment service group task.

Experimental and control program profiles remained quite stable during the next 6 months. Control patients and staff reported less emphasis on Involvement, Spontaneity, and Practical Orientation in the follow-up phase profile, however, indicating a further deterioration in this program. The remarkable stability that a treatment milieu can attain once a structured program has been implemented is revealed in the final profile for the experimental program, obtained more than 2 years later. The overall program orientation remained basically identical during this interval. The overall stability of the experimental program from the initial to the final testing (a period of more than 3 years) is indicated by the intraclass profile correlations of .73 for patients and .96 for staff. This stability was achieved even though different patients and staff were continually coming into the program and, of course, responding to the WAS.

Staff opinions were also solicited several times on a 12-item questionnaire. The experimental program staff generally showed a more positive view than the control program staff. During the active research phase, differences of opinion were especially pronounced regarding patient hopefulness, morale, enthusiasm, and beliefs about program effectiveness. The control program staff finally switched to the belief that the experimental program would have better results than their own program. The total proportion of patients who worked full-time or part-time during their hospitalization was approximately four times higher in the experimental program. Thus the combination of slow patient turnover, a gradually accumulating group of chronic patients, and a comparatively small proportion of patients who worked or took training during their hospitalization resulted in the more pessimistic views of the control staff. Various other differences between the two programs are discussed in more detail by Daniels (1970).

Assessment as Self-Analysis and Quality Control

The preceding comparisons illustrate possible applications of social systems assessment of treatment environment—for example, direct comparison of treatment programs, relating the effects of specific program components to treatment outcome, and monitoring program changes over time. The WAS provided an additional systematic description of the treatment environment in the two programs, a description that closely corresponded to the different emphases in the programs. By comparing patient and staff groups with each other and over time, similarities and differences between programs and groups were identified. The greater emphasis on the Treatment Program dimensions in the experimental program and on the System Maintenance dimensions in the control program (especially in the early phase of the study) reflected the experimental program's emphasis on task groups, confrontation, practical performance, and adult status as well as the control program's emphasis on the maintenance of a traditional treatment system. During this time phase, both programs had generally "favorable" treatment environments and approximately equal discharge rates. Later changes in the control program were accompanied by a decrease in discharge rates and a decline in staff enthusiasm about their program's effectiveness.

There was a high degree of congruence between the WAS findings and such other findings regarding the two treatment programs as staff opinions about their programs, staff rankings of the importance of different treatment components, and analyses of the communications in the community meetings. For example, the experimental program community meetings emphasized problem solving and task orientation; they were highly structured, patient dominated, and decision oriented, The control program community meeting—unstructured forums for imparting information —were staff dominated and oriented toward discussing group and personal problems.

Better posthospitalization work adjustment was displayed by patients discharged from the experimental program. A 12- to 18-month follow-up showed 44% less accumulated rehospitalization for the experimental program and better work outcome: 136.5 versus 115.3 equivalent 8-hour days worked on the average during the first 360 days after discharge and 270.3 versus 136.4 days worked on the first full-time job. However, somewhat better symptom improvement resulted in the control program: 54.1% of the experimental patients and only 36.4% of the control patients experienced high anxiety at 12- to 18-month follow-up. In this connection it should be noted that the experimental program, while emphasizing support and practical orientation, also stressed anger, aggression, and confrontation. This program was relatively demanding and anxiety provoking, even though a generally satisfying environment was maintained and patients felt that the program was enhancing their personal development.

This detailed example indicates that regular social system assessment can serve a valuable monitoring or "quality control" function. Congruence between patient and staff groups and/or between actual and ideal environments is an important factor in effective systems operation. Repeated measures of social system process over time provide the opportunity for self-analysis at both individual program and institution levels. Regular feedback of process data not only helps monitor the evolution and function of a system over time, it can be utilized to spot crises and to bring about desired changes in program goals.

PSYCHOSOCIAL TREATMENT MILIEU ANALYSES

In Chapter 4 the clinical utility of the WAS was discussed in terms of detailed profile interpretations of single individual programs. A number of investigators, both in this country and in the United Kingdom, have used the WAS to describe and compare different types of treatment programs. One of the most detailed program descriptions employing the WAS as an outside tool for evaluation is that of the psychiatric ward at the University of Oregon Medical School, as discussed in Chapter 4 (Grant and Saslow, 1971).

A Peer Confrontation Program

Van Stone and Gilbert (1972) described an experimental program at the Palo Alto VA hospital which was stimulated partly by Synanon and partly by the drug and alcohol addiction units at Mendocino State Hospital in California. Housed on an open ward, the program had about 30 male patients who were seeking help because of alcoholism, drug abuse or addiction, gambling, sexual deviation, repeated conflicts with the law, or other self-defeating life styles. Patients' ages ranged from 20 to 60, the median being in the early 40s. At the time of testing there were only three paid staff members: two counselors (one had been a nursing aide, the other was a former addict recruited from the *Peer* program) and the director, a social worker with 19 years of experience in prison and parole work and in the treatment of alcoholism.

The basic treatment principles were as follows: (1) An individualized, negotiated treatment contract was made between each potential member and his peers. Approximately one-half of the applicants to the program were rejected as unwilling to commit themselves to make a radical change in their life style. (2) The development of personal growth and of a capacity for close relationships was strongly stressed. (3) A member-controlled social structure was established, and graduated responsibility, status, and jobs were designated for each member. Paid staff had no more and no fewer privileges than other members. (4) The primary psychological intervention was by way of the peer confrontation group, a kind of therapy group in which each member is presented with candid personal facts regarding every observable behavior or attitude recognized by the group as being self-defeating or dishonest. If the member attempts to explain away or deny an observation, he is ridiculed, browbeaten, shouted down, and insulted by his fellow members.

As might be expected, the WAS profile obtained on this ward was quite different from average (see Figure 5.5). Even though the program was poorly staffed by the usual criteria, the treatment environment was highly unusual, and there was almost exact agreement between patients and staff on its characteristics. Emphasis on all three Relationship dimensions was substantially above average, as was the emphasis on all four Treatment Program dimensions. The emphasis on Order and Organization and Program Clarity was moderately above average, whereas that of Staff Control was well below average. The profile reveals a high degree of involvement and cohesion, with considerable emphasis on patient

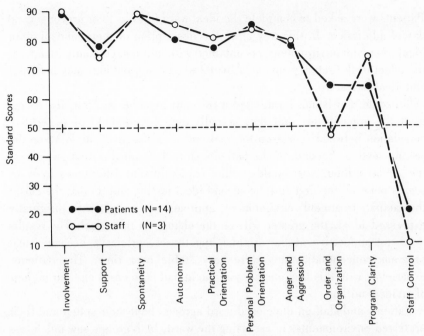

Figure 5.5   WAS Form C profiles for patients and staff on peer confrontation program.

independence and self-responsibility, practical down-to-earth problem solving, as well as self-understanding and the open expression of anger and aggression. The results are generally consistent with the program description as presented by Van Stone and Gilbert, except that neither patients nor staff perceived high Staff Control—perhaps because the "high authoritarian social structure" was essentially totally patient controlled. More details about the program can be found in their article.

Two Drug Treatment Programs

Teasdale and Isham (1969) utilized the WAS in the drug-dependence clinical research and treatment unit at the Bethlem Royal Hospital in London. The unit consists of two programs: one a 10-bed closed ward for the treatment of intravenous drug users (mainly dependent on opiates), the other an 11-bed open ward for the treatment of all other types of drug users (mainly dependent on stimulants or barbiturates). As a result of a number of incidents with individual patients on the closed ward, members of the staff developed an informal hypothesis that "whatever patients actually get in the way of ward management, they will usually want the opposite."

Patients were asked to complete the ideal ward form on their first or second day of admission. In this way an initial description of their concept of an ideal treatment environment was obtained with minimal contamination from the effect of the actual program. About 2 weeks later patients took both real and ideal forms.

Teasdale and Isham formulated a two-part hypothesis. First, if patients want the opposite of what they actually get, there should be a negative correlation between scores on the real and ideal forms of the WAS on the second testing. Second, if the patients shift their ideal milieu away from the actual milieu, one would predict (a) significant differences in WAS scores between the first and the second ideal testing and (b) that the closer the actual treatment environment approaches the patient's originally expressed ideal, the greater will be the change in that ideal. The results were not supportive of the original hypotheses, primarily because ideal program conceptualizations were very stable over time. The patients' experience with this treatment environment had little effect on their notions of an ideal milieu.

Patients and staff on the closed ward agreed about their actual and their preferred environments. In assessing the ward, both groups saw much less emphasis on Involvement, Autonomy, and Practical Orientation than they ideally wished. The open ward was regarded more positively and as closer to the ideal than was the closed ward. The authors point out that ward milieu differences occurred even though the senior staff were common to both programs and both programs were located in the same building.

Other Program Comparisons

In other relevant studies, Kleinsasser (1969) constructed a WAS profile for an entire psychiatric hospital and discussed its overall treatment milieu in comparison to our American reference group norms, and Ballard (1971) has compared the treatment environments of four psychiatric wards in a state hospital in Texas. Westmaas (1971) studied several different wards in a private hospital which had recently shifted its emphasis to group as opposed to strictly individual approaches. He found that the hospital had a distinctive treatment environment characterized by an unusually high degree of emphasis on Involvement, Support, and Personal Problem Orientation as perceived by staff and patients alike, although there were some differences from ward to ward even in the same building. Feedback of results was helpful to staff in stimulating self-analysis and in suggesting areas for attention and change.

In a comparison of five different VA hospital programs, Kish (1971) noted that ward treatment teams were concerned about the effectiveness of their treatment environment and thus needed feedback for evaluation purposes. One ward utilized a social-psychological approach, a second was oriented more traditionally toward drugs and activities, and a third, an alcoholism treatment unit, utilized an educational approach centered on Alcoholics Anonymous. On the other two wards treatment depended more on the preference and judgment of individual staff members; no attempt was made to develop an official treatment philosophy. Kish reported that the areas of WAS emphasis on the first three wards were generally consistent with their treatment programs. For example, both patients and staff on the alcoholism unit saw the milieu as emphasizing Involvement, Practical Orientation, and Personal Problem Orientation. These qualities seemed to be consistent with a program stressing participation in Alcoholics Anonymous, using group therapy to promote self-understanding, and aiming to rehabilitate the alcoholic socially and vocationally.

In an interesting aside, Kish comments that patients and staff perceived high emphasis on order and neatness in the ward that was oriented toward social-psychological treatment. This observation led to an examination of transactions made through notes, which were the main device for communication between the treatment team and the patient groups. When it was revealed that 30 to 50% of the notes were concerned with such matters as unmade beds and dusty lockers, the emphasis on order was lessened. Other disparities between staff and patient perceptions were also discussed, and changes of emphasis were suggested and implemented. Kish points out that the ward teams expressed considerable interest in their WAS profiles, believing the findings to be useful for self-evaluation. The feedback was of particular value to those wards having a consistent treatment program and philosophy, and this result is directly consistent with our experience. The feedback was less helpful on the two wards on which the treatment orientation was more individualized and on which staff had not developed a coherent treatment philosophy. Kish recommends the administration and analysis of the WAS as a useful additional service that a hospital psychology department can provide to ward treatment teams.

Finally, Lewis et al. (1971) are utilizing the WAS in a detailed, ongoing study to help evaluate milieu therapy in a multidisciplinary investigation of six wards in three institutions. In the milieu approach, each experience to which the patient is exposed is considered to be potentially therapeutic; however, Lewis et al. note the exact methods employed to achieve treatment goals are usually poorly detailed. What actually happens in different treatment milieus is generally unclear, since the number of different potentially therapeutic influences impinging upon a patient during even one hospital day is enormous. Therefore, these authors organized an intensive milieu study. Only preliminary results have been obtained thus far, and the authors have reported that the WAS has not differentiated unequivocally among the six wards under study, although some differences have appeared. The project is currently continuing, but the authors state with some dismay that many staff show considerable ambivalence toward hearing about the results of the milieu assessment and that at times "it was more difficult to get appointments to discuss the results of certain tests than it had been to get appointments to administer them" (p. 11).

EVALUATING PROGRAM CHANGE

Establishing an Active Milieu Program

Several investigators have utilized the WAS in assessing the effects of program changes. For example, Cleghorn (1969) used the WAS to discriminate between two programs and to observe the effect of changing one of these programs during a 6-month period. Patients in one program had increased responsibility, and high value was placed on group functioning, self-understanding, appropriate behavior, and relevant emotional interchanges about problems with nursing personnel. The morale in this program was good, and the staff were eager for more liberal changes. No attempt was made to modify the treatment milieu in this program.

The experimental ward was identical to the control ward both in size and in physical characteristics. Only the public patients participated in the ward programs, and the private practitioners frequently disallowed group therapy involvement for their patients. The ward had a bad reputation among residents, who felt that they were exploited by the private practitioners there and that they were taught little on the assignment. The nurses also felt that assignment to the ward was distasteful, and it required considerable support on the part of the nursing director to keep them employed there.

The differences between the WAS profiles on the two wards were approximately as expected. Both patients and staff perceived the experimental program as substantially lower on all three Relationship dimensions, particularly Involvement and Spontaneity. They also saw it as much lower on Personal Problem Orientation, and staff saw it as lower on Practical Orientation. The differences on the System Maintenance dimensions were relatively minor.

When Cleghorn took over as ward chief he initiated ward meetings for all patients. Patients began to take initiatives in forming committees to welcome new patients and to govern their behavior in the program. The general level of anxiety and depression among both patients and staff declined. Most members of the attending staff made an attempt to cooperate with the new program.

Substantial changes occurred in patients' and staff's perception of this program during the subsequent 2 months. Staff perceived relatively large increases in emphasis on all three Relationship dimensions, but patients perceived only slight increases. On the other hand, patients reported substantial increases in emphasis on the Treatment Program dimensions of Autonomy and Personal Problem Orientation, whereas staff perceived such increases as slight. However, patients and staff agreed on the direction of change, since they both perceived more emphasis on all six of the dimensions. Also, patients in the experimental program saw more positive change (i.e., increased emphasis) on all three Relationship and on all four Treatment Program dimensions than did patients in the control program. Exactly the same finding held true for staff. These changes were consistent with the kinds of modifications Cleghorn was attempting to institute. The study provides a nice illustration of the use of the WAS in documenting planned ward milieu changes.

Training Staff in Group Therapy Techniques

In a similar type of study, Leviege (1969) investigated the effect of 5 months of training psychiatric nurses and technicians in group therapy. He compared three state hospital admission wards of similar size and staffing. The staff on the experimental ward participated in a formal group therapy training course; the staff on a second ward were informally trained in group techniques by the ward psychiatrist; the staff on a third ward received no group training. On the experimental ward the group training included all the staff members (physicians, psychologist, social worker, rehabilitation therapist, supervising nurses, psychiatric technicians, etc.). The training emphasized self-understanding and the development of insight into personal feelings. Lecturing was minimized, and direct "here and now" encounter techniques were used.

Leviege hypothesized that staff who engaged in this training would develop a more positive treatment environment in their programs than staff who did not. The WAS was given to patients and staff about 2 months after the completion of the group training. There were substantial differences between the experimental program and the program on which staff had had no group training. Patients and staff on the experimental ward perceived much more emphasis on the Relationship dimensions of Involvement and Spontaneity and on the Treatment Program dimensions of Autonomy and Personal Problem Orientation. They also perceived significantly more emphasis on Order and Organization and significantly less emphasis on Staff Control. Patients and staff in the program that had informal group therapy training, as conducted by the ward psychiatrist, saw their milieu somewhat more positively than patients and staff in the control program and somewhat more negatively than patients and staff in the experimental program.

The results must be interpreted with caution because no WAS pretest data were available. However, given the close similarity of the three admission wards utilized, it appears that either formal or (to a somewhat lesser extent) informal group therapy training may have important effects on a program's overall treatment milieu. The results are generally consistent with those obtained by Cleghorn in the study discussed previously. It must be noted that the objective characteristics of size and staffing of Leviege's three programs should have militated against his actual findings. The experimental program had the largest number of patients ($N = 50$) and the smallest number of full-time staff ($N = 14$), whereas the other two programs had 31 and 36 patients and 17 and 16 full-time staff members, respectively. On the basis of these size and staffing differences, a somewhat more positive treatment milieu would have been predicted, both in the control program and in the program for which there was only informal group training.

Instituting a Token Economy

In an attempt to evaluate a different type of milieu change, Gripp and Magaro (1971) utilized the WAS to help specify the effects of developing a token-economy program as compared with untreated control programs. They instituted a staff training program that was similar to Leviege's group therapy training program, although of course it concentrated on establishing a quite different type of treatment milieu.

Forty-five female patients were selected on the basis of being chronically ill, disruptive, or combative, but without organic involvement. Their age range was 17 to 66, the median being 44 years. Their overall length of hospitalization ranged from 1 to 37 years, with a median of 16 years. This was clearly a difficult and chronic state hospital patient population. Of the three control wards, two were similar to the experimental ward in terms of physical structure and patient population. The third control ward was located in a more recently constructed wing of the hospital; the patients there were disturbed but were not quite as chronic. The experimental ward was located in an old wing of the hospital and was physically run-down and dreary in appearance. It contained four dormitories of various sizes, sleeping from four to fifteen patients each, and seven single rooms, one reserved for seclusion and another remodeled to serve as an operant conditioning chamber for research purposes. Gripp and Magaro describe the ward as a typical state hospital back ward, adding that little could be done to alter its physical atmosphere.

The specific staff involved, the specific training procedures, the details of the token-economy program, and the variety of behavioral rating scales utilized to monitor patient behavior changes are described in detail by Gripp and Magaro. Of particular interest here is that the WAS was administered to the nursing staff on the experimental and the three control wards both prior to the initiation of the program and 6 months after the program was begun. The results indicated that the treatment environment of the token-economy ward changed significantly on 6 of the 10 WAS dimensions. Significant increases were observed on the Relationship dimensions of Involvement and Spontaneity ($p < .01$) and on the Treatment Program dimensions of Autonomy and Practical Orientation ($p < .005$). Significant decreases occurred on the System Maintenance dimensions of Order and Organization and Staff Control ($p < .01$). As would be expected with a token-economy ward, the biggest differences occurred on the Autonomy and Practical Orientation subscales. There were some differences in staff perceptions over time on each of the three control wards; however, all significant differences were in the negative direction (e.g., staff on all three control wards perceived significantly less emphasis on Autonomy on the second than on the first WAS administration).

Thus very substantial differences may result in the general treatment environment of a chronic state hospital ward when a token-economy program is initiated. The results also showed more improvement in the behavior of the patients assigned to the token-economy program than in those remaining on or transferred to control programs. The staff on the token-economy ward felt that the program was a more congenial and therapeutic place in which to work. They reported a greater sense of responsibility, accomplishment, and hopefulness for the patients as compared with their earlier feelings. Staff on the control wards may have felt more negative about their treatment environments because they were comparing them with the more positively functioning token-economy program.

Changing from Uniforms to Street Clothes

Three studies have obtained results indicating that only moderate if any changes in overall treatment environments are related to whether nursing staff wear uniforms or street clothes. In unpublished data of our own, the WAS was given to patients and staff on each of four wards just prior to and again one month after nursing personnel changed from wearing uniforms to wearing street clothes. We found no consistent changes coincident with the new practice, although the one-month time period for retesting may have been too short.

Guido and Haberland (1971) studied two wards with the real and ideal forms of the WAS. The two forms were initially administered in January 1970. Nursing staff on both wards changed from wearing uniforms to street clothes (on all three shifts) one week later. Staff on the other wards in the hospital retained their uniforms. In May 1970 both forms of the WAS were readministered to all patients and all nursing staff. Unfortunately the authors felt they could not compare the experimental with the control wards because of unexpected changes on the control wards during the 4-month interval. Thus they simply identified changes on the two experimental wards. Both patients and staff perceived slightly more emphasis on the three Relationship dimensions, and the patients also perceived some increased emphasis on Autonomy and Personal Problem Orientation. Since most of the changes were not statistically significant, Guido and Haberland concluded that allowing nursing staff to wear street clothes has no functional value on patient care.

In a final study on this issue, Klein et al. (1972) organized a three-stage project in which staff members wore traditional white uniforms, changed to wearing street clothes, and then returned to wearing uniforms. Attitudes toward and perceptions of self, others, and the program in general were assessed during each stage. Initially there was a 3-week baseline (stage one), followed by a 6-week period (stage two) during which nursing staff wore street clothes. During the last 3-week period (stage three) the nursing staff returned to wearing traditional white uniforms. The study was conducted on a 28-bed, milieu-oriented ward of a university hospital where the average length of stay of patients was approximately 28 days. The ward was heavily staffed with nurses, nursing assistants, nursing students, psychiatric residents, medical students, administrative staff, and activities personnel.

Klein et al. assessed 94 separate variables regarding possible changes. The results on the vast majority of such variables remained surprisingly stable regardless of changes in nursing staff dress. The changes that did occur in patient responses were generally "negative"; that is, patients felt slightly more secure and less anxious when the nursing staff wore uniforms. Patients rated themselves and other patients as less distant and perceived themselves as better models for their own behavior at stage one than at stage two. They also had more confidence in the staff members, rated them as emotionally healthier, as easier to discuss sexual concerns with, and as easier to identify at stage one. On the WAS the patients perceived the treatment environment as characterized by greater Involvement and greater Order and Organization during stage one.

The data for staff indicated that they also found the changes to and from street clothes to be disruptive; moreover, they experienced disappointment and an apparent loss of self-esteem when required to return to wearing uniforms. Staff members rated nursing staff as most difficult to identify at stage two, when they were wearing street clothes, and they perceived the treatment environment as characterized by less Program Clarity at that time. There was increased disruption on the ward, decreased interpersonal contact and involvement, and increased reliance on the use of medication as a treatment modality during stage three; however, these changes were most likely related to a turnover in residents and staff that was occurring at the time. Klein et al. concluded that there was no clear evidence that wearing street clothes facilitated closer personal therapeutic engagements with patients. It is possible, however, that the comparatively short time interval of stage two (6 weeks), and the subsequent necessity for the nurses to revert to wearing uniforms precluded any larger or more permanent change.

The results of these studies indicate that the WAS is sensitive to treatment environment changes as perceived by both patients and staff. Relatively large changes may occur when the entire treatment program is changed, as in the studies of Cleghorn, Leviege, and Gripp and Magaro. Change in the three Relationship dimensions—probably signifying increased patient and staff morale, increased perception of helpfulness and supportiveness, and increased personal openness and expressivity—occurred in all three studies. Changes in the Treatment Program dimensions are more directly related to the specific type of change that is instituted. Thus Leviege found relatively large increases in Personal Problem Orientation and Anger and Aggression in a program on which group therapy training was given to staff, whereas Gripp and Magaro recorded substantial increases in Autonomy and Practical Orientation in a token-economy program. On the other hand, not all attempts are sufficient to bring about either large or long-term milieu change. In a very chronic state hospital back ward, for example, Maier (1970) found relatively little change attendant on what was unfortunately a minimal resocialization training program. Such simple changes as having nurses wear street clothes instead of uniforms or adding clerks to a ward (Oregon Mental Health Division, 1971) also fail to produce changes in the treatment milieu. When substantial changes are made in the overall program, both patient and staff WAS perceptions usually accurately reflect such alterations.

INNOVATIVE APPLICATIONS

A number of investigators have applied the WAS in novel ways and/or in assessing the environments of institutions other than psychiatric hospitals. For example, Bancke (1969) used the WAS to assess the treatment environment of a chronic disease hospital. The 10 subscales clearly and predictably differentiated among staff perceptions of the environment at a main hospital, an annex, and a pavillion. Bancke also found no significant differences between registered nurses and licensed practical nurses, and she learned that younger staff members (aged 25 to 32 years) did not perceive the environment differently from older staff members (aged 49 to 55 years).

In a larger but still incomplete study, Davis and Maroney (1971) utilized an adaptation of the WAS to evaluate the psychosocial milieus of VA spinal cord injury units. They collected data from more than 500 patients and 450 staff. They preliminarily identified four factors that permitted differentiation among the units, labeling them as follows: (1) active treatment program, (2) dissatisfaction with ward, (3) guardedness, and (4) lack of cooperation among patients. Attempts to relate these data to outcome criteria differentiating among the units are currently being made.

In a different use of the WAS, Penwarden (1970) modified the items to reflect concern with staff rather than patients. In effect he attempted to develop a Work Environment Scale for staff. For example, the item "Patients are careful about what they say when staff are around" was changed to "Staff are careful about what they say when supervisors are around." Penwarden studied three programs in a provincial medical hospital and tested the hypothesis that personnel satisfaction and involvement varies with variation in the organizational climate. One program was an integrated geriatrics ward reputed to have low staff morale. The second was a chronic medical ward treating mainly geriatric patients and regarded as a smoothly running unit. The third program was an active, treatment-oriented male admission ward reputed to be one of the best wards in the hospital.

The results indicated that satisfaction and involvement varied significantly among the three programs. The head nurses on the two wards with greater satisfaction and involvement both spent more time in nursing care activities, thus presenting images of being members of the ward team as well as supervisors. The head nurse on the third ward was seen primarily as a supervisor entrenched in the formal organization of the hospital, since she participated little in actual nursing care activities. Penwarden's main conclusion was that the style of leadership of the head nurse has a significant effect on the morale of the nursing staff. The ward with the lowest WAS Involvement, Spontaneity, Autonomy, and Order and Organization scores also had the lowest mean staff job satisfaction scores. The other results were generally as expected, indicating that the WAS items could reasonably be modified for use in assessing the work environment of program staff.

In another application in a quite different setting, Henchy (1970) adapted the items of the WAS to measure the press of an outpatient psychiatric clinic. Since this adaptation in a sense measures the work environment of the staff, it represents an approach similar to Penwarden's. Henchy proposed that the press of an outpatient clinic would have strong effects on how staff act toward patients and on how well the clinic serves the community. He speculated that a measure of clinic press might also explain why one clinic has an appreciably larger staff turnover than another. Henchy also assessed the personality types of individual staff members by utilizing Stein's Self Description Inventory. The instruments were administered to the staff of a small outpatient psychiatric clinic in New York City.

Since no significant relationships appeared between the personality types and their perceptions of clinic press, Henchy concluded that a measurable atmosphere existed independent of the personality of the viewer. He hypothesized that those serving different functions and roles would perceive different demands from the environment. None of the between-staff differences were significant, although psychiatrists and psychiatric social workers perceived the most emphasis on Involvement and Autonomy, whereas psychologists perceived the least. The specific findings are preliminary because only one clinic was used and a small number of staff were involved, but the results point to the potential utility of adapting the WAS for the measurement of the social milieus of outpatient clinics.

The major conclusions to be derived from these studies are that the WAS items have some cross-cultural applicability, that they are relevant to assessing the environments of medically oriented wards (e.g., a chronic disease hospital, spinal cord injury units), and that they can be adapted to describing the work environments of psychiatric staff in hospitals and in outpatient clinics. In our own research we have independently derived perceived environment scales for use in various social environments (e.g., correctional facilities, military training companies, junior high and high school classrooms, and university student living groups). All this work indicates that the conceptual organization underlying the WAS has broad utility in a substantial range of different social environments (see Chapter 14).

REFERENCES

Ballard, M. Personal communication, 1971.

Bancke, L. Staff and patient perception of ward atmosphere at Drake Memorial Hospital. Unpublished paper. Drake Memorial Hospital, Cincinnati, Ohio, May, 1969.

Cleghorn, J. Comparison of two psychiatric wards for six months. Unpublished paper. McMaster University, Ontario, Canada, 1969.

Daniels, D. The Dann Services Program. Department of Psychiatry, Stanford University School of Medicine, Palo Alto, 1970.

Davis, J.. & Maroney, R. Personal communication, 1971.

Grant, R. & Saslow, G. Maximizing responsible decision making, or how do we get out of here? In Abroms, G. & Greenfield, N. (Eds.). The new hospital psychiatry. Academic Press, New York, 1971.

Gripp, R. & Magaro, P. A token economy program evaluation with untreated control ward comparisons. *Behavior Research and Therapy,* **9**: 137–139, 1971.

Guido, J.. & Haberland, J. A study of nursing staff attire in county psychiatric wards. Paper presented at the California State Psychological Association Conference, January 1971.

Henchy, T. A measure of the press of an outpatient clinic. Unpublished paper. New Hope Guild Center, Brooklyn, N.Y., 1970.

Kish, G. Evaluation of ward atmosphere. *Hospital and Community Psychiatry,* **22**: 159–161, 1971.

Klein, R., Pillsbury, J., Bushey, M., & Snell, S. Psychiatric staff: Uniforms or street clothes? *Archives of General Psychiatry,* **26**: 19–22, 1972.

Kleinsasser, D. Social atmosphere of Fort Logan psychiatric teams: A comparison with other hospitals. Unpublished paper. Fort Logan Mental Health Center, Colorado, 1969.

Leviege, V. Group relations: Group therapy with mentally ill offenders. M.A. thesis, Fresno State College, Fresno, Calif., 1969.

Lewis, D., Beck, P., King, H., & Stephen, L. Some approaches to the evaluation of milieu therapy. *Canadian Psychiatric Association Journal,* **16**: 203–208, 1971.

Maier, L. A resocialization program on state mental hospital wards serving long-term patients. Ph.D. dissertation, Catholic University of America, 1970.

Oregon Mental Health Division. Report on staffing adjustments at Oregon State Hospital. Unpublished paper. State of Oregon, 1971.

Penwarden, G. Nursing staff morale on mental wards. Bachelor's thesis, Queen's University, N.Y., 1970.

Teasdale, J. & Isham, H. Use of the Ward Atmosphere Scale in a drug dependency treatment unit. Unpublished paper. University of London, 1969.

Van Stone, W. & Gilbert, R. Peer confrontation groups—What, why, and whether. *American Journal of Psychiatry,* **129**: 583–589, 1972.

Westmaas, R. A study of social atmosphere on Pine Rest Christian Hospital intensive treatment units. Unpublished paper. Pine Rest Christian Hospital, Grand Rapids, Mich., 1971.

Chapter Six

STRUCTURAL AND ORGANIZATIONAL PROGRAM CHARACTERISTICS

MULTIPLE METHODS OF ASSESSING ENVIRONMENTS

In this chapter we examine the relationships of patient and staff perceptions of their treatment environment to other more usual ways of describing and differentiating among psychiatric programs. In the broadest sense we deal with the question of the relationships among different ways of characterizing environments. Chapter 1 presented a brief review of six major categories of environmental dimensions. Our concern here is with how variables in these different categories relate to each other; for example, to what extent do perceptions of environments provide information that is not more easily obtained by objective structural variables? Results discussed in Chapter 3 indicate that knowing whether a ward is in a state, VA, or university teaching hospital tells relatively little about the treatment environment on that ward. The detailed program comparison presented in Chapter 5 shows that wards of essentially identical size, staffing, patient background, and architectural characteristics *may* have very different treatment environments. On the other hand, there is some relation between structural characteristics of programs such as size and staffing and their treatment environments.

Two of the types of dimensions by which environments have been characterized are particularly relevant here. First are the dimensions of organizational structure and functioning, such as size and staffing ratios. Usually psychiatric programs have been compared in terms of readily observable indices of this sort—number of patients, number of staff, whether there are open or locked doors, whether there are community meetings, the kind of occupational or recreational therapy program, and so on. Most of the classical work on organizational characteristics in different institutions has utilized such dimensions (March, 1965).

Typical examples include work on the properties of organizational structure in industrial institutions in relation to job attitudes and job behavior (Porter and Lawler, 1965), and work characterizing colleges and universities along dimensions such as affluence (wealth), size, private versus public, masculinity versus femininity, realistic (technical) emphasis, and homogeneity (Astin, 1962). Data about perceived environmental characteristics such as obtained by the College and University Environment Scales (Pace, 1969) give information that is congruent with but adds substantially to information presented by more objective institutional variables also differentiating among universities.

For example, Astin (1968) and Creager and Astin (1968) were concerned with comprehensive descriptions of college and university environments, particularly in relation to their effects on student development. In this connection they estimated the relationships among some of the commonly used administrative or institutional variables (e.g., geographical region) and college environment factors. They obtained 70 administrative and environmental variables and used them in describing 244 four-year colleges. Of particular interest here is that the authors included eight "college image" factors that were derived from the perceptions of students in the university environment. Only two of the eight college image factors had substantial correlations with other institutional variables, indicating that these image factors represent relatively unique ways of describing institutions.

These findings are consonant with data reported by Stern (1970) on the relationships between the College Characteristics Index and more objective indices differentiating among universities, and those reported by Centra, Hartnett, and Peterson (1970) relating the Institutional Functioning Inventory (IFI) to published institutional data such as number of books in the library, library books per student, and faculty–student ratio. The general conclusion of this line of studies is that objective structural or institutional dimensions characterizing environments provide information congruent but not identical to that obtained from techniques assessing perceived environment and social climate characteristics.

The second category of relevant dimensions concerns the average personal and behavioral characteristics of the inhabitants of the milieu.

Various factors related to the characteristics (e.g., average age, ability level, socioeconomic background, educational attainment) of the individuals inhabiting a particular environment can be considered to be situational variables insofar as they partially define relevant characteristics of the environment (e.g., Sells, 1963). This idea is based on the suggestion made by Linton (1945) that most of the social and cultural environment is transmitted through other people. As pointed out in Chapter 1, this implies that the character of an environment is dependent on the nature of its members and that the dominant features of an environment depend on the typical characteristics of its members.

This logic is represented by the Environmental Assessment Technique (EAT), in which it is assumed that the college environment depends on the personal characteristics of the students, faculty, administration, and staff of the institution (Astin and Holland, 1961). The EAT was based on the assumption that the major portion of the student's environment was determined by the characteristics of his fellow students. Accordingly, the environment was defined in part in terms of six personal orientations based on the proportion of students in six broad areas of study. Similar approaches have been utilized by Astin (1968) in the Inventory of College Activities (ICA) and by Centra (1968) in the Questionnaire on Student and College Characteristics (QSCC).

Centra (1970) administered the QSCC to upper class students at more than 200 institutions. He compared three different methods of assessing the college environment—student perceptions, student self-reports, and objective institutional data—by use of multimethod factor analysis, a technique that removes method variance by focusing on correlations between rather than within different methods of measurement. Centra concluded that "each method seems to tap *some* information not predictably obtained by other methods. Quite likely then there are certain kinds of information that can be obtained by only one method, even when it appears that two or more methods assess the same domain" (Centra, 1970, p. 39).

Thus these studies indicate that different methods of evaluating institutional environments must be used together. Various types of information about the environment may also have differential utility. Information about social climate may be most relevant for facilitating short-term environmental change. Information on the characteristics of the milieu inhabitants may be most relevant for providing prospective inhabitants with information about the stimuli they are likely to encounter in the environment. For example, it may be important for a student to learn that students in his chosen university spend approximately 15 hours a week studying, since that will give the new student some specific ideas about the kinds of behaviors he will probably need to engage in. Finally, information about more objective institutional characteristics may be most applicable to relatively quick comparisons among institutions and to overall planning of long-term changes.

THE WARD INFORMATION FORM (WIF)

Following this logic we obtained data on organizational policy and patient behavior characteristics of wards. We used the Ward Information Form (WIF) developed by Kellam et al. (1966) in a study of 27 psychiatric admission wards. The WIF dimensions were also related to treatment outcome, as discussed in Chapter 8. The four WIF variables we used were: (1) ward census, (2) staff–patient ratio, (3) adult status, and (4) disturbed behavior. Ward census was simply defined as the number of patients on the ward at the time of testing. This was identical to total ward size, since almost every ward was filled to capacity. All full-time day staff were included in computing the staff–patient ratio.

Kellam et al. based the adult status dimension on the hypothesis that "A patient on a ward which allowed possession of more symbols of adulthood would not tend to regress as severely as a patient who was treated on a ward which allowed possession of fewer" (1966, p. 563). Data are gathered on ward policy variables such as whether patients have free access to the bedrooms, the lavatories, and the showers, how freely patients are allowed to smoke, and how significantly patients regulate the use of various items such as television, radio, telephone, books and magazines, and game tables. Also included is information about specific admission procedures, such as whether newly admitted patients are given a bath and whether they have their hair examined and their clothes or glasses and dentures stored. The exact items and scoring are given in Kellam et al. (1966).

The disturbed behavior dimension is based on questions about bizarre and aggressive behaviors. A score is derived for each ward by determining the percentage of patients on the ward during a 30-day period who exhibited each of a number of different types of behaviors. The "bizarre" behaviors include incontinence, smearing feces, talking to voices, lying or sitting on the floor, collecting or hoarding trash, and having to be dressed, fed, or bathed by the staff. The "aggressive" behaviors include damaging or destroying property, being assaultive to other patients, and attempting suicide.

Information on these WIF variables was obtained for 143 of the 160 wards in the American normative sample and for the 36 wards in the British sample. The intercorrelations among the four WIF variables were generally low, except for significant negative relationships between ward size and staff–patient ratio, indicating that large wards are more poorly staffed.

SIZE AND STAFF—PATIENT RATIO

Correlations were computed between the 10 WAS subscale means and the WIF dimensions over the 143 American and the 36 British wards, separately for patients and staff. The results for size and staff–patient ratio appear in Tables 6.1 and 6.2. The data of Table 6.1 suggest that the greater the number of patients on a ward, the less emphasis patients see on the Relationship dimensions of Support and Spontaneity and the more emphasis they see on Staff Control. As the staff–patient ratio increases, patients perceive more emphasis on Support and Spontaneity and less on Staff Control. These findings are virtually identical in the American and British samples. The correlations are of moderate magnitude, indicating that size and staffing have limited relationships to perceived treatment environments. In addition, several of the treatment environment dimensions (e.g., Involvement), all four Treatment Program dimensions, and Order and Organization and Program Clarity are essentially uncorrelated with size and staffing, at least in terms of patient perceptions.

According to Table 6.2 (results for staff), as ward size increases, staff see less emphasis on the Relationship dimensions of Support and Spontaneity and the Treatment Program dimensions of Personal Problem Orientation and Anger and Aggression, and greater emphasis on Order and Organization. The results were similar in the British sample, except that British staff did not see less emphasis on Personal Problem Orientation or Anger and Aggression on larger wards. As staff–patient ratio increases, staff find more emphasis on Support and Anger and Aggression and less on Order and Organization and Staff Control. The results for British staff are generally similar except that British staff perceive greater emphasis on Spontaneity, also, as the staff–patient ratio increases.

Thus certain dimensions of treatment environment are more highly related to size and staffing than others. The Relationship dimensions of

TABLE 6.1 CORRELATIONS BETWEEN PATIENT WAS SUBSCALE MEANS AND SIZE AND STAFF—PATIENT RATIO

WAS Subscales	N = 143 American Wards		N = 36 British Wards	
	Number of Patients	Staff–Patient Ratio	Number of Patients	Staff–Patient Ratio
Involvement	−.04	.04	.04	.07
Support	−.25**	.30**	−.21	.26
Spontaneity	−.33**	.25**	−.49**	.51**
Autonomy	−.06	−.04	−.25	−.16
Practical Orientation	.00	.14	−.13	.08
Personal Problem Orientation	−.13	.05	−.19	.30
Anger and Aggression	−.16*	.06	−.02	.16
Order and Organization	.05	.02	.05	−.10
Program Clarity	.00	.10	−.09	.05
Staff Control	.48**	−.45**	.36*	−.39*

* $p < .05$.

** $p < .01$.

TABLE 6.2 CORRELATIONS BETWEEN STAFF WAS SUBSCALE MEANS AND SIZE AND STAFF—PATIENT RATIO

WAS Subscales	N = 143 American Wards		N = 36 British Wards	
	Number of Patients	Staff–Patient Ratio	Number of Patients	Staff–Patient Ratio
Involvement	−.02	.00	−.17	.23
Support	−.21**	.28**	−.34*	.42**
Spontaneity	−.27**	.13	−.26	.48**
Autonomy	−.12	−.10	−.28	.10
Practical Orientation	.07	.00	−.23	.26
Personal Problem Orientation	−.22**	.09	−.09	.30
Anger and Aggression	−.32**	.23**	−.12	.37*
Order and Organization	.31**	−.17*	.29	−.26
Program Clarity	.00	.10	.02	.05
Staff Control	.09	−.28**	−.09	−.16

* $p < .05$.

** $p < .01$.

Support and Spontaneity are consistently negatively related to ward size and consistently positively related to staff–patient ratio for both patient and staff perceptions in both American and British samples. As size increases and/or staff–patient ratio decreases, there are decreases in the encouragement of patients to be helpful and supportive toward other patients and in the supportiveness of staff to patients. Moreover, patients are less strongly encouraged to act openly and to freely express their feelings. Both American and British patients, but not staff, feel that staff use more measures to keep them under necessary controls on large and/or more poorly staffed wards.

The actual magnitude of the differences between large and small wards is between 1 and 2 mean raw score points, indicating that there are important differences related to size but that the differences are of moderate magnitude. These results are quite consistent with those we obtained in our earlier subsample of 55 VA wards (Moos, 1972). Size and staffing were uncorrelated in this initial study, but the actual magnitudes of the relationships between size and staffing and treatment climate were somewhat larger than those reported here.

Specific items to which patients and staff on larger wards answered true significantly ($p < .01$) more often than patients and staff on smaller wards include "Doctors have very little time to encourage patients," "Patients rarely help each other," "Nurses have very little time to encourage patients," and "The staff discourage criticism." Patients and staff on large wards were more likely to answer false to the following items: "Patients are encouraged to show their feelings," "Patients can wear what they want," "Patients can leave the ward without saying where they are going," "Patients here are encouraged to be independent," and "This ward emphasizes training for new kinds of jobs."

Two additional analyses were performed on the American data. First the extent of agreement between patients and staff (as assessed by intraclass correlations between patient and staff subscale means) was correlated with size and staffing. Agreement was significantly negatively related to staff–patient ratio ($r = -.33$; $p < .01$), indicating that patient–staff consensus about the milieu is higher in programs that are more heavily staffed.

The last analysis investigated whether there was greater disagreement among patients and/or among staff in larger and more poorly staffed programs. In checking this hypothesis, the standard deviations of each of the 10 subscales were correlated with size and staffing, separately for patients and staff. Ward size was positively related to all 10 patient and all 10 staff subscale standard deviations, and in each case 6 of the correlations were statistically significant, 5 at the .01 level. Thus as program size increases there is less agreement within both the patient and the staff groups about the characteristics of the treatment milieu. However, none of the significant correlations was above .40, indicating again that the effect of size is moderate rather than substantial. Although correlations were calculated for staffing ratios, there was no relation between staffing and the extent of agreement about the treatment milieu within either the patient or the staff group.

Conceptualizing the Effects of Size and Staffing

Our results are in overall agreement with previous findings in other environments, ranging from correctional institutions such as cottages for young offenders, to educational institutions such as high schools and universities, and to business organizations. Indik (1963) and Thomas and Fink (1963) have reviewed the early literature on the effects of organization and group size. For example, accident rates, duration of absences due to accidents, and sickness rates rise as factory size increases; absence rates in hospitals rise as hospital size increases; tardiness is more frequent in larger organizations; and morale and satisfaction are significantly higher in small than in large work units (Revans, 1958; Hewitt and Parfit, 1953). Smigel (1956) found that people prefer to steal from, and are more approving of others stealing from, large, impersonal firms rather than small, cohesive organizations. Other data suggest that as size increases, the heterogeneity of the individuals in the system also increases, and personal intimacy, solidarity, and cohesion decrease. Thomas and Fink concluded that group size "has significant effects on aspects of individual and group performance, on the nature of interaction and distribution of participation of group members, on group organization, on conformity and consensus and on member satisfaction" (p. 383).

In a detailed study of high school environments, Barker and Gump (1964) found that students in small schools reported more satisfactions relating to the development of competence, to being challenged, to engaging in important actions, to being involved in group activities, and to achieving moral and cultural values than students in large schools. Wicker (1969) generalized these results to Methodist churches. Comparing one small and one large church, he found that members of the small church participated in more different kinds of activities, had more leadership positions, spent more time in activities, attended church more often, and contributed more money. He also collected archival data on 104 additional churches and learned that worship service attendance, church school attendance, women's organization membership, and women's organizations' contributions each bore a significant negative relation to church size.

Pace (1969) found more friendliness, cohesiveness, group orientation and politeness, consideration, and thoughtfulness on small than on large college campuses. Astin (1968) reported significant negative correlations between size of entering class and both classroom involvement and familiarity with the instructor. Centra (1970) identified a size–cliquishness factor characterizing small institutions in which students reported heavy involvement in campus government and campus publications, in religious activities, in vocal music groups, and in community service. Centra, Hartnett, and Peterson (1970), utilizing faculty perceptions of institutional functioning, reported significant positive relationships between size (enrollment) and the following factors: (1) human diversity (i.e., the degree to which faculty and student body are heterogeneous in their backgrounds and attitudes), (2) concern for improvement of society (i.e., a desire to apply knowledge and skills in solving social problems and prompting social change), (3) concern for advancing knowledge (i.e., the amount of emphasis placed by the institution on research and scholarship), and (4) meeting local needs (i.e., the efforts to provide educational and cultural opportunities for adults in the surrounding area). There was a significant negative relationship between size and perceived concern for undergraduate learning. However, these relationships suggest that large size may have some beneficial correlates.

Some recent work has focused on correctional institutions and psychiatric hospitals. Ullmann (1967) computed partial correlations for 30 psychiatric hospitals, relating four different measures of hospital effectiveness to size and staffing. He found that small size was significantly associated with high early release rate, even with staffing held constant, and that high staffing was significantly associated with three different measures of turnover, again with size held constant. He concluded that *both* small size and high staffing had independent demonstrable value and that each had specific effects on different measures of hospital effectiveness.

In another study, Lasky and Dowling (1971) calculated the daily maintenance costs per patient, percentage of releases, and staff–patient ratios for the 50 states and the District of Columbia over a 5-year period. Highly significant correlations appeared between maintenance costs and release rates, between maintenance costs and staff–patient ratio, and between staff–patient ratio and release rates. Higher expenditures and more staff were significantly associated with greater patient turnover. Linn (1970) studied 12 state mental hospitals and also found that both small size and high staffing were positively related to patient turnover.

Thus there is substantial evidence that size and staffing independently relate to some indices of mental hospital effectiveness, particularly patient turnover rates. However, there is relatively little information about *how* these organizational variables affect the psychosocial or treatment environment. We have much to learn, in other words, about the intermediate variables that actually affect the relevant patient behaviors. Thomas and Fink (1963) point out that many investigators implicitly assume that size itself has an immediate effect on behavior and therefore, the relevant intervening variables are almost never measured. Recently there has been more speculation about the intervening variables, however, and this issue is discussed by Linn, by Ullmann, and by Knight (1971) for correctional institutions and psychiatric hospitals, and by Barker and Gump and Indik for other types of organizations.

In one exchange of views on this point, Cohen and Struening (1964) related hospital social atmosphere types to the length of time discharged patients spent in the community, the data being adjusted for prognosis. They found that authoritarian–restrictive staff attitudes were negatively related to community tenure, whereas other types of hospital atmospheres were positively related to community tenure. Ullmann (1965) argues that these results can be "explained" by differences in size and staffing among the hospitals studied. Cohen and Struening (1965) cogently reply that size and staffing are not psychological variables that directly bear on patients and that their only importance is due to their effects on staff attitudes, which do bear directly on patients.

In an interesting corroborative study, Becker (1969) developed a staff–patient attention ratio, which was the total number of minutes per week spent in formal meetings by each staff member divided by the number of patients on the unit. Becker posited and found a positive relation between this staff–patient attention ratio and patient outcome. He felt that this ratio expressed staff–patient interaction in a much more realistic manner than the staff–patient ratio alone.

Jesness (1972) compared the parole performance of delinquent boys assigned to an intensive treatment program functioning in a 20-boy living unit with that of boys assigned to an identically staffed, less intensive program functioning in a 50-boy living unit. In an intriguing finding, he noted that boys classified as "neurotic" in the experimental program showed a parole violation rate of only 30%, versus 61% for those "neurotic" boys assigned to a larger living unit. On the other hand, the "nonneurotic" boys showed relatively similar parole violation rates in the two programs. Jesness called attention to certain variables that may have mediated the relationships between size and staffing and parole violation. For example, boys in the small unit had almost five times as much contact with staff as did boys in the large unit. The small program was described as more informal; moreover, it seemed to reflect a stronger emphasis on the use of reason and more willingness of staff to offer support. There was a greater need to assure conformity and to establish tighter limits and more stringent punishments in the larger unit. Also, staff in the larger unit tended to admire those attributes in the boys which did not interfere with program operation—lack of complaining, lack of dependency, conformity, and so on. Thus there was less emphasis on Relationship dimensions and more on System Maintenance dimensions on the larger unit.

We also found that both size and staffing were highly correlated with correctional unit social climate as perceived by residents (Moos, 1968). Larger and more poorly staffed units were seen as having less emphasis on Relationship dimensions such as Involvement, Support, and Spontaneity and Treatment Program dimensions such as Autonomy and Practical Orientation, but more emphasis on Submission (Staff Control).

These results indicate that the effects of size and staffing are very similar on psychiatric wards and in correctional units. Our data are the first directly relating size and staffing to the actual treatment environments in such institutions. Linn concluded from his study that size and staffing were negatively related to each other and that both were related to the amount of time that physicians spent on the ward, to the frequency of patient–staff interaction, and to high patient involvement in treatment programs. In a further finding relevant to the issue of mediating variables, we found (as summarized in Chapter 7, but see also Moos and Houts, 1970) that patients on wards displaying more emphasis on Support and Spontaneity and less emphasis on Staff Control are generally more satisfied and like the other patients and the staff more.

Thus the evidence indicates that increased size and/or decreased staffing has several effects: (1) it creates pressures toward a more rigid structure,

(2) it increases staff need to control and manage, (3) it decreases the degree of patient independence and responsibility and the amount of support and involvement which staff are able to give patients, (4) it leads to less spontaneous relationships among patients and between patients and staff, and (5) it results in somewhat less emphasis on understanding patients' personal problems and the open handling of their angry feelings. Knight (1971) has presented an excellent discussion of almost exactly the same effects with particular reference to inmates in correctional institutions. He concludes that large size alone creates organizational pressures toward custodial rather than treatment operations, suggesting also that the custodial atmosphere may itself help to create "unreceptive" behavior, which justifies the need for further regimentation. He fears that large size may initiate a "vicious circle" that specifically reinforces System Maintenance staff behaviors, particularly Staff Control

Conceptualizing the reasons for the effects of large size and poor staffing is important because their generally negative effects can sometimes be ameliorated by changing certain aspects of the social environment. In our sample there were examples of large, relatively well-staffed programs and small, relatively poorly staffed programs which had active coherent treatment programs. There was even one VA ward that was both large (156 patients) and relatively poorly staffed (staff–patient ratio of 1:11) but nevertheless had a positively perceived treatment milieu; that is, patients and staff agreed that there was above-average emphasis on all three Relationship and all four Treatment Program dimensions. In addition, even though size and staffing both relate significantly to certain dimensions of treatment environments, the highest correlations account for only about 25% of the variance. Some dimensions, furthermore, particularly those connected with the Treatment Program, are relatively independent of size and staffing in both our American and British samples. Detailed studies of means of counteracting the potential negative effects of large size and/or poor staffing should be valuable, especially since strong institutional pressures and increasingly stringent financial limitations and cost effectiveness analyses often make it impossible to mount small, well-staffed programs. Clinical case studies of large and/or relatively poorly staffed wards that manage to maintain cohesive treatment programs with low dropout, high release, and/or high community tenure rates would be most helpful.

The literature contains some suggestions in this regard. Ullmann has pointed out that negative effects of large hospitals may be partially alleviated by a unit system in which the hospital is functionally divided into smaller sections. In an analogous way, some very large wards may benefit from organizing patients and staff into smaller treatment teams. Porter and Lawler (1965) have hypothesized that the effects of large size in industrial organizations may be partly or wholly counteracted by designating small-sized subunits. Since patient–staff agreement is negatively related to size, and since the extent of disagreement within both the patient and the staff groups is positively related to size, the tendency toward less well developed treatment programs and greater "cultural disorganization" and misperception on large wards seems clear. In this connection Knight has emphasized the probability of "pluralistic ignorance" or shared misunderstandings that may occur on larger wards because of the reduced group cohesion and the weaker patient–staff relationships. Dividing a large treatment unit into patient–staff treatment teams or other small groups led by patient-elected or volunteer leaders might enhance communication and cohesion.

Relatively little experimental work explicitly tests specific hypotheses about how size affects attitudinal and behavioral outcomes. In one example, Indik (1965) postulated that low participation rates may not be necessary effects of increased size. Using correlations and partial correlations, he made a very intriguing comparison of four explanations linking size to member participation by way of three different sets of organizations, namely, 32 package delivery organizations, 36 automobile sales dealerships, and 28 voluntary educational–political organizations. The most strongly supported explanation was that in larger organizations there are more potential and necessary communication linkages among the members; therefore, adequate communication is less likely to be achieved, resulting in a reduced level of interpersonal attraction among members and lower member participation rates. Indik also found that organization size affects the techniques available for use in the organization in controlling member behavior. Specifically, there is less reliance on interpersonal control methods and more reliance on impersonal (i.e., bureaucratic and inflexible) forms of control. Increased size led to less personal forms of control and reduced participation rates in all three types of organizations studied; however, the relationships were not strong.

Indik concluded that organization size does not inherently determine member participation rates. He believes that this is an indirect effect serving to reveal the "impact of a social structural variable like size on the psychological environment of the organizational member and thus on member behavior" (Indik, 1965; p. 349). The author also states that the negative effects of large size can be avoided through the control of organizational processes. He suggests that the manager of a large organization could take steps to ensure high rates of internal communication, thereby facilitating interpersonal attraction and maintaining motivation to participate.

Barker's behavior setting theory suggests that large treatment units would benefit from an increased number of behavior settings in which patients and staff alike could assume roles of responsibility and authority. The theory also predicts that extremely high staffing levels on very small treatment units might have the somewhat unexpected effect of increasing staff absenteeism and decreasing the amount of responsibility of each staff member because of the relative overmanning of the available behavior settings. On the other hand, a small, highly staffed program could compensate for these effects by increasing the number of available behavior settings.

In summary, a great deal more work is required on the effects of size and staffing in program environments, especially since staffing represents by far the greatest cost in running treatment-oriented institutions. Issues of cost effectiveness and public accountability (Fox, 1968) demand very careful research in this area. Of particular importance are the specification of the variables that mediate the effects of size and staffing and the collection of specific examples and case studies of treatment units in which these effects have been minimized.

A PROGRAM POLICY DIMENSION: ADULT STATUS

To review, Kellam et al. (1966) proposed a concept of an adult status dimension as assessing the degree to which patients on wards were "allowed to maintain basic symbols of adulthood." We felt that this constituted a very basic program policy dimension, particularly since it was linked to Goffman's (1961) description of the "total institution." Many investigators have discussed a dimension of this sort, which is usually believed to discriminate between "good" and "bad" treatment institutions. King and Raynes (1968) and Wing and Brown (1970) have examined similar dimensions with their measures of inmate management and ward restrictiveness, as discussed in Chapter 1.

Adult status scores were obtained for the 143 American wards that had been utilized in the previous analysis on size and staffing. The theoretical range of scores is 0 to 100%, but the actual range obtained was only 28 to 100%. The mean score was 76%, indicating some skewness in the distribution. Nevertheless, the adult status scores were intercorrelated with patient and staff mean scores on the 10 WAS subscales. The results (Table 6.3) indicate that in programs with higher adult status patients and staff agreed in perceiving more emphasis on the Relationship dimension of Spontaneity and the Treatment Program dimensions of Autonomy, Personal Problem Orientation, and Anger and Aggression. Patients also perceived less emphasis on Staff Control in high adult status programs. The actual differences between high and low adult status programs are between 1 and 2 mean raw score points.

TABLE 6.3 CORRELATIONS BETWEEN PATIENT AND STAFF SUBSCALE MEANS AND WIF ADULT STATUS

WAS Subscales	N = 143 American Wards	
	Patients	Staff
Involvement	.14	.15
Support	.13	.12
Spontaneity	.34**	.28**
Autonomy	.23**	.29**
Practical Orientation	.06	−.08
Personal Problem Orientation	.31**	.26**
Anger and Aggression	.32**	.35**
Order and Organization	−.11	−.08
Program Clarity	−.07	.14
Staff Control	−.32**	−.12

* $P < .05$.
** $P < .01$.

These results bring out significant but moderate relationships between the program policy dimension of how much adult status staff allow patients to assume and the amount of emphasis in the treatment environment on certain dimensions. Perhaps just as important, adult status is not related to the emphasis on the Relationship dimensions of Involvement and Support, on the Treatment Program dimension of Practical Orientation, or on the System Maintenance dimensions of Order and Organization and Program Clairty. As with size and staffing, thus, there are quite specific relationships between this dimension and treatment environment.

Our earlier study on 55 VA wards (Moos, 1972) indicates that the current correlations between adult status and treatment environment may be somewhat attenuated, possibly because of the skewness in the adult status scores. In the 55 VA wards the mean adult status score was 65%, with a range of 30 to 100%. The pattern of relationships between adult status and treatment environment was essentially identical to that shown in Table 6.3, but the actual correlations were substantially higher; for example, correlations of .59 and .54 between staff-perceived Autonomy and Anger and Aggression, respectively, and adult status. On the other hand, size was negatively correlated with adult status on the 55 wards, and therefore the higher correlations may have been partly due to the effects of ward size.

In further analyses neither the extent of patient–staff agreement nor the intraward standard deviations of either patients or staff on the 10 WAS subscales was significantly correlated with adult status. Thus high adult status does not imply greater agreement between patients and staff or among patients or staff. The adult status scores on the 36 British wards were extremely skewed (more than half being greater than 90%), indicating that this dimension, as currently assessed by the WIF, does not adequately discriminate among British psychiatric programs.

It is unfortunate that systematic data were not collected on a wider range of program policy characteristics. Like size and staffing, the perceived treatment environment can be thought of as a set of mediating variables through which program policy characteristics such as adult status have specific attitudinal and behavioral effects. Systematic assessments of treatment environments in programs with varying policy characteristics can help to determine the actual effects of these policy dimensions. Some program policy changes may not in themselves have important effects on treatment environments (e.g., the addition of a ward clerk or deciding whether nurses will wear uniforms or street clothes, as discussed in Chapter 5). On the other hand, the effects of certain policy dimensions may be more important than we have supposed. These considerations indicate the need to evaluate program policy and perceived environment dimensions in further studies of the effects of hospital-based treatment programs.

A PATIENT CHARACTERISTICS DIMENSION: DISTURBED BEHAVIOR

Information was also obtained on the extent of disturbed behavior of the patients on the 143 American wards. This score was derived from an estimate of the number of patients who exhibited a variety of "sick" behaviors during the 30-day period prior to the administration of the WAS. The correlation between the bizarre behavior items (incontinence, smearing feces, talking to voices, etc.) and such aggressive behavior items as assaultiveness was substantial; thus the different indices were combined into one disturbed behavior score (see Kellam et al., 1966). Intercorrelations were calculated between patient and staff WAS subscale means and this disturbed behavior score over the 143 wards. The results (Table 6.4) indicate that patients and staff agree in perceiving less emphasis on the Treatment Program dimensions of Autonomy, Personal Problem Orientation, and Anger and Aggression on high disturbed behavior wards; in addition, staff perceive less emphasis on the System Maintenance dimensions of Program Clarity and Staff Control on the high disturbed wards. These findings are generally consistent with those obtained in our earlier subsample of 55 VA wards (Moos, 1972). The magnitude of the differences between low and high disturbed behavior wards was between 1 and 2 mean raw score points.

TABLE 6.4 CORRELATIONS BETWEEN PATIENT AND STAFF SUBSCALE MEANS AND PATIENT DISTURBED BEHAVIOR

WAS Subscales	WIF Disturbed Behavior $N = 143$ American Wards		Behavior Incidents $N = 23$ State Hospital Wards	
	Patients	Staff	Patients	Staff
Involvement	−.11	−.12	−.61**	−.36
Support	.14	.00	−.21	−.07
Spontaneity	−.06	−.02	−.29	−.39
Autonomy	−.31**	−.26**	−.23	−.18
Practical Orientation	−.09	−.07	−.53**	−.45*
Personal Problem Orientation	−.20*	−.28**	−.31	−.23
Anger and Aggression	−.28**	−.23**	−.10	−.19
Order and Organization	.02	.13	−.33	−.42*
Program Clarity	−.06	−.32**	.01	−.36
Staff Control	−.07	−.20*	.12	.11

* $p<.05.$
** $p<.01.$

Disturbed behavior was unrelated to the degree of patient–staff agreement or the degree of agreement within either the patient group or the staff group. There was a highly skewed distribution of disturbed behavior scores on the 36 British wards, implying that the specific incidents included do not adequately discriminate among these programs. In this connection it should be noted that the range of disturbed behavior scores in the 143 American wards was extremely wide, varying from 0 (no disturbed behavior occurring in the past 30 days in any of the nine categories) to many wards having scores exceeding 100%, indicating an average of at least one disturbed behavior incident per patient.

In our study on 23 wards in one state hospital (described in greater detail in Chapter 7), the actual number of behavior incidents was tabulated for each ward over a 4-month interval during which the WAS was also administered to both patients and staff. There was a heavy preponderance of aggressive and assaultive behavior incidents rather than of bizarre behavior, in distinction to the usual situation on most of the other psychiatric wards we studied. Correlations were calculated between the average number of behavior incidents for each ward and the patient and staff perceptions of the ward's treatment milieu. The results appearing in Table 6.4 indicate that patients saw lower emphasis on Involvement and Practical Orientation on wards that had more behavior incidents, and staff saw lower emphasis on the Relationship dimensions of Involvement and Spontaneity, the Treatment Program dimension of Practical Orientation, and the System Maintenance dimensions of Order and Organization and Program Clarity on these wards. The relationships occurred even though the number of behavior incidents was basically uncorrelated with size and staffing.

Thus moderate to substantial relationships exist between average patient behavioral characteristics (i.e., disturbed behavior, behavior incidents) and treatment environment. These relationships are generally in the predicted direction in that there is less emphasis on the Relationship and Treatment Program dimensions on wards where patients engage in more disturbed and/or aggressive behavior. Although there was an overall consistency in the results, there were some important differences in the magnitude of the relationships in our two samples. Such discrepancies are probably attributable to the special nature of the study using all 23 wards in one hospital that had more assaultive and aggressive patients rather than psychotically disturbed patients.

Relationships between the average personal and behavioral characteristics of milieu inhabitants and perceived organizational climate have been most extensively studied in colleges and universities. The results suggest that these two sets of variables are moderately but not substantially related. For example, Pace (1969) presents a large number of correlations between CUES and average student characteristics such as recollections of career plans as freshmen, career plans as seniors, major field of studies in college, plans to attend graduate school, self-ratings of political and religious preferences, and various types of values about college. Reported correlations, which vary between .30 and .60, support the conclusion that the characteristics of students are generally congruent with the characteristics of the school they attend. For example, there are positive relationships between the scholastic aptitude of the entering freshmen and the Scholarship scale score of the college, between the esthetic interests of the entering students and the Awareness scale score of the college, and between the religious interests of students and the Propriety and Community scale scores of a college. Illustratively, planning to enter graduate school is related negatively to the Practicality, Community, and Propriety scores and positively to the Scholarship score. Thus there is some evidence that students select (or are selected by) colleges whose social environments are appropriate for them. Generally corroborative evidence is found in the work of Astin (1968) and Centra (1970). Each of these authors, however, also concludes that measures of perceived environments identify at least some unique characteristics differentiating among colleges and universities. Similar work relating perceived treatment environments to various average behavioral characteristics of patients and/or staff on psychiatric wards has yet to be carried out, although Ellsworth and Maroney (1972) have related average patient perception of ward scores to patients' mean age and chronicity.

EFFECTS ON IDEAL WARD CONCEPTUALIZATIONS

An issue that has not been systematically investigated in any of the environments for which perceived organizational climate scales have been derived involves the relations between structural and organizational characteristics and value systems about preferred or ideal environments. Clinical evidence presented in Chapter 4 indicates that staff values about an ideal treatment milieu may change and become more consonant with the actual treatment milieu. Other studies have also revealed substantial changes of individual values and attitudes as a function of individual experiences in different environments. Most of this work has been done in colleges and universities (see particularly Sanford, 1962; Feldman and Newcomb, 1970). Thus there is every reason to believe that the values of patients and staff might differ as a function of their experiences in programs with different treatment environments.

We were fortunate to obtain some data bearing on this issue in our intensive 23-ward state hospital study, since all patients and staff involved filled out Form I of the WAS. Ward size was not related to either patient or staff ideal ward conceptualizations. However, patients on more poorly staffed wards ideally wanted significantly ($p < .05$) less emphasis on the Relationship dimensions of Involvement and Support and on the System Maintenance dimensions of Order and Organization and Program Clarity. In addition, ($p < .01$) they ideally wanted less Spontaneity, Autonomy, Practical Orientation, and Personal Problem Orientation and more Staff Control than patients who were on more highly staffed wards. Thus the staff–patient ratio has substantial effects on the way in which patients imagine ideal wards. This assumes that patients were not self-selected into wards of different staffing on the basis of their real treatment environment conceptualizations, which is reasonable although unproven.

There were no significant relationships between staff–patient ratio and the 10 WAS Form I means for staff. In addition, no relationships existed between adult status or disturbed behavior (as measured by the WIF) and patient or staff ideal ward conceptualizations. There were, however, some very intriguing relationships between these notions and the actual number of behavior incidents on the ward. Behavior incidents were unrelated to patient views of ideal wards, but they were highly related to those of staff, particularly in relation to four subscales. Staff functioning on wards with a high number of behavior incidents ideally wanted much less emphasis on the Relationship dimension of Spontaneity and on the Treatment Program dimensions of Autonomy and Practical Orientation, but they wanted much more emphasis on Staff Control. Since it is unlikely that staff were differentially selected for these wards on the basis of their values about ideal treatment environments, their exposure to a ward in which patients engage in certain types of behaviors seems to have had an important impact on their treatment environment preferences.

One last finding is relevant here. One way of punishing program patients who engaged in assaultive behavior was to put them in seclusion. We obtained information on the total number of patients in seclusion and on the average number of days in seclusion per patient. We assumed that this average reflected the general severity of ward policies; however, it was totally unrelated to either patient or staff real ward perception. It was also unrelated to staff views of ideal wards, but it was positively ($p < .05$) correlated with patient preferences for emphasis on Involvement, Support, and Program Clarity. Thus when ward policy is more severe, patients react by wanting more staff support and involvement and greater clarity regarding program policies and procedures.

The data indicate that the staff–patient ratio may have an important effect on patients' values about ideal wards and that patient behavior may significantly affect staff values about ideal wards. Thus staff behavior has an effect on patient views of ideal wards, whereas patient behavior has an effect on staff views of ideal wards. These preliminary results, which require replication, are nevertheless quite intriguing, especially because they are related to important issues such as the changing kinds of treatment environments that are likely to be maximally satisfying for patients and staff with differing prior experiences on other wards.

REFERENCES

Astin, A. W. An empirical characterization of higher educational institutions. *Journal of Educational Psychology*, **53**: 224–235, 1962.

Astin, A. W. *The college environment*. American Council on Education, Washington, D.C., 1968.

Astin, A. W. & Holland, J. L. The environmental assessment technique: A way to measure college environments. *Journal of Educational Psychology*, **52**: 308–315, 1961.

Barker, R. G. & Gump, P. V. *Big school, small school*. Stanford University Press, Stanford, Calif., 1964.

Becker, R. E. Staffing level and treatment effectiveness. *British Journal of Psychiatry*, **115**: 481–482, 1969.

Centra, J. Development of the Questionnaire on Student and College Characteristics. Research Memorandum 68–11. Educational Testing Service, Princeton, N.J., 1968.

Centra, J. The college environment revisited: Current descriptions and a comparison of three methods of assessment. Research Memorandum 70–44. Educational Testing Service, Princeton, N.J., 1970.

Centra, J., Hartnett, R., & Peterson, R. Faculty views of institutional functioning: A new measure of college environments. *Educational and Psychological Measurement*, **30**: 405–416, 1970.

Cohen, J. & Struening, E. Opinions about mental illness: Hospital social atmosphere profiles and their relevance to effectiveness. *Journal of Consulting Psychology*, **28**: 291–298, 1964.

Cohen, J. & Struening, E. Simple-minded questions and twirling stools. *Journal of*

Consulting Psychology, **29**: 278–289, 1965.

Creager, J. & Astin, A. Alternative methods of describing characteristics of colleges and universities. *Educational and Psychological Measurement*, **28**: 719–734, 1968.

Ellsworth, R. B. & Maroney, R. Characteristics of psychiatric programs and their effects on patients' adjustment. *Journal of Consulting and Clinical Psychology*, **39**: 436–447, 1972.

Feldman, K. A. & Newcomb, T. M. *The impact of college on students*, Vol. 1. Jossey-Bass, San Francisco, 1970.

Fox, P. D. Cost-effectiveness of mental health: An evaluation of an experimental rehabilitation program. Doctoral dissertation, Stanford University, Stanford, Calif., 1968.

Goffman, E. The moral career of the mental patient. In *Asylums*, Doubleday, Garden City, N.Y., 1961.

Hewitt, D. & Parfit, J. A note on working morale and size of group. *Occupational Psychology*, **27**: 38–42, 1953.

Indik, B. P. Some effects of organization size on member attitudes and behavior. *Human Relations*, **16**: 369–384, 1963.

Indik, B. P. Organization size and member participation. *Human Relations*, **18**: 339–350, 1965.

Jesness, C. J. Comparative effectiveness of two institutional treatment programs for delinquents. *Child Care Quarterly*, **1**: 119–130, 1972.

Kellam, S. G., Shmelzer, J., & Berman, A. Variation in the atmospheres of psychiatric wards. *Archives of General Psychiatry*, **14**: 561–570, 1966.

King, R. D. & Raynes, N. V. An operational measure of inmate management in residential institutions. *Social Science and Medicine*, **2**: 41–53, 1968.

Knight, D. The impact of living-unit size in youth training schools. Unpublished manuscript. California Youth Authority, Division of Research and Development, Sacramento, 1971.

Lasky, D. I. & Dowling, M. The release rates of state mental hospitals as related to maintenance costs and patient–staff ratio. *Journal of Clinical Psychology*, **27**: 272–277, 1971.

Linn, L. S. State hospital environment and rates of patient discharge. *Archives of General Psychiatry*, **23**: 346–351, 1970.

Linton, R. *The cultural background of personality*. Century, New York, 1945.

March, J. (Ed.). *Handbook of organizations*. Rand-McNally, Chicago, 1965.

Moos, R. The assessment of the social climates of correctional institutions. *Journal of Research in Crime and Delinquency*, **5**: 174–188, 1968.

Moos, R. Size, staffing and psychiatric ward treatment environments. *Archives of General Psychiatry*, **26**: 414–418, 1972.

Moos, R. & Houts, P. Differential effects of the social atmospheres of psychiatric wards. *Human Relations*, **23**: 47–60, 1970.

Pace, R. *College and University Environment Scale*, Technical manual, 2nd ed., Educational Testing Service, Princeton, N.J., 1969.

Peterson, R., Centra, J., Hartnett, R. & Linn, R. *Institutional Functioning Inventory:* Preliminary technical manual. Educational Testing Service, Princeton, N.J., 1970.

Porter, L. W. & Lawler, E. E. Properties of organization structure in relation to job attitudes and job behavior. *Psychological Bulletin*, **64**: 23–51, 1965.

Revans, R. W. Human relations, management and size. In Hugh-Jones, E. M. (Ed.). *Human relations and modern management*, North Holland, Amsterdam, 1958, pp. 177–220.

Sanford, N. Higher education as a field of study. In Sanford, N. (Ed.). *The American college: A psychological and social interpretation of the higher learning.* Wiley, New York, 1962, pp. 31–73.

Sells, S. Dimensions of stimulus situations which account for behavior variance. In Sells, S. (Ed.). *Stimulus determinants of behavior.* Ronald Press, New York, 1963, pp. 1–15.

Smigel, E. O. Public attitudes toward stealing as related to the size of the victim organization. *American Sociological Review*, **21**: 320–327, 1956.

Stern, G. *People in context: Measuring person environment congruence in education and industry.* Wiley, New York, 1970.

Thomas, E. H. & Fink, C. F. Effects of group size. *Psychological Bulletin*, **60**: 371–384, 1963.

Ullmann, L. P. A discussion of hospital social atmosphere profiles and their relevance to effectiveness. *Journal of Consulting Psychology*, **29**: 277–278, 1965.

Ullmann, L. P. *Institution and outcome: A comparative study of psychiatric hospitals.* Pergamon Press, Oxford, 1967.

Walberg, H. J. Class size and the social environment of learning. *Human Relations*, **22**: 465–475, 1969.

Wing, J. & Brown, G. *Institutionalism and schizophrenia*, Cambridge University Press, Cambridge, 1970.

Wicker, A. W. Size of church membership and members' support of church behavior settings. *Journal of Personality and Social Psychology*, **12**: 278–288, 1969.

Chapter Seven

THE EFFECTS OF TREATMENT ENVIRONMENTS: MORALE, SELF–ESTEEM, AND COPING BEHAVIOR

INTRODUCTION AND THEORETICAL RATIONALE

In our conceptualization, social environments are active and directed with respect to their inhabitants. People have plans or personal agendas that impel their behavior in specific directions. Environments have programs that organize and shape the behavior of their inhabitants. A number of dimensions differentiating among physical and social environments have important consequences for individual behavior, as discussed in Chapter 1. The studies reported here and in Chapter 8 assessed the differential effects of the treatment environments of psychiatric programs. This chapter deals with the effects of the treatment environments on morale, personal development, initiatives, and styles of helping behavior.

The particular pattern of press in an environment creates a group atmosphere or social climate which, as Lewin (1951a) has pointed out, needs to be thought of as having demonstrable effects. For example, Lewin showed that the aggressive behavior of two girls tended to change commensurate with the social atmosphere of the group. After transferring from one group to another, each girl rapidly displayed the level of conduct that had characterized the other girl's behavior before the change (1951a, p. 212). Lewin theorized that individual members of a group tend to fall in line with the norms of that group. Thus an individual in a group that inhibits the expression of aggression will tend to express little aggression, whereas the same individual in a group that facilitates the expression of aggression will tend to express a high amount of aggression.

Lewin, Lippitt, and White (1939) and Lippitt and White (1943) have reported that different group climates affect group behavior on variables such as spontaneity, the number of friendly remarks made by group members to one another, the degree to which normal sociability is inhibited, and the general amount of satisfaction or dissatisfaction within the group. The theory is that social climates have effects on individual behavior by creating "induced forces" and possibly new needs, which in turn impel behavior in particular directions that are shaped by these social climates (Lewin, 1951b).

Our research followed this logic. We hypothesized that patients in climates emphasizing high staff–patient and patient–patient interaction (Involvement, Support), patient independence (Autonomy), and freedom of emotional expression and understanding each individual's problems (Spontaneity, Personal Problem Orientation) would be more satisfied, would like one another and the staff more, and would feel that the program was having a greater impact on their personal development. Thus the prediction was that the Relationship and the Treatment Program dimensions would correlate positively with "positive" patient reactions. No specific predictions were made for the System Maintenance dimensions of Order and Organization or Program Clarity, although the expectation was that they would also relate positively to patient satisfaction and personal development. Finally, it was proposed that Staff Control would relate negatively to patient satisfaction and personal development. It was also predicted that different treatment environments would differentially facilitate specific initiatives and coping styles.

AN INITIAL STUDY ON EIGHT PROGRAMS

Three extensive studies were completed in the area of treatment environments just described. In the first study a sample of eight programs was composed of four VA hospital wards of relatively acute patients (three all-male wards and the other male and female) and four state hospital wards (two located in one hospital and two in another; two that were regionalized and two that were not). Three of the state hospital wards were male and one was female. Each of the two regionalized wards had a wide variety of patients who were on the ward because of their geographical area of origin rather than because of their particular symptoms. Of the other two wards, one was mainly for the treatment of alcoholic patients and the other, which had a representative variety of patients, was a moderately intensive acute treatment service. The mean age of the patients on the eight wards ranged from 32 to 50, and their median length of stay was from 2 to 39 weeks. The wards themselves varied in size from 10 to 80 and in patient–staff ratio from 3.8 to 13.5 patients per staff member. The eight wards were generally representative of the programs in the three hospitals studied.

Three questionnaires were given to patients. The first questionnaire was the WAS. The second questionnaire, designed to measure patient morale and general reactions to the ward, consisted of six questions asking patients to rate their general satisfaction with the ward (6-point scale), how much they liked the patients and staff on the ward, how anxious they felt while on the ward, and the extent to which they felt that their experiences on the ward had given them a chance to test their abilities and to increase their self-confidence (5-point scales). The third questionnaire was the Ward Initiative Scale (WIS), discussed below.

Styles of Coping Behavior

The WIS was originally developed by Houts and Moos (1969) to measure the initiatives taken by patients on psychiatric wards. Psychiatric treatment programs attempt to facilitate or inhibit specific initiatives through the treatment environment they create. It thus seemed important to develop methods of assessing patient initiatives in response to different programs.

An initial 217-item questionnaire was given to 246 patients on 11 heterogeneous psychiatric wards. All items especially confusing to less educated and chronic patients were discarded, as were all items that correlated positively with the Crowne-Marlowe Social Desirability Scale. The remaining 98 items were subjected to one-way analysis of variance to determine the degree to which they differentiated among the 11 wards. There were 70 items discriminating at the $p < .20$ level, and these were sorted into eight categories based on similar content and similarity to the WAS subscales, plus a miscellaneous category that was later discarded. Two of the subscales were dropped in subsequent analyses because of low internal consistency and/or low test–retest reliability.

The remaining five subscales were labeled as follows: Affiliation with Patients, Autonomy toward the Staff, Revealing Self to Others, Aggression, and Submission to the Staff. The item scores were summed into five subscale scores, and one-way analyses of variance were repeated for each of the subscale scores, which all discriminated significantly ($p < .05$) among the wards. An additional subscale intended to measure social desirability responses was constructed from items that correlated significantly with the Crowne-Marlowe Social Desirability Scale. Nine items were selected on the basis of high correlations with and similar content to the Crowne-Marlowe. Additional information about the development of the WIS, test–retest reliability, and correlates of the subscales with patient background variables is supplied in the paper by Houts and Moos (1969).

The items in the WIS are indicative of concrete initiatives that can be taken by patients on wards. For example, intiatives in the area of Affiliation with Patients are inferred from items such as "I try to become friends with the other patients on the ward," "I try to find out about new people who come onto the ward," and "If I am interested in a conversation I will join in and give my opinions." Initiatives in the area of Autonomy toward the Staff are inferred from the following items: "I ask my doctor if he thinks I am getting better," "I tell my doctor what I want him to do for me," and "I try to make clear to the staff that I have special problems." Initiatives in the area of Revealing Self to Others are inferred from the following items: "I try to share my personal problems with patients" and "I tell the staff about my feelings." Finally, initiatives in the area of Submission to the Staff are inferred from such items as "I try to talk about things that the staff thinks are important" and "I do things that the staff ask me to do even if I don't like to."

Patient Morale and Personal Development

The total sample on the eight wards was composed of 186 patients. The first two tests were scored for each patient and the following scores were obtained for further analyses: (1) 10 subscale scores for the 10 WAS dimensions and (2) 6 scores on the items measuring general satisfaction and personal development variables. Ward means were obtained for each of these 16 scores.

One-way analyses of variance (between-ward variations versus within-ward variations) indicated that all 10 WAS subscale scores differentiated significantly ($p < .05$) among the wards. Since, however, the average ward scores on the three Relationship dimensions were significantly intercor-related, the Support and Spontaneity subscales were dropped from further analyses. The six general satisfaction and personal development variables were also intercorrelated across wards. General satisfaction and liking for patients were highly intercorrelated, as were the questions about whether patients could test their abilities and increase their self-confidence. Thus these two sets of variables were each combined into one.

TABLE 7.1   RANK–ORDER CORRELATIONS OVER WARDS ($N = 8$) BETWEEN WAS SUBSCALES AND PATIENT REACTIONS

WAS Subscale	General Satisfaction	Liking for Staff	Anxiety	Personal Development
Involvement	.79**	.67**	−.07	.66*
Autonomy	.70**	.58*	.40	.36
Practical Orientation	.77**	.56	−.09	.35
Personal Problem Orientation	.82***	.76**	.43	.21
Anger and Aggression	−.27	−.12	.64*	−.31
Order and Organization	.67**	.52	−.35	.34
Program Clarity	.51	.55	.63*	.14
Staff Control	−.49	−.52	−.22	−.42

* $p < .10$.
** $p < .05$.
*** $p < .01$.

Rank-order correlations were calculated across wards between the WAS subscale scores and the general satisfaction and personal development variables. The results (Table 7.1) indicate the following tendencies. (a) Involvement, Autonomy, Practical Orientation, Personal Problem Orientation, and Order and Organization were each positively correlated with general satisfaction. Program Clarity and Staff Control were positively and negatively correlated with this variable, respectively, although the correlation was not significant. Essentially the same pattern of relationships was found between the WAS subscales and the extent of patient liking for staff. (b) Involvement was positively correlated with the extent to which patients felt that what they were doing on the ward enhanced their abilities and their self-confidence. Several other subscales were also positively related to these variables (e.g., Autonomy, Practical Orientation, and Order and Organization, although none of these relationships was statistically significant). (c) Both Anger and Aggression and Program Clarity were positively correlated with anixety. Autonomy and Personal Problem Orientation were positively but not significantly correlated with anxiety.

These results suggest that each of the Relationship and Treatment Program dimensions (excluding Anger and Aggression) and the System Maintenance dimension of Order and Organization is highly related to patient general satisfaction (which in turn is closely connected to the patients' liking for one another) and patient liking for staff. These dimensions are also related to the degree to which patients feel that they can test their abilities and enhance their self-confidence in the program, although the relationships are somewhat less salient. Emphases on the expression of Anger and Aggression and, rather surprisingly, on an active, clear treatment program, are related to greater patient anxiety.

Patient Initiatives

Next correlations were calculated to determine the relationships between the WAS subscales and the WIS subscales. When the five WIS subscales were intercorrelated, significant correlations were noted between the Affiliation and Autonomy subscales; thus the Autonomy subscale was dropped from further analyses.

TABLE 7.2   RANK–ORDER CORRELATIONS OVER WARDS ($N = 8$) BETWEEN WAS AND WIS SUBSCALES

WAS Subscales	Affiliation	Self-Revealing	Aggression	Submission
Involvement	−.09	.31	.60	−.66*
Autonomy	−.30	.17	.33	−.68**
Practical Orientation	−.30	−.25	−.16	−.09
Personal Problem Orientation	−.10	.31	.60*	−.66*
Anger and Aggression	−.79**	.14	.74**	−.49
Order and Organization	.61*	−.32	−.19	.15
Program Clarity	−.55	.61*	.46	−.89***
Staff Control	−.05	.05	−.16	.10

* $p<.10$.
** $p<.05$.
*** $p<.01$.

From Table 7.2 which presents the correlations over wards ($N = 8$) between the WAS and the WIS scores, we can note the following points.

(1) Patients on wards that have more emphasis on Involvement and/or

Personal Problem Orientation see themselves as taking more Aggression and fewer Submission initiatives.

(2) Patients on wards that have high emphasis on Autonomy see themselves as taking fewer Submission initiatives.

(3) Patients on wards that have high emphasis on Anger and Aggression see themselves as taking more Aggression and fewer Affiliation initiatives.

(4) Patients on wards that emphasize Order and Organization see themselves as taking more Affiliation initiatives.

(5) Patients on wards with more emphasis on Program Clarity see themselves as taking more Self-Revealing but fewer Affiliation and Submission initiatives.

Thus it appears that patients on wards with varying treatment environments perceive themselves as taking quite different types of initiatives in order to cope with the particular milieu of the ward. High emphasis on Involvement and/or Personal Problem Orientation is associated (a) with high patient levels of general satisfaction and patient liking for one another and for staff and (b) with more initiatives in expressing anger and aggression and fewer initiatives in expressing submission to staff. The results also clarify the reason for the positive relationship between the emphasis on Anger and Aggression and Program Clarity and patient anxiety. More emphasis on Aggression is related to fewer initiatives in expressing affiliation. More emphasis on Program Clarity relates to more initiatives in being self-revealing, but again fewer affiliation initiatives. Thus as Aggression and Program Clarity increase, the amount of support (in terms of affiliation initiatives) decreases, producing an increase in patient anxiety. In these wards, the WAS dimension of Program Clarity was also related to an active, directed attempt to motivate patients to "get moving" and get out of the hospital, thereby raising their anxiety.

To estimate how much the tendency to answer items in socially desirable directions might have mediated the relationships among the three tests, correlations were calculated across the eight wards between the social desirability subscale of the WIS and all the other variables. Partial correlations were also calculated for all significant results in Table 7.2. These partial correlations were very similar to the initial correlations, indicating that the foregoing results were not primarily mediated by social desirability, especially since none of the WAS subscales was itself significantly correlated with social desirability (see Moos and Houts, 1970).

A REPLICATION STUDY ON 23 PROGRAMS

Our initial study presented some intriguing findings. Different social climates indeed have differential effects on the people who live and function within them. The importance of these effects, particularly on patient morale, indicated that a replication study was desirable. In addition, since the original eight wards were located in three different hospitals, there was a confounding of interward and interhospital differences. Thus an attempt was made at replicating the relationships by studying 23 different programs in one state hospital. It was felt that this design would allow for the further control of extraneous variables.

Setting and Subjects

The state hospital chosen was a particularly suitable institution for a study of this type, since it provided for the care and treatment of male patients committed directly from the courts. The population was about evenly divided between those patients committed as "sex offenders" and those committed as "criminally insane." The typical patient had a history of criminal activity prior to hospital commitment. His behavioral problems were often directly related to physical or social deprivation and frequently included alcoholism and drug addiction. His maladjustment was often characterized by aggressive behavior, long periods of depression, hallucinatory experiences, paranoid ideation, and/or episodic periods of intellectual and emotional confusion.

Most patients were committed after they had been tried and found guilty of various antisocial acts. Some patients were legally committed to the hospital for an indeterminant period, which averaged about 16 months. The trials of other patients had ended with a verdict of not guilty on the grounds of insanity. These patients were treated until the staff determined that they could be returned to court, no longer mentally ill. Finally, certain patients had been accused of a crime, but no determination of their guilt or innocence had been made because they were judged unable to stand trial. After treatment, such patients are returned to court for completion of criminal proceedings.

This is clearly a somewhat unusual hospital, and in one sense the results may be less generalizable to other hospitals. In another sense, however, the setting was unique and particularly favorable in that there was almost total cooperation from the entire hospital; moreover, the patient population on the 23 wards constituted a relatively homogeneous group, at least as contrasted with the variety of patients to be found in other state hospitals. The wards were all of moderate to large size, varying from a low of 40 to a high of 90 patients. The patient–staff ratio showed somewhat more variation than ward size, ranging from a low of 3.1 patients per staff member to a high of 19.0 patients per staff member.

Cooperation in this study was excellent: more than 80% of the available patients on the 23 wards completed three different questionnaires within less than 10 days. The tests were administered by way of a hospital closed-circuit television system, patients staying on their wards and answering the questions on IBM sheets. In addition to being efficient, this procedure assured minimal discussion and comparison of the different questionnaires during the actual process of data collection. The three questionnaires were the WAS, the six morale questions and the WIS. A total of 978 patients adequately completed all the questionaires.

Patient Morale and Personal Development

One-way analyses of variance for patients indicated that all WAS subscales significantly differentiated among the 23 wards; again, however, significant positive correlations over wards occurred among the three Relationship variables. Intercorrelations over wards among the satisfaction and personal development variables were also similar to those found in the previous study, and thus the same sets of variables were combined in further analyses.

Intercorrelations over wards ($N = 23$) were calculated between the WAS subscales and patient reactions to the ward. Table 7.3, which shows these correlations. allows us to make several observations. (a) The Relationship dimension of Involvement and the Treatment Program dimensions of Autonomy, Practical Orientation, and Personal Problem Orientation were positively related to general satisfaction, patient liking for staff, and the extent to which patients felt they could enhance their personal development. (b) The System Maintenance dimensions of Order and Organization and Program Clarity were positively related to general satisfaction and patient liking for staff, whereas Staff Control was negatively related to both these variables. Order and Organization was also positively related to personal development, whereas Staff Control bore a negative relation to this variable. (c) The only significant relationship between the WAS subscales and anxiety was a negative correlation with Program Clarity; that is, as Program Clarity increased, anxiety decreased.

TABLE 7.3   CORRELATIONS OVER WARDS (N = 23) BETWEEN WAS SUBSCALES AND PATIENT REACTIONS

WAS Subscales	General Satisfaction	Liking for Staff	Anxiety	Personal Development
Involvement	.77***	.52***	.06	.71***
Autonomy	.45**	.46**	−.13	.37*
Practical Orientation	.48***	.26	.12	.55***
Personal Problem Orientation	.75***	.65***	−.01	.65***
Anger and Aggression	.28	.39*	−.27	.21
Order and Organization	.70***	.33*	−.05	.47**
Program Clarity	.58***	.33*	−.42**	.27
Staff Control	−.62***	−.73***	.29	−.49**

* $p < .10.$
** $p < .05.$
*** $p < .01.$

Since a fairly large number of patients occupied each of the 23 wards, a further analysis was feasible. One possible explanation of the results relating treatment environments to patient reactions is that individual response tendencies such as positive or negative halo mediate the correlations between the two tests, which were taken by the same individuals. To control for these influences, we randomly divided the patients in each ward into two equal samples, by putting patients who had odd subject numbers into one sample and patients who had even subject numbers into the other. New means were calculated for the WAS subscales and the patient morale questions for each of the two samples of patients on each of the 23 wards. Correlations over wards ($N=23$) between the WAS subscales and the patient morale questions were then calculated separately for the two random samples. One set of correlations was calculated between the WAS subscale means of the odd-numbered patient sample and the patient morale results of the even-numbered sample, and the other set was calculated between the even-numbered patients' WAS subscale means and the odd-numbered patients' morale results. These correlations could not be mediated by individual response set tendencies.

The results were almost identical to those previously obtained. In Table 7.3 there are 21 significant correlations between WAS subscales and patient morale questions. Of these 21 relationships, 15 showed significant correlations in *both* the odd and even pairs of the split sample. Four of the 21 relationships were replicated in only one of the two split samples, although revealing correlations that were in the same direction but not quite significant in the other sample. Only two of the significant correlations in Table 7.3 (those between Order and Organization and liking for staff, and Program Clarity and Anxiety) were not replicated to a statistically significant degree in either of the two split samples.

Thus these results strongly substantiate the conclusion that important relationships exist between program treatment environment and patients' morale and general reactions. As a rule, patients are more satisfied, like the staff and one another more, and feel that they can enhance their personal development better in programs emphasizing Involvement, Autonomy, Practical Orientation, Personal Problem Orientation, and Order and Organization. Patients feel less satisfied, like the staff less, and feel less able to enhance their abilities in programs strongly emphasizing Staff Control.

TABLE 7.4   CORRELATIONS OVER WARDS (N = 23) BETWEEN WAS AND WIS SUBSCALES

WAS Subscales	WIS Subscales			
	Affiliation	Self-Revealing	Aggression	Submission
Involvement	.46**	.48***	.38*	−.37*
Autonomy	.06	.15	.26	−.41**
Practical Orientation	.53***	.43**	.23	−.08
Personal Problem Orientation	.38*	.51***	.22	−.23
Anger and Aggression	−.03	.38*	.67***	−.58***
Order and Organization	.14	.05	−.04	−.14
Program Clarity	−.02	−.13	.17	−.10
Staff Control	−.34*	−.32	−.43**	.57***

* $p<.10.$
** $p<.05.$
*** $p<.01.$

Patient Initiatives

Table 7.4 shows the correlations for patients over the 23 wards between the WAS subscales and the same four WIS subscales that were utilized in the analyses in the previous study. Emphasis on Involvement was positively related to initiatives in the areas of Affiliation, Self-Revealing, and Aggression and negatively related to initiatives in the area of Submission to the Staff. Emphasis on Practical Orientation and/or Personal Problem Orientation was positively related to both Affiliation and Self-Revealing initiatives. Emphasis on Autonomy was negatively related to Submission initiatives, as was a high emphasis on Anger and Aggression. In addition, emphasis on Anger and Aggression was positively related to both Self-Revealing and Aggression initiatives. Finally, emphasis on Staff Control was positively related to Submission and negatively related to both Affiliation and Aggression initiatives.

The pattern of relationships between program treatment environment and patient initiatives is quite clear. As the emphasis on Relationship and Treatment Program dimensions increases, patients take more initiatives in areas such as Affiliation and Self-Revealing. They also take fewer initiatives in Submitting to the Staff. Thus as the "press" toward personal development increases, the degree of patient-perceived initiatives in these areas tends to increase. Conversely, as the emphasis on Staff Control increases, the degree of patient-perceived initiatives in this area (i.e., Submission) increases. There exists an important generalization effect in that the increasing emphasis on Staff Control has the related effect of decreasing the emphasis on personal development initiatives.

Correlations were again calculated between the WAS subscale means of the odd-numbered patients and the WIS subscale means of the even-numbered patients, and vice versa. The correlations obtained were again almost identical to those appearing in Table 7.4. All 15 of the 15 significant correlations in Table 7.4 were also statistically significant in either or both of the split analyses. Thus the findings replicate, even when the assessments of program environment and of patient initiatives are carried out on different subsamples of patients.

Correlations were calculated across 23 wards between the Crowne-Marlowe Social Desirability Scale and all the other variables. There were significant negative correlations between five of the WAS subscales and the Crowne-Marlowe: as the emphasis on Involvement, Autonomy, Personal Problem Orientation, Anger and Aggression, and Program Clarity increased, the average patient social desirability score decreased. There appears to be a sophistication element for patients on wards with active treatment programs, for these patients are too "wise" to answer items on the Crowne-Marlowe in the socially desirable direction. These results indicate that the relationships between treatment environment and patient morale and initiatives were not mediated by social desirability response sets.

AN OVERVIEW OF THE TWO STUDIES

A comparison of the results of the two studies shows that the findings were almost entirely replicated, as summarized in Table 7.5. (a) The Relationship dimension of Involvement was positively related to patient general satisfaction and personal development, as well as to Self-Revealing and Aggression. It was negatively related to initiatives in Submitting to the Staff. (b) Essentially, the same relationships held for the Treatment Program dimension of Personal Problem Orientation. Autonomy and Practical Orientation were positively related to general satisfaction and personal development, and Autonomy was also negatively related to Submission to the Staff initiatives. (c) Anger and Aggression was positively related to Self-Revealing and Aggression initiatives and negatively related to Affiliation and Submission initiatives. (d) Patient anxiety is the one dimension that functioned quite differently in the two studies.

With respect to item (d), we should note that patients in the first study felt greater anxiety when staff organized an active, directed, clear treatment program and also when they emphasized the expression of personal problems and angry feelings and increased the amount of patient independence and responsibility. Thus as pressure was put on patients to "perform," they became more anxious. These results did not replicate in the second study, in which the relationships between Anger and Aggression and Program Clarity and Anxiety were exactly the opposite, that is, anxiety decreased as the emphasis on these two dimensions of treatment environment increased. These differences probably occurred because the patients in the first study were psychiatrically sicker and more disturbed than the patients in the second. Whereas the sicker patients were made more anxious by an active treatment-oriented program, the healthier patients welcomed it.

These findings are similar to those of Manasse (1965), who concluded that chronic schizophrenics may have lower self-regard owing to their participation in an active work-oriented day treatment program, and those of Fox (1968), who learned that male VA patients on a work-oriented ward (the experimental program, discussed in Chapter 5, which was high in emphasis on Clarity and Anger and Aggression) worked more but felt more anxious than their counterparts on a control ward. Certain kinds of pressure on patients may simultaneously increase performance, anxiety, and stress.

The relationships between the System Maintenance dimensions and

TABLE 7.5 SUMMARY OF THE EFFECTS [a] OF THE TREATMENT ENVIRONMENTS ON PATIENTS

WAS Subscales	Patient Reactions			Patient Initiatives				
	Gen'l Satis-faction	Liking for Staff	Anxiety	Personal Develop-ment	Affil-iation	Self-Reveal-ing	Aggres-sion	Sub-mission
Involvement	++	++		++		+	++	− −
Autonomy	++	++		+				− −
Practical Orientation	++	+		+				
Personal Problem Orientation	++	++		+		+	+	−
Anger and Aggression					−	+	++	−
Order and Organization	++	+		+	+			
Program Clarity	+	+	I	−	−		−	−
Staff Control	−	−						+

[a]Key to symbols:

++ strong positive relationship.

+ moderate positive relationship.

− − strong negative relationship.

− moderate negative relationship.

I inconsistent relationship.

162

patient reactions were relatively consistent. General satisfaction and liking for staff were positively related to Order and Organization and Program Clarity, and negatively to Staff Control. Staff Control was negatively related to personal development and to affiliation and aggression initiatives, and positively related to submission initiatives.

Thus according to the overall results, patients' satisfaction and their liking for other patients and for staff may be a general reaction that can be tied to a variety of different program elements. This may be important, since patient–patient contacts are a major therapeutic influence, at least for certain types of patients (Keith-Spiegel and Spiegel, 1967).

Hence there are numerous alternative ways for staff to change the social climate; therefore, any one may have the effect of increasing patients' liking for one another and thus the extent of patient–patient contact and mutual therapeutic influence. Staff in programs emphasizing Involvement, Autonomy, Practical Orientation, and Personal Problem Orientation tended to be well liked by patients. The significance of this variable is in the relationship between liking for staff, contact with staff, and amount of therapeutic benefit which staff is likely to achieve (Truax and Carkhuff, 1968).

One of the major therapeutic influences involves allowing patients to test their abilities and to enhance their self-confidence. In these studies, Involvement, three of the Treatment Program dimensions, and Order and Organization were significantly related to the variables named, indicating that different treatment environments may have greater differential effects in these areas than has been previously demonstrated.

To sum up, when Relationship and Treatment Program areas (excluding Anger and Aggression) are emphasized, patients feel more satisfied, like the staff more, and believe that the program contributes more toward their personal development. The same conclusions hold for the System Maintenance dimensions of Order and Organization, whereas exactly the reverse effects are noted for Staff Control. Figure 7.1 illustrates these results by comparing patient profiles for two different wards. Compared with patients on ward 228, patients on ward 215 see their treatment environment as higher on each of the three Relationship dimensions as well as on the Treatment Program dimensions of Autonomy, Personal Problem Orientation, and Anger and Aggression. In addition, the patients on ward 215 percieve less emphasis on Staff Control. For example, more than 90% of the patients on ward 215 agreed that "Patients tell each other about their personal problems" and "Personal problems are openly talked about."

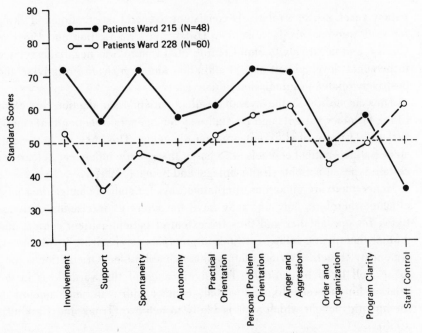

Figure 7.1   Comparison of patient perceptions on wards 215 and 228.

More than 80% agreed that "This is a lively ward," "The patients are proud of this ward," "Discussions are pretty interesting on this ward," and "Patients often do things together on the weekends."

The patients on ward 215 were significantly more satisfied with their ward, liked the other patients and the staff more, and felt that the ward was more likely to contribute to their personal development than did the patients on ward 228. In addition, the patients on ward 215 saw themselves as taking significantly more initiatives in the areas of Self-Revealing and Aggression and significantly fewer Submission initiatives. The two wards are physically similar; they have similar size and staffing and highly similar patient populations. However, they reveal two quite different treatment environments, which are associated with relatively pervasive differential effects on the patients.

STYLES OF HELPING BEHAVIOR

The third study, carried out in collaboration with Jack Sidman, assessed the relation between treatment environment and helping behavior. It is implied by the two previous studies that different treatment environments have differential effects partly because they make it more likely that certain types of helping behavior will occur. The various methods or styles of helping actually utilized by patients and staff in psychiatric programs have received little detailed study. Styles of helping behavior constitute the "mediating mechanism" or social matrix through which treatment environment affects treatment outcome. Our hypothesis was that different treatment environments would produce demonstrably different types of patient and staff helping styles.

The relationship between patient perception of treatment environment and patient and staff styles of helping behavior was explored across nine different state hospital wards. A Helping Scale was developed by compiling lists of different helping behaviors. These lists were generated in several different ways: (1) by asking therapists of varying schools to describe the specifics of their therapy techniques, (2) by talking to patients on several wards about what they regarded as specific examples of helping behaviors, and (3) by referring to an earlier study of college student helping behavior (Sidman, 1968). After the resulting items had been pretested on a small group of patients, those which had extreme item splits or proved to be incomprehensible to a number of patients were either reworded or excluded. The final item pool consisted of 70 items, worded in terms of patient or staff helping behavior. Each item was to be checked on a 7-point scale measuring the frequency with which each of the helping behaviors occurred on the ward (Sidman and Moos, 1973).

The Helping Scale was administered to 226 patients on nine wards approximately one week after WAS data were collected. The factor analyses were performed separately on the 70 patient and the 70 staff helping items, and three parallel factors discriminating significantly among the nine wards emerged in both analyses. The factors were as follows:

1.   A friendship factor; for example "One patient tries to show another that he cares about him," "One patient praises another," and "One patient tells another to relax."

2.   A directive teaching factor; for example, "One patient helps another by getting him to follow a schedule," "One patient helps another to practice new ways of dealing with difficult situations," and "One patient rewards another patient for doing things on his own."

3.   A supportive enhancement of self-esteem factor; for example, "One patient treats another as a competent and responsible person" and "One patient helps another patient accomplish something he wants to do."

The mean factor scores were related to the 10 WAS subscale means across all the wards using the Spearman rank-order correlation technique. The significant results for patient helping behaviors indicated (a) that patients saw more patient helping activity in the areas of friendship and enhancement of self-esteem on wards emphasizing Involvement, Support, Practical Orientation, and Order and Organization and (b) that patients saw more of the directive teaching type of helping activity on wards with more emphasis on Staff Control.

The results for staff helping behaviors led to the following observations: (a) Patients saw more staff helping by way of friendship behavior on wards that put greater emphasis on Involvement, Practical Orientation, Order and Organization, and Program Clarity and less emphasis on Anger and Aggression. (b) Patients saw more staff helping behavior of the directive teaching type on wards high on Involvement, Spontaneity, Practical Orientation, and Program Clarity. (c) Patients saw more supportive enhancement of the self-esteem type of help on wards high in Support and Order and Organization.

The results of the two earlier studies pointed to relationships between program treatment environment and both the general reactions of patients and their preferred initiatives. The study under discussion generalizes this finding to include patient perceptions of patient and staff helping styles. The earlier studies indicated that patients were more satisfied and liked one another and the staff more on wards emphasizing Involvement, Autonomy, Practical Orientation, Personal Problem Orientation, and Order and Organization. In one study, patients on wards that emphasized Anger and Aggression tended to feel greater anxiety; here the emphasis on Anger and Aggression was negatively related to helping behavior, particularly to staff friendship and the directive teaching type of helping. This supports the notion that some wards with active treatment programs oriented toward the open expression of anger may make patients more uncomfortable, actually resulting in a decrease in the amount of helping behavior. In this connection, we found a positive correlation between staff perception of Anger and Aggression and patient dropout rate (Moos and Schwartz, 1972).

These relationships serve to designate possible mediating variables between treatment environment and treatment outcome. Some of the WAS variables that are related to objective indices of treatment outcome (see Chapter 8) are also related to patient and staff helping styles. For example, patient-perceived Practical Orientation was related to release rate in two independent studies of treatment outcome. In this study Practical

Orientation was positively related to patient friendship and enhancement of the self-esteem type of helping and to staff friendship and the directive teaching type of helping. These helping activities, as engaged in by patients and staff, may be related partly to the rapid turnover rate typifying wards with a high emphasis on Practical Orientation.

The three studies have implications for planning evaluations comparing different treatment programs. Some of the mediating variables that differentiate among different program environments and their effects are measurable, and this may help us to understand why programs do or do not have differential effects. Patient morale, liking for other patients and staff, opportunities for personal development, and initiatives and helping behavior constitute important mediating variables. Treatment programs characterized by different treatment philosophies and methods may or may not actually create different psychological climates and reward different types of initiatives or helping styles.

Finally we confront the intriguing possibility of relating measures of program effectiveness and individual outcome data to both the WAS and morale, initiatives and helping style variables. The range of predictability of the effects of psychiatric treatment could be substantially increased by obtaining measures of the psychological environments in which the patient is living in the hospital, as well as measures of the similarity between in- and out-of-hospital environments. Such predictions should especially improve once it becomes possible to assess systematically different coping and helping styles occuring in and out of hospital.

RELEVANT RESEARCH IN OTHER ENVIRONMENTS

In this section we review selected research in other environments, aiming to provide a context within which our work on psychiatric programs can be interpreted. First some work in psychiatric and correctional milieus is presented, and an attempt is made to integrate the results with relevant research in individual and group psychotherapy. Literature on both social and task-oriented groups and results of selected studies conducted in industrial and educational environments are also discussed.

As we mentioned in Chapter 1, one of the basic assumptions of therapeutic community milieus is that the social environment has a significant influence on behavioral maladaptions and disorders. Relevant demonstrations are found in the work of Hobbs (1966), who developed an alternative institutional model for the reeducation of emotionally disturbed children, and in the project by Donahue, Gottesman, and Coons (1968), who demonstrated that even chronic "backward" geriatric patients can be helped to resume a more independent life and to work if they experience a community-oriented hospital milieu. Also important in this respect is the work reviewed earlier by Sanders, Smith, and Weinman (1967), who gathered evidence of the effectiveness of socioenvironmental treatment for certain groups of patients. Cumming and Cumming (1962) have presented a theoretical rationale, based on developments in ego psychology, to explain some of the effects of milieu therapy.

We have assessed the differential effects of the social climates of 16 correctional units (Moos, 1970). The study was organized very similarly to those reported in this chapter; that is, residents took three different scales. These were the Correctional Institutions Environment Scale (CIES), assessing nine dimensions of the social environments of correctional institutions; a Resident Reaction Scale, assessing residents' reactions to the unit on the same six questions that were utilized in the ward studies; and a Resident Initiative Scale, assessing the initiatives residents perceive themselves as taking in the areas of Affiliation, Self-Revealing, Aggression, and Submission.

In these correctional units for example, the relationships between the unit social environment and resident satisfaction were low. On the other hand, there were significant positive relationships between how much the residents liked the staff and the amount of emphasis on the Relationship dimensions of Involvement and Spontaneity and the Treatment Program dimensions of Autonomy and Personal Problem Orientation. These dimensions of the social environment were also related to the residents' feelings about how much the unit contributed to the development of their abilities and to their self-confidence. Emphasis on Involvement, Spontaneity, Autonomy, and Personal Problem Orientation was also positively related to residents' perceptions of their initiatives in the areas of Affiliation and Self-Revealing. The relationships were considerably stronger than those found on psychiatric wards.

The results indicate that the social climates in both psychiatric and correctional programs have important effects on individual behavior; these effects, however, seem to derive from different aspects of the climate and to relate to different dependent variables. Although the conclusion that different social climates have differential effects may generalize from one type of institution (psychiatric wards) to another (correctional units), the exact relationship between specific dimensions of climate and specific dependent variables differ as a function of the overall characteristics of the institution. Since residents in correctional units are being held against their will, it is reasonable to suppose that the social climate of such units is not related to resident satisfaction. On the other hand, most correctional units, including the 16 we studied, have a very strong emphasis on learning vocational and job-oriented skills. Thus the climate of correctional units is highly related to residents' perceptions of the opportunities for personal development. The specific relationships between social climate dimensions and differential effects of living groups are mediated by the overall characteristics of these living groups (e.g., whether they are in " total" institutions).

Individual and Group Psychotherapy

Relevant work in individual and group psychotherapy has focused almost exclusively on Relationship dimensions. Truax and Carkhuff (1967) and Truax and Mitchell (1971) marshal cogent evidence supporting the existence of certain prepotent therapist variables or qualities that are relevant in a wide variety of different kinds of psychotherapy. Three characteristics of an effective therapist have emerged from the divergent viewpoints: (1) an effective therapist is nondefensive and authentic or genuine; (2) an effective therapist is able to provide a nonthreatening, safe, trusting, or secure atmosphere through his own acceptance or nonpossessive warmth for the client; and (3) an effective therapist is able to have a high degree of accurate empathic understanding of the client on a moment-by-moment basis. Truax and Mitchell state that "these ingredients of the psychotherapeutic relationship are aspects of human encounters that cut across the parochial theories of psychotherapy and appear to be common elements in a wide variety of psychoanalytic, client-centered, eclectic or learning-theory approaches to psychotherapy" (p. 302).

The evidence indicates that insofar as these therapist qualities are present in a relationship, positive personality change is likely to follow, whereas to the extent that they are lacking, negative change or personality deterioration may occur. Indeed, therapists or counselors who are accurately empathic, nonpossessively warm, and genuine seem to work effectively with their clients regardless of the training or theoretical orientation of the former; and such effectiveness is observed with a wide variety of clients, varying from hospitalized schizophrenics to college underachievers and juvenile delinquents. In a significant early paper that led to most of this research, Rogers (1957) asserted that these dimensions of the relationship were the necessary and sufficient conditions for positive personality change.

These dimensions appear to us to be conceptually analogous to our three Relationship dimensions. Empathy, warmth, and genuineness assess the overall quality of the relationship between the patient and therapist, exactly as Involvement, Support, and Spontaneity assess the general quality of the relationships among patients and between patients and staff in a ward milieu. Yalom (1970) has proposed an analogy between cohesiveness in group therapy and the concept of the "relationship" in individual therapy. He assumes that the relationship in psychotherapy and cohesiveness in group therapy constitute necessary but *not* sufficient conditions for positive personality change, stating: "It is obvious that the group therapy analog of the patient–therapist relationship is a broader concept encompassing the patient's relationship to his group therapist, to the other group members and to the group as a whole" (p. 37).

There is some evidence that group cohesiveness is associated with positive personality change in group members. Dickoff and Lakin (1963) found that group cohesiveness has important therapeutic value and is essential for the continuation of a group. Most of their patients felt that the primary mode of help in group therapy was obtained through mutual support. Patients who rejected their group often complained of not having experienced meaningful social contact with other group members. Dickoff and Lakin concluded that cohesiveness is of therapeutic value and that it is essential for the continuation of a group.

Kapp et al. (1964) found that self-perceived personality change correlated significantly both with the members' feelings of involvement in their group and with their assessment of total group cohesiveness. Other evidence relating group cohesiveness to a number of positive effects on patients inside and outside therapy groups are reviewed by Yalom (1970) and Goldstein et al. (1966). In one additional study, Truax (1961) examined the effects of group cohesiveeess on depth of patient intrapersonal exploration. He used three psychotherapy groups and randomly selected 3-minute samples of verbal interaction from recordings of 42 successive therapy sessions. He found significant positive correlations between ratings of group cohesiveness and judged intrapersonal exploration as obtained from ratings made by independent observers.

Thus the evidence indicates that the qualities of the relationship in individual therapy and in group therapy (as conceptualized by cohesiveness) are strongly related to positive evaluation of treatment and to positive personality change. The results on the Relationship dimensions in our ward milieu studies are strikingly similar. Wards on which relationships are perceived as being involving, supportive, and spontaneous, have patients who are more satisfied, who like one another and the staff more, who believe that their ward experiences are relevant to their personal development, and who engage in more self-revealing, more open expression of anger, and less submission to the staff. Positive relationship qualities are as essential in mediating positive personality change in ward milieus as they are in individual and group psychotherapy.

Our formulation of Treatment Program and System Maintenance dimensions suggests relevant sets of dimensions along which different individual and group therapies could be compared fruitfully. Rather than global characterizations of psychotherapy as client centered or as oriented toward behavior modification, different types of psychotherapies could be compared in terms of their relative emphases on Autonomy, Practical Orientation, Personal Problem Orientation, and Anger and Aggression. The System Maintenance dimensions, which seldom receive heavy emphasis in psychotherapy (except in Adlerian and directive therapy), may be far more important than has been previously thought. A conceptualization of Relationship Dimensions, Treatment Program dimensions, and System Maintenance dimensions is highly relevant for comparisons of different kinds of individual and group psychotherapy. The comparison of different types of psychotherapy on similar dimensions would facilitate studies of the comparative effects of different types of treatment. We have developed a Group Environment Scale (GES) for assessing the characteristics of group psychotherapy in terms of these three types of dimensions (Moos and Humphrey, 1973). The GES significantly discriminates among psychotherapy groups and promises to be useful in developing a more comprehensive characterization of the similarities and differences in various group psychotherapies.

Selected Further Studies in Other Milieus

The body of literature in social and task-oriented groups indicating that group characteristics and/or climate affect the mood and behavior of individuals functioning within the group is too large to permit a systematic review here. A few examples can be mentioned, however. In an interesting study, Faigin (1958) made observations in two Israeli nurseries and showed that dependent passive behavior was more common among children who resided in a highly structured nursery than among children who lived in a less highly organized center. This directly corroborates our findings on the effects of Staff Control. Gump, Schoggen, and Redl (1957) reported that assertive behavior and aggressive behavior occurred more frequently during swimming than during crafts among preadolescent boys attending summer camp. However, helping reactions occurred more frequently during crafts than during swimming, indicating that ties exist between the activity that is dominant in the setting and important individual reactions such as helping behavior.

The potential utility of our concepts of Relationship, Personal Development, and System Maintenance dimensions appears from a careful analysis of the descriptions of the "democratic," "authoritarian," and "laissez-faire" climates in the Lewin studies mentioned earlier. Although authoritarian leadership at times produced highly aggressive groups; at other times it led to very apathetic groups. This effect may be less related to authoritarian leadership than to the positive or negative reinforcement accorded the expression of anger and aggression in the particular group. Another finding was that cohesiveness or "we-feeling" was lower in the authoritarian groups than in the other groups. However, the authoritarian group climates usually involved distant, cold leadership; thus some of the effects described by Lewin et al. may be related to a lack of emphasis on the Relationship dimensions rather than to a strong emphasis on authoritarianism or leader control. The findings of these and other group studies would be much clearer if a more differentiated assessment of the characteristics of the respective groups had been made.

Some relevant research has also been carried out in industrial and educational environments. A wealth of literature in industrial environments substantiates the relationships between the quality of personal interactions in the work environment, particularly in connection with supervisor behavior, and different dimensions of job satisfaction (e.g., Friedlander and Margulies, 1969; Lyons, 1971). A recent review of some of this literature, as well as a discussion of the complexity of individual and situational determinants of job satisfaction, is given in Ronan (1970). Schneider and Bartlett (1970) have developed an 80-item Agency Climate Questionnaire that assesses the social climates of life insurance agencies. They characterized general satisfaction as one of the agency climate dimensions and found that it was highly correlated with the extent of perceived managerial support, managerial structure, new employee concern, and agent independence in both agent and managerial samples.

In an intriguing further study Schneider (1973) found that bank customers decide to switch their accounts on the basis of generalized perceptions they have of the bank. The investigators utilized a 13-item Climate Questionnaire and obtained data from 674 account holders in two retail and two commercial banks. They found that items descriptive of employee behavior had the highest correlations with customer intention to switch and that the strongest correlates (negative) of switch tendency in all four banks were obtained with two items that defined the relationship between the bank employees and the bank customers—namely, "The bank employees bend over backward to provide good service" and "The atmosphere in my bank is warm and friendly." These broad impressions or perceptions of the climate, which must be based on specific events and experiences of bank customers, were more strongly related to switching intentions than were the specific events and experiences themselves.

A small sample of former account holders (i.e., individuals who had switched their accounts) indicated that the same two items also significantly discriminated between the perceptions of people who actually switched their accounts and those who did not. Account holders who had switched their accounts for service-related reasons perceived the bank and its employees significantly more negatively than did customers still maintaining their accounts. In an important additional analysis, Schneider found that the more objective characteristics of customers (size of account, type of account, distance from bank, length of time with bank, sex, number of bank services used) and of the bank itself (waiting time, size of accounts, procedure for queuing customers) were unrelated to climate perceptions.

Pace (1969) presents a number of relationships between CUES scale scores and student attitudes and activities. Most relevant here is the finding that colleges high on CUES Community and Awareness subscales have a high proportion of students who feel a strong emotional attachment to the college. In addition, it was rare for students to report not having participated in any extracurricular activities in college environments that were high on CUES Community. Finally, Peterson et al. (1970) relate the subscales of the Institutional Functioning Inventory (IFI) to seven different factors of student protest in a sample of 50 institutions. A number of relationships are presented, but it was most interesting to learn that student radicalism as a protest factor was highly correlated with the IFI subscales of Human Diversity and Concern for Improvement of Society. The other relationships found are generally predictable ones—for example, the absence of senior faculty and the quality of instruction were protest issues in institutions with a low perceived emphasis on Undergraduate Learning, and classified research was a protest issue in institutions with a high degree of emphasis on Concern for Advancing Knowledge.

In summary, the dominant findings of the effects of social climates concern what we have termed Relationship dimensions. A variety of research has strongly substantiated the critical importance of these dimensions in individual and group psychotherapy, in social and task-oriented groups, and in industrial and educational environments. The Relationship dimensions appear to exert similar influence across different types of institutions; however, much less is known about the differential effects of the Personal Development and the System Maintenance dimensions. These types of dimensions have been less widely used in studies of group and institutional effects. More critically, when they have been used (e.g., in the studies of authoritarian leadership conducted by Lewin), Relationship dimensions have not been systematically assessed. Thus, as pointed out earlier, some of the presumed negative effects of certain leader styles *may* be more highly related to a lack of emphasis on Relationship dimensions than to an emphasis on leader control and similar variables.

This point is also relevant to Stern's conceptualizations of Relationship dimensions as anabolic (i.e., growth-enhancing) and System Maintenance dimensions as catabolic (i.e., growth-inhibiting), respectively. Although the dimension of Staff Control appeared to be catabolic in this sense in our studies, the dimensions of Order and Organization and Program Clarity were largely, although not totally, anabolic. In addition, the emphasis on Anger and Aggression, which is regarded by psychiatric staff as a personal development press, had largely catabolic effects. Future research will need to assess the effects of more relationship-oriented "benevolent" control on different types of individuals in institutions. The evidence on the growth-inhibiting effects of System Maintenance dimensions, especially Control, is as yet unclear, particularly in institutions other than universities. The most unambiguous conclusion is that satisfying human relationships in all milieus studied to date facilitate personal growth and development and are in this sense anabolic. However, insofar as "love is not enough," the effects of Personal Development and System Maintenance dimensions merit further study.

REFERENCES

Cumming, J. & Cumming, E. *Ego and milieu.* New York, Atherton, 1962.

Dickoff, H. & Lakin, M. Patients' views of group psychotherapy: Retrospections and interpretations. *International Journal of Group Psychotherapy,* **13:** 61–73, 1963.

Donahue, W., Gottesman, L. E., & Coons, D. Milieu therapy and the long-term geriatric mental patient. *Mental Health Program Reports,* 2. Government Printing Office, 1968, Washington, D.C. (PHS Publication No. 1743).

Faigin, H. Social behavior of young children in the kibbutz. *Journal of Abnormal and Social Psychology,* **56:** 117–129, 1958.

Fox, P. D. Cost-effectiveness of mental health: An evaluation of an experimental rehabilitation program. Ph.D. dissertation, Stanford University, 1968.

Friedlander, F. & Margulies, N. Multiple impacts of organizational climate and individual value systems upon job satisfaction. *Personnel Psychology,* **22:** 171–183, 1969.

Goldstein, A., Heller, K., & Sechrest, L. *Psychotherapy and the psychology of behavior change.* Wiley, New York, 1966.

Gump, P., Schoggen, P., & Redl, F. The camp milieu and its immediate effects. *Journal of Social Issues,* **13:** 40–46, 1957.

Hobbs, N. Helping disturbed children: Psychological and ecological strategies. *American Psychologist,* **21:** 1105–1115, 1966.

Houts, P. & Moos, R. The development of a Ward Initiative Scale for patients. *Journal of Clinical Psychology,* **25:** 319–322, 1969.

Kapp, F., Gleser, G., Brissenden, A., Emerson, R., Winget, J., & Kashdan, B. Group participation and self-perceived personality change. *Journal of Nervous and Mental Disease,* **139:** 255–265, 1964.

Keith-Spiegel, P. & Spiegel, D. Perceived helpfulness of others as a function of compatible intelligence levels. *Journal of Counseling Psychology,* **14:** 61–62, 1967.

Lewin, K. Frontiers in group dynamics. In Cartwright, D. (Ed.). *Field theory and social science.* New York, Harper & Row, 1951a.

Lewin, K. Behavior and development as a function of the total situation. In Cartwright, D. (Ed.). *Field theory and social science.* New York, Harper & Row, 1951b.

Lewin, K., Lippitt, R., & White, R. Patterns of aggressive behavior in experimentally created 'social climates.' *Journal of Social Psychology,* **10:** 271–299, 1939.

Lippitt, R. & White, R. The "social climate" of children's groups. In Barker, R. (Ed.). *Child behavior and development.* New York, McGraw-Hill, 1943.

Lyons, T. F. Role clarity, need for clarity, satisfaction, tension and withdrawal. *Organizational Behavior and Human Performance,* **6:** 99–110, 1971.

Manasse, T. Self-regard as a function of environmental demands in chronic schizophrenics. *Journal of Abnormal Psychology,* **70:** 210–213, 1965.

Moos, R. Differential effects of the social climates of correctional institutions. *Journal of Research in Crime and Delinquency,* **7:** 71–82, 1970.

Moos, R. & Houts, P. Differential effects of the social atmospheres of psychiatric wards. *Human Relations*, **23:** 47–60, 1970.

Moos, R. & Humphrey, B. *Group Environment Scale technical report.* Social Ecology Laboratory, Department of Psychiatry, Stanford University, Palo Alto, Calif., 1973.

Moos, R. & Schwartz, J. Treatment environment and treatment outcome, *Journal of Nervous and Mental Disease*, **154:** 264–275, 1972.

Pace, R. College and University Environment Scale. Technical manual, 2nd ed. Educational Testing Service, Princeton, N.J., 1969.

Peterson, R., Centra, J., Hartnett, R., & Linn, R. Institutional Functioning Inventory. Preliminary technical manual. Educational Testing Service, Princeton, N.J., 1970.

Rogers, C. The necessary and sufficient conditions of therapeutic personality change. *Journal of Consulting Psychology*, **21:** 95–103, 1957.

Ronan, W. Individual and situational variables relating to job satisfaction. *Journal of Applied Psychology Monograph*, **54:** 1–31, 1970.

Sanders, R., Smith, R., & Weinman, B. *Chronic psychoses and recovery.* Jossey-Bass, San Francisco, 1967.

Schneider, B. The perception of organizational climate: The customer's view. *Journal of Applied Psychology*, in press, 1973.

Schneider, B. & Bartlett, C. Individual differences and organizational climate. II: Measurement of organizational climate by the multi-trait multi-rater matrix. *Personnel Psychology*, **23:** 493–512, 1970.

Sidman, J. Empathy and helping behavior in college students. Doctoral dissertation, University of Colorado, Boulder, 1968.

Sidman, J. & Moos, R. On the relation between psychiatric ward atmosphere and helping behavior. *Journal of Clinical Psychology*, **29:** 74–78, 1973.

Truax, C. The process of group therapy: Relationships between hypothesized therapeutic conditions and intrapersonal exploration. *Psychology Monographs*, **75** (whole no. 511), 1961.

Truax, C. & Carkhuff, R. *Toward effective counseling and psychotherapy: Training and practice.* Aldine, Chicago, 1967.

Truax, C. & Mitchell, K. Research on certain therapist interpersonal skills in relation to process and outcome. In Bergin, A. & Garfield, A. (Eds.). *Handbook of psychotherapy and behavior change: An empirical analysis.* Wiley, New York, 1971.

Yalom, I. *The theory and practice of group psychotherapy.* Basic Books, New York, 1970.

Chapter Eight

THE EFFECTS OF TREATMENT ENVIRONMENTS: TREATMENT OUTCOME

Rudolf H. Moos, Charles Petty, and Robert Shelton

Only a few previous studies have related treatment environment and treatment outcome. Indeed, until recently there have been no standard techniques by which the treatment environments of different psychiatric programs could be readily assessed and compared. Cohen and Struening (1964), studying 12 VA hospitals with the Opinions about Mental Ilness questionnaire, found that in the five hospitals in which staff were less authoritarian–restrictive, patients spent more total time in the community as assessed 6 and 12 months after admission than did patients treated in the seven hospitals in which the staff tended to endorse authoritarian–restrictive attitudes. Gurel (1964), also working in VA hospitals, learned that smaller hospitals released patients earlier but were not necessarily more effective in reducing patients' symptoms.

Ullmann (1967) studied 30 different VA hospitals and found that smaller and better staffed hospitals tended to have the highest turnover rates. It should be noted that the units of analysis in these investigations were entire hospitals. As discussed in Chapters 4 and 5, treatment milieus vary widely from ward to ward in the same hospital; thus the conclusions that size, staffing ratios, and staff attitudes are related to release rates may or may not generalize to studies in which the unit of analysis is the individual ward.

Two recent studies have related the characteristics of individual psychiatric programs to treatment outcome. Kellam et al. (1967) assessed eight dimensions of program atmospheres on 12 admission wards in four emergency receiving hospitals. The 202 study patients were mainly diagnosed schizophrenic, and the outcome measures utilized included global improvement ratings, changes in interview behavior, and changes in ward behavior which occurred during the first 6 weeks of drug treatment. The results were complex and somewhat inconsistent; however, certain characteristics differentiated between effective and ineffective programs. Patients on wards that had high patient–patient and staff–patient contact improved most on six of the 24 symptom and behavior scales; patients who showed the least improvement in five different symptom and behavioral adjustment areas came from wards that gave patients high adult status.

Kellam et al. concluded that interward differences on patient behavior variables (e.g., social cluster size) were stronger predictors of improvement than more objective ecological variables such as ward census and patient–staff ratio. The specific finding that schizophrenic patients improved least on high adult status wards is contrary to a priori expectations; however, two possible complicating factors must be considered. First, since hospital adjustment is generally unrelated to community adjustment, as has been well documented by Ellsworth et al. (1968), Kellam's findings may be specifically limited to the effects of program characteristics on in-hospital adjustment measures. Second, it is not at all clear whether ward policy measures of adult status (free access to showers and bedrooms, privacy in bathrooms, etc.) are necessarily accompanied by increased patient responsibility in other areas (determining one's own program, taking independent leadership initiatives, etc.). Autonomy and adult status only showed moderate positive relationships in our American normative sample (see Chapter 6).

Ellsworth et al. (1971) have recently completed an excellent study in which 19 units in five VA hospitals were assessed with the patient and staff Perception of Ward (POW) scales. They found that efficient (high-turnover) wards were perceived more negatively by nursing staff, who felt, for example, that they received less praise for work and that the professional staff were less well motivated. The highest release rate units also tended not to promote patient autonomy. These findings gave the impression that the efficient units were run by professional staff who did not take the time to involve either patients or staff in responsible roles but focused instead on admitting and discharging patients. Effective programs (those with low return rates), on the other hand, were characterized as having motivated professional staff and active participant roles for both nursing staff and patients. Nursing staff on these wards saw themselves as participating in treatment planning and receiving praise for their work. Significantly, wards with the highest nursing staff ratios also had the poorest community tenure rates for admissions and for resident patients. The authors concluded that the program dimensions associated with high community tenure rates were quite different from those related to high release rates.

TREATMENT OUTCOME CRITERIA

We related treatment environment as perceived by patients and staff to treatment outcome, as assessed by dropout rates, release (discharge) rates, and community tenure rates. Release rate is an important outcome criterion for at least three reasons: (1) leaving the treatment program is the first step the patient must take in order to adjust to his community environment; (2) it is important to return the patient to the community as soon as possible, since the longer a person remains in the hospital, the lower are his chances for later release; and (3) as part of the danger of extended hospital stay, a patient may learn new patterns of behavior in the ward setting which are rewarded there but which are maladaptive and socially unacceptable in the community environment. Release rate is a measure of a program's efficiency in returning patients to the community. Community tenure rate is one measure of the success released patients have in the community. The longer a patient stays in the community before (and if) he returns to the program, the more successful the program is based on this outcome criterion. Dropout rate is less often used in outcome studies, although it reflects a program's inability to be effective with at least a certain proportion of its patients.

We used the following methods to calculate the three outcome criteria:

1. *Dropout rate.* The total number of patients in each program who (*a*) eloped (simply left the program without permission) or (*b*) were formally discharged at their own request Against Medical Advice (AMA) during the study period, was divided by the overall patient census.

2. *Release rate.* The total number of patients released from each program during the study period was divided by the overall patient census. This total included only people who were released under the following circumstances: on Trial Visit (TV), as having received Maximum Hospital Benefits (MHB), or assigned to receive posthospital care (PHC). Patients who eloped or were discharged were not included.

3.   *Community tenure rate.* We calculated the percentage of patients released from a given program who were still in the community at the end of a stipulated period of time (i.e., 6 months for the first outcome study or 3 months for the second).

Since both outcome studies were done at VA hospitals, where every admission or discharge is routinely reported in the patient's permanent file, a relatively accurate record of releases, readmissions, and dropouts is assured, except for a small proportion of released patients who are later admitted to non-VA hospitals.

STUDY ONE: EIGHT SMALL VA WARDS

In the first study, eight male wards in one VA hospital were utilized. Seven of the wards were quite small (averaging 24 patients per ward), the eighth being somewhat larger (42 patients). The staffing ratios were similar from ward to ward, although the smaller wards had slightly fewer patients per staff member.

Both patients and staff were used in the portion of the study involving the evaluation of treatment environment. All staff who worked in direct contact with patients on each ward were asked to participate, and about 85% did so. The participating patients were all those who were willing to cooperate and who were able to respond to paper-and-pencil questionnaires. About 53% of these patients adequately completed the WAS. There were no significant differences in the proportion of patients who completed the questionnaire on the different wards. Completed questionnaires were obtained from 111 patients and 88 staff members.

Subjects for the follow-up portion of the study included 175 patients who were released from the hospital during a 6 month period following administration of the WAS. An additional 46 patients either eloped or left the hospital during this 6 month period. These 46 patients were not followed up, and they were not counted as readmissions if they returned to the hospital. The number of patients still in the community after the 6-month follow-up period was divided by the total number of patients who had been discharged from that ward to obtain the *community tenure rate.* The dropout rate varied from 0.04 to 0.45, the release rate varied from 0.38 to 1.59, and the community tenure rate varied from 0.11 to 0.76.

The x^2 test was used to examine the hypothesis that dropout, release, and community tenure rates on the eight wards were proportionate to ward population size, using corrected ward census values as the theoretical expected frequency for each ward. The x^2 values were all significant (release and dropout rate, $p < .001$; community tenure, $p < .05$), indicating that dropout, release, and community tenure rates differed significantly from ward to ward. The three outcome criteria were moderately interrelated–release rate correlated .51 with dropout rate and .43 with community tenure. Dropout rate was not correlated with community tenure.

The background characteristics of the total patient cohort on each ward were compared to determine whether any significant differences existed in the patient populations being studied. Briefly, the patients were all male; their average age was about 40 years; more than 80% were single, widowed, or divorced; more than 65% were diagnosed schizophrenic; and the vast majority had been previously hospitalized, most more than once. Median length of stay in the hospital was the only variable that significantly differentiated among the wards, indicating that the wards were closely comparable.

STUDY TWO: SEVEN LARGE VA WARDS

In the second study, we utilized seven large male wards in another VA hospital. Patients were randomly assigned to the wards, and there was a continuing policy of rotating new admissions unselectively among the wards. If readmission became necessary; patients were returned to the ward from which they had been released. The ward census varied from a low of 73 to a high of 129 patients, whereas the patient–staff ratio varied from a low of 3.7 to a high of 5.6. Other ward and patient background characteristics of the seven wards were closely comparable (for more detailed descriptions, see Moos and Schwartz 1972). For example, 62% of all released patients were diagnosed schizophrenic; this varied only from 57 to 72%. Furthermore, the percentage of released patients who were married averaged 38% and varied only from 30 to 43%.

Again both patients and staff were used in the portion of the study involving the evaluation of treatment environment. All staff who worked in direct contact with patients on each ward were asked to participate, and about 70% did so. Only about 45% of the patients adequately completed the WAS; yet once more there were no significant differences in the proportion of patients who completed the questionnaire on the different wards.

Subjects used in the follow-up included 725 patients who were released from the hospital during a 3-month period ranging from about 5 weeks prior to testing to 5 weeks after testing. Of these, 285 patients were released on trial visit, 343 were discharged on maximum hospital benefit status, and 97 were released to posthospital care. In addition, the number of patients who eloped and the number of patients who left the hospital AMA were enumerated for each ward. During the 3-month period, 269 patients eloped and 118 were discharged AMA.

Dropout, release, and community tenure rates were calculated as in the first study. The dropout rate varied from 0.32 to 0.79, the release rate from 0.76 to 1.67, and the community tenure rate from 0.78 to 0.89. Both the dropout and the release rates differed significantly from ward to ward. The community tenure rate did not quite significantly differentiate among the wards. The three outcome criteria were again moderately interrelated; that is, release rate correlated −.54 with dropout rate and .61 with community tenure. Dropout rate was not correlated with community tenure.

THREE TREATMENT OUTCOME SCALES

We attempted to derive three WAS subscales that would consistently relate to the three objective treatment outcome criteria. The basic question was whether there were consistent characteristics of treatment milieus that would correlate with rates of dropout, release, and community tenure in both studies.

Each of the WAS items is answered either true or false. First the percentage true was calculated for each item for each of the wards in the two studies, separately for patients and staff. Next each of the items was correlated with each of the three treatment outcome criteria. These were Spearman rank-order correlations in which the wards in each study were rank-ordered on each of the outcome variables and on the percentage of patients or staff who answered the item in the true direction.

A substantial number of items displayed moderate to high correlations with the different outcome criteria. For example, patient perceptions on 30 items in the first study and on 29 items in the second study correlated .40 or greater with ward dropout rates. Staff perceptions on 43 items in the first study and 48 items in the second study correlated .40 or greater with dropout rates. The next step was to search for the best combination of items which would correlate with each of the outcome measures for both patient and staff perceptions. It was possible to construct three nonoverlapping scales that were highly correlated with the three outcome criteria for patients and staff in both studies.

The Dropout Scale

Table 8.1 shows the rank-order correlations between the 15-item dropout scale and the three treatment outcome criteria. Patient and staff perceptions on this scale are significantly correlated with dropout rates in the two studies, but neither is significantly correlated with release rates or with community tenure rates in either study. Thus the dropout scale is uniquely related to dropout rate.

TABLE 8.1   RANK–ORDER CORRELATIONS OVER WARDS BE- TWEEN DROPOUT SCALE AND TREATMENT OUTCOME CRITERIA

	Eight Small Wards			Seven Large Wards		
	Dropout Rate	Release Rate	Community Tenure	Dropout Rate	Release Rate	Community Tenure
Patients	.90**	.19	−.45	.82*	−.43	.50
Staff	.97**	.41	−.36	.86**	−.46	.29

* $p<.05$.
** $p<.01$.

In Table 8.2 the items on the dropout scale are grouped by similar content areas. The scoring direction for each item in the dropout scale is given.

From Table 8.2 we can infer that patients and staff see wards with high dropout rates as low in the Relationship dimensions of Involvement and Support and low in the Treatment Program dimensions of Autonomy, Order and Organization, and Program Clarity. A close examination of the items in this scale gives a fairly clear picture of the milieu of a program with a high dropout rate. The program has few social activities, there is no particular emphasis on involving patients in the program, and since patients' activities are not well planned, they have much free time with little or no guidance. It is difficult for patients to form social clusters with other patients. Staff do not go out of their way to help patients and are not interested in learning about patients' feelings. Staff also discourage criticism from patients and are unwilling to act on patients' suggestions. Patients often gripe about or criticize the staff, perhaps because the

TABLE 8.2   DROPOUT SCALE ITEMS AND SCORING KEY

Scored Direction	Item
True	It's hard to get a group together for card games or other activities.
True	The ward has very few social activities.
False	Patients are pretty busy all the time.
False	Staff go out of their way to help patients.
False	Most patients follow a regular schedule each day.
True	Many patients look messy.
False	Patients' activities are carefully planned.
True	Things are sometimes very disorganized around here.
False	On this ward everyone knows who's in charge.
False	This is a very well organized ward.
False	The staff act on patient suggestions.
True	The staff discourages criticism.
False	Staff are mainly interested in learning about patients' feelings.
True	Patients often gripe.
True	Patients often criticize or joke about the ward staff.

program is perceived (by patients *and* staff) as poorly organized, and patients have no regular schedule that is followed each day. The program gives the impression of being rather unfriendly, and it seems that patients do not really feel comfortable or at ease, that social contacts are hard to make, and that the staff are probably unhappy with the environment and/or with one another. It is important to note that patients and staff alike agreed in perceiving these items to be characteristic of programs with high dropout rates; specifically, rank-order correlations over wards between patient and staff dropout scale scores were .93 for the eight small wards and .61 for the seven large wards.

The Release Rate Scale

Table 8.3 shows the rank-order correlations between the release rate scale and the three treatment outcome criteria. Again, patient and staff perceptions are significantly related to release rate in both studies. Except for the correlation between staff perceptions and community tenure in the eight small wards, the correlations between the release rate scale and the other outcome criteria are nonsignificant. However, staff perceptions on the release rate scale are negatively correlated with community tenure in the other study. Thus the release rate scale is uniquely related to release rates. Patient and staff release rate scale scores correlated .86 for the eight small wards and .79 for the seven large wards, indicating a high degree of agreement on the perceived characteristics of the treatment environments of high release rate programs.

TABLE 8.3   RANK–ORDER CORRELATIONS OVER WARDS BE-TWEEN RELEASE RATE SCALE AND TREATMENT OUTCOME CRITERIA

	Eight Small Wards			Seven Large Wards		
	Dropout Rate	Release Rate	Community Tenure	Dropout Rate	Release Rate	Community Tenure
Patients	.04	.83**	.46	−.50	.82*	−.54
Staff	−.08	.76*	.74*	−.39	.82*	−.21

* $p < .05$
** $p < .01$

Of the 14 items on the release rate scale, (see Table 8.4) five come from the Practical Orientation subscale. Programs with high release rates typically emphasize making plans for leaving the hospital, training patients for new kinds of jobs, and making concrete plans before departing from the hospital. There is a fair amount of staff control, insofar as the patient must follow a schedule that has been arranged for him. Staff are personally interested in the patients and tell them when they are making progress, although staff are not always aware of what patients need or want. There is relatively little emphasis on expressiveness: when patients disagree with one another, they do not usually involve staff and they rarely argue among themselves. Significantly, neither patients nor staff perceive particularly high support on such wards. The item "Patients are rarely asked personal questions by the staff" is probably more related in this context to information gathering than it is to Personal Problem Orientation. It is interesting that even though these wards are practical and "unexpressive," patients and staff agree that "The patients are proud of this ward." Thus

TABLE 8.4   RELEASE RATE SCALE ITEMS AND SCORING KEY

Scored Direction	Item
False	There is very little emphasis on making plans for getting out of the hospital.
True	This ward emphasizes training for new kinds of jobs.
True	New treatment approaches are often tried on this ward.
True	Patients are encouraged to plan for the future.
True	Patients must make plans before leaving the hospital.
True	Staff tell patients when they are getting better.
True	Once a schedule is arranged for a patient the patient must follow it.
True	When patients disagree with each other, they keep it to themselves.
False	The staff know what the patients want.
False	Patients say anything they want to the doctors.
True	Nobody ever volunteers around here.
True	Patients on this ward rarely argue.
True	The patients are proud of this ward.
False	Patients are rarely asked personal questions by the staff.

there is a certain kind of pride and involvement in a high release rate program, although the focus is on practical decisions and information gathering in a somewhat unexpressive context.

THE COMMUNITY TENURE SCALE

The rank-order correlations between the community tenure scale and the three treatment outcome criteria (Table 8.5) indicate that patient and staff perceptions are significantly correlated with community tenure criteria in the two outcome studies. Neither patient nor staff perceptions correlated with the other two outcome criteria in either study, except for a significant negative correlation between patient perceptions and dropout rate in the study on eight small wards. However, patient perceptions on the community tenure scale were positively correlated with dropout rate in the other study. Thus, as with the dropout and the release rate scales, the community tenure scale is uniquely related to community tenure. There was a high level of agreement between patient and staff community tenure scale scores for each study—.90 for the eight small wards and .86 for the seven large wards.

TABLE 8.5 RANK–ORDER CORRELATIONS BETWEEN COMMUNITY TENURE SCALE AND TREATMENT OUTCOME CRITERIA

	Eight Small Wards			Seven Large Wards		
	Dropout Rate	Release Rate	Community Tenure	Dropout Rate	Release Rate	Community Tenure
Patients	−.70*	.00	.82**	.36	−.18	.71*
Staff	−.41	.33	.97**	.14	.00	.79*

* $p < .05.$
** $p < .01.$

The items listed in Table 8.6 describe a program emphasizing the free and open expression of feelings and emotions, particularly angry feelings. Staff think it is a healthy thing to argue, and they are seen arguing among themselves, sometimes even starting arguments in group meetings. Patients are expected to share their personal problems and feelings with each other and with staff. Thus programs that are most successful in keeping patients out of the hospital stress a personal problem orientation and an open expression of anger. This emphasis occurs in a particular kind of context that, as the other items indicate, embodies autonomy and independence, a practical orientation, order and organization, and a reasonable degree of staff control. For example, patients are transferred from the ward if they do not obey the rules, but they are treated with respect by the staff and are encouraged to be independent. On several dimensions, programs that keep patients out of the hospital longest function somewhat similarly to high release rate programs; that is, they emphasize Order and Organization, Practical Orientation, and some Staff Control. On the other hand, these programs are quite different from high release rate programs on the dimension of "expressiveness." High community tenure programs encourage, whereas high release rate programs inhibit, the open, spontaneous expression of feelings, including angry feelings.

TABLE 8.6   COMMUNITY TENURE SCALE ITEMS AND SCORING KEY

Scored Direction	Item
False	Staff never start arguments in group meetings.
True	On this ward staff think it is a healthy thing to argue.
True	Patients are expected to share their personal problems with each other.
True	Patients are encouraged to show their feelings.
True	Staff sometimes argue with each other.
False	A lot of patients just seem to be passing time on the ward.
False	There is very little emphasis on what patients will be doing after they leave.
True	Patients are encouraged to learn new ways of doing things.
True	Patients will be transferred from this ward if they don't obey the rules.
True	Patients are rarely kept waiting when they have appointments with staff.
True	The staff set an example for neatness and orderliness.
True	Patients here are encouraged to be independent.

In summary, three treatment outcome scales were developed, using patient and staff perceptions of treatment environment in two independent studies. Both patient and staff perceptions on the three scales significantly correlated with the outcome criterion for that scale and did not correlate with the outcome criterion for either of the other two scales. Patients and staff showed extremely high agreement on the specific characteristics of their programs.

The final analysis was performed to provide information on the relationship between (a) objective ward characteristics and patient background characteristics and (b) the three outcome scales and the three outcome criteria. The patient and staff scales and the treatment outcome criteria were correlated, separately, with ward size and staffing in each of the two studies. Only five of the resulting 36 rank-order correlations were statistically significant, and no significant correlation was replicated in both studies.

In the first study, we calculated the proportion of married patients, the proportion of patients diagnosed schizophrenic, and the median length of previous hospital stay; for each ward, both for the total patient cohort and for the released patients only. Rank-order correlations were calculated over wards between the three patient background characteristics and both the treatment outcome scales and the treatment outcome criteria. There were no significant correlations either for the total patient group or for the group of released patients.

In the second study, the only information available was on the proportions of released married patients and released patients diagnosed schizophrenic. These two variables were correlated with the outcome scales and the outcome criteria, and only two of the resulting 18 correlations were statistically significant. The proportions of patients married and diagnosed schizophrenic were related positively and negatively, respectively, to patient perceptions on the release rate scale. Although it would have been better if we had been able to collect data on the entire patient cohort in the second study (including chronicity), the results fail to indicate consistent relationships between the ward or patient characteristics measured and either the outcome scales or the outcome criteria. Thus the correlations between the outcome scales and actual treatment outcome were not mediated by these characteristics.

EXAMPLES OF EFFECTIVE AND INEFFECTIVE PROGRAMS

The results just enumerated are made more meaningful by specific examples of contrasting wards in each of the two outcome studies. Figures 8.1 and 8.2 show the WAS Form C profiles for patients and staff on wards E-1 and H-1, respectively. Ward E-1 had the highest proportion of patients who stayed in the community for 6 months after release and the third highest release rate, whereas ward H-1 had the lowest community tenure rate and the third highest dropout rate.

Patients on ward E-1 perceived the treatment milieu as significantly

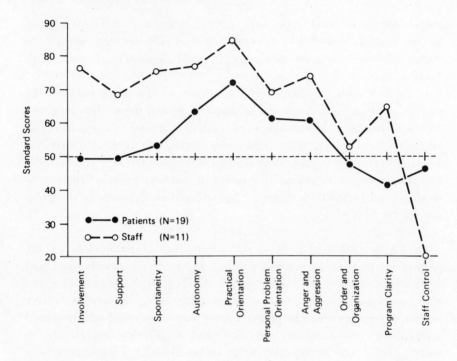

Figure 8.1   WAS Form C profiles for patients and staff on ward E-1.

above average on all four Treatment Program dimensions and somewhat below average on the three System Maintenance dimensions. Staff saw the ward as very high on the Relationship and Treatment Program dimensions. Staff also felt that the program was clear and explicit and ran with relatively little direction from them. The treatment milieu on ward H-1 was quite different. Patients perceived average emphasis on Autonomy and Anger and Aggression, but they saw much less emphasis on the other two Treatment Program dimensions. They also reported moderate emphasis on Staff Control. Thus the patients felt that the staff generally controlled the program but they did not believe that the program was particularly clear and explicit nor that there was a concentrated effort to prepare them for release or to deal with their personal problems. Compared with ward E-1, patients on ward H-1 perceived the Relationship and System Maintenance dimensions (except Staff Control) in much the same terms, but they differed markedly in their perception of the Treatment Program dimensions.

Staffs on wards H-1 and E-1 also saw their respective programs quite

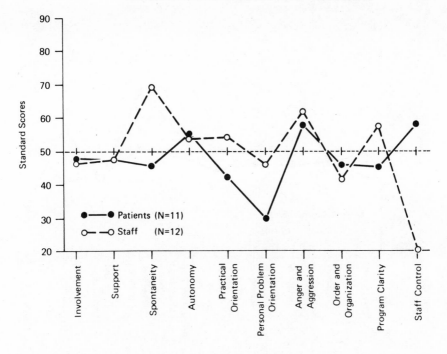

Figure 8.2   WAS Form C profiles for patients and staff on ward H-1.

differently. These differences were most apparent in the Relationship dimensions of Involvement and Support and in all four Treatment Program dimensions. The staff of ward H-1 agreed in general with patient perceptions of the ward milieu, Spontaneity and Staff Control being the two major exceptions. Thus in study one the highest (ward E-1) and the lowest (ward H-1) community tenure rate wards had quite different treatment milieus according to patients and staff alike.

The two wards differed sharply from the average of our 160 American wards on the community tenure scale. Mean patient and staff scores on the three treatment outcome scales for the 15 VA wards were relatively similar to the overall means of the three outcome scales obtained on our total normative sample of 160 American Wards. This indicated that our 15 study wards constituted a relatively representative sample, in terms of treatment milieus, of the entire American normative group. Nevertheless, patients on ward E-1 scored 1.5 standard deviations above average, and staff scored 2 standard deviations above average on the community tenure scale. In

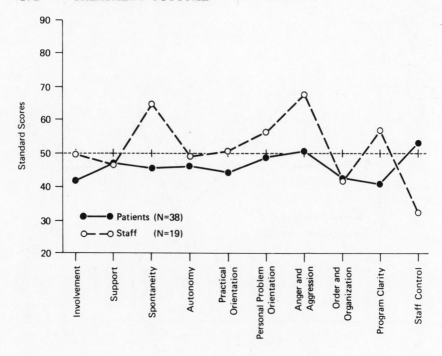

Figure 8.3 WAS Form C profiles for patients and staff on ward A-2.

contrast, both patients and staff on ward H-1 scored approximately 1.5 standard deviations below average on the community tenure scale.

For example, 68% of the patients and 82% of the staff on ward E-1 agreed that "Patients are expected to share their personal problems with each other." Only 9% of the patients and 36% of the staff on ward H-1 agreed with this statement. Furthermore, 63% of the patients and 100% of the staff on ward E-1 agreed that "Staff sometimes argue with each other," whereas only 36% of patients and 58% of staff on ward H-1 agreed with the same statement. There were also large differences between the two wards on most of the other community tenure scale items. Illustratively, patients and staff on ward E-1 agreed much more often to the following items: "On this ward staff think it is a healthy thing to argue," "Patients are encouraged to show their feelings," "Staff sometimes argue with each other," "Patients will be transferred from this ward if they don't obey the rules," and "Patients here are encouraged to be independent."

Figures 8.3 and 8.4 represent the WAS Form C profiles for patients and

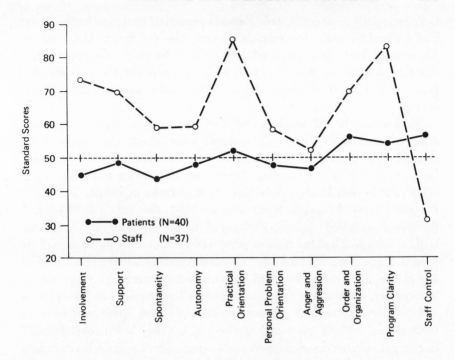

Figure 8.4   WAS Form C profiles for patients and staff on ward G-2.

staff on two contrasting wards in our second outcome study. Ward A-2 had the highest dropout rate and the second lowest release rate, whereas ward G-2 had the lowest dropout rate and the highest release rate. The profile for ward G-2 indicates that patients saw the treatment milieu as somewhat above average in emphasis on four dimensions: Practical Orientation, Order and Organization, Program Clarity, and Staff Control. Thus by patient perceptions this ward had a relatively structured and specific program in which staff exercised a high amount of control and took a practical, "no nonsense" approach to treatment. Staff saw ward G-2 as extremely high on Practical Orientation, Order and Organization, and Program Clarity; in addition, they judged the program to be substantially above average in Involvement and Support. By staff perceptions ward G-2 obtained the highest scores on all five of these dimensions (as compared with the other six wards in this study), and it obtained the lowest score on Anger and Aggression, as well.

The treatment milieu on ward A-2 was quite different from that on ward

G-2, especially as seen by staff. Patients perceived moderate emphasis on Staff Control but much less emphasis on the other two System Maintenance dimensions. Thus the patients felt that the staff controlled the program but that the program itself was not very clear and explicit. The patients also believed that the emphasis on Practical Orientation was moderately below average.

Staffs on wards A-2 and G-2 saw their respective programs in radically different manners. These differences were most apparent on the Relationship dimensions of Involvement and Support, on the Treatment Program dimensions of Practical Orientation and Anger and Aggression, and on the System Maintenance dimensions of Order and Organization and Program Clarity. In specific contrast to ward G-2, the staff on ward A-2 had the lowest perceived emphasis on each of the five dimensions on which the staff on ward G-2 had the highest perceived emphasis; in addition, staff on ward A-2 saw more emphasis on Anger and Aggression than did the staff on any of the other six wards. Staff on ward A-2 reported high emphasis on Spontaneity, but this was in the context of the low emphasis on Involvement and Support. Thus staff encouraged the free and open expression of feelings, particularly anger and aggression, but they failed concomitantly to give patients necessary support and to emphasize a practical orientation; moreover, they did not provide a clear and explicit ward treatment program.

Again, as would be expected, wards A-2 and G-2 contrasted sharply in terms of their actual scores on the dropout and release rate scales; staff on A-2 scored more than 2 standard deviations above the mean on the dropout scale, whereas staff on ward G-2 scored 2 standard deviations below. In terms of specific item examples, patients and staff on ward A-2 (highest dropout rate) answered false considerably more often to the following items: "Most patients follow a regular schedule each day," "This is a very well organized ward," and "Staff go out of their way to help patients." On the other hand, both patients and staff on ward G-2 answered true much more often to the following items on the release rate scale: "Patients are encouraged to plan for the future," "Patients must make plans before leaving the hospital," and "Once a schedule is arranged for a patient, the patient must follow it." Again, these item examples are given to convey a somewhat more specific flavor of the sharply contrasting milieus on wards A-2 and G-2.

OVERVIEW OF RESULTS

Perceived ward climate is related very consistently to different indices of treatment outcome. In addition, specific characteristics of the treatment environments of relatively small and relatively large male VA psychiatric programs· are differentially related to different criteria of treatment outcome.

Patients and staff saw wards with high dropout rates as low in Involvement, Support, Order and Organization, and Program Clarity. Staff were seen as discouraging criticism and as generally unresponsive to patient influence. Patients tended to gripe and criticize or joke about staff. Significantly, patients and staff agreed about such unfavorable program characteristics. The relationships noted between dropout rates and treatment environment are consistent with those of Spiegel and Younger (1972), who found that ward elopement rates were significantly negatively related to the amount of personnel concern for patients, ward morale, and warmth of ward climate.

Some possible variables mediating between overall treatment milieu and dropout rate are suggested by our results in Chapter 7. Involvement, Autonomy, Personal Problem Orientation, and Order and Organization are positively related to patient satisfaction, to how much patients like other patients and staff, and to perceived opportunities for personal development. Since all these dimensions are also negatively related to dropout rate, programs with high dropout rates are more likely to have patients who are generally dissatisfied, who do not particularly like one another, and who feel that they have limited opportunities to enhance their self-confidence. In addition, programs lacking emphasis on Involvement and Order and Organization have less helping activity in the areas of friendship, enhancement of self-esteem, and directive teaching.

Dropout rates are seldom used as indicators of treatment outcome. Programs with high dropout rates are probably relatively ineffective with at least a certain proportion of patients, however, and this proportion is surprisingly high for many programs. For example, the number of patients who either eloped or were discharged against medical advice on our seven large wards during the 3-month study period was 387, versus 725 patients who were actually released. Thus out of 1312 patients who left the hospital during the 3-month study period, nearly one-third simply dropped out of the program or insisted on being discharged against the advice of their doctors. This proportion was much less for the eight small wards; even there, however, one out of the five patients who left the hospital departed without a medical release. The rates on the eight small wards ranged from 0.04 to 0.45 for a 6-month period whereas the rates on the seven large wards ranged from 0.32 to 0.79 for a 3-month period. Ward dropout rates must be used as an additional treatment outcome criterion in subsequent studies, and patients who drop out of treatment should be followed longitudinally whenever possible.

Programs with high release rates seem to place strong emphasis on practical orientation but not on the open, spontaneous expression of feelings. These wards are perceived as well organized and explicit and clear in their program policies. Patients and staff agree that there is a certain pride and involvement on high release rate wards, even though—or perhaps because—they focus on practical decision making and information gathering within a somewhat unexpressive context.

Relating these results to those of Chapter 7 indicates that the patients on high release rate wards are probably more satisfied, like other patients and staff more, and feel that the program helps increase their abilities and self-confidence. Patients on these wards would probably see a high amount of helping activity in the areas of friendship, enhancement of self-esteem, and directive teaching—exactly the reverse of the situation on high dropout rate wards.

The results relating treatment environment and release rate are generally consistent with those of Ellsworth et al. (1971), who found that high release rate wards tended not to promote patient autonomy and were perceived somewhat more negatively by staff. All the studies agree that wards that are most successful in releasing patients specifically prepare the patients for release from the hospital and emphasize new and practical ways of doing things. The studies also agree that high release rate wards do not emphasize Relationship dimenions; that is, they do not encourage patients to become involved with the ward or to act openly and express their feelings toward other patients and staff.

Finally, wards that are successful in keeping patients out of the hospital emphasize Autonomy and Independence, a Practical Orientation, Order and Organization, and a reasonable degree of Staff Control. They also emphasize Personal Problem Orientation and the free and open expression of Anger. These wards apparently functioned similarly on several dimensions to high release rate wards: specifically, both kinds of wards emphasized Order and Organization, Practical Orientation, and to some extent Staff Control. On the other hand, the former were quite different from high release rate wards on the dimension of "expressiveness". The open, spontaneous expression of feelings tended to be encouraged by high community tenure wards and inhibited by high release rate wards. From the results in Chapter 7 we can infer that the patients on high community tenure wards are generally satisfied, like other patients and staff, feel they can enhance their self esteem in the program, and perceive a high amount of friendship and the enhancement of self-esteem type of helping activity.

The results just summarized are also quite consistent with those of earlier studies concerned with the characteristics of programs most successful in keeping patients out of the hospital. Kellam et al. (1967) learned that patients did better on wards with larger social clusters and high staff-patient contact. Ellsworth et al. found that units with high community tenure were those in which nursing staff saw themselves as active participants and the professional staff as motivated and non-dominant.

In terms of our tripartite categorization of Relationship, Treatment Program and System Maintenance dimensions, programs with high dropout rates have little emphasis in either the Relationship or the System Maintenance area. Programs with high release rates are relatively strong in System Maintenance and in the Treatment Program area of Practical Orientation. In addition, they are perceived as having moderate emphasis on the Relationship area of Involvement. Programs that keep patients out of the hospital longest place a high degree of emphasis in the Relationship and System Maintenance dimensions and also in the Treatment Program dimensions, particularly Autonomy and Practical Orientation.

Although we looked for consistencies in results for large and small wards, it should be noted that the difference in the general sizes of the two groups of wards studied may play a role in the approach and success of their treatment programs. Careful comparison of the contrasting profiles from the two outcome studies illustrates what may be a difference in general treatment orientation between the two groups of wards. Indeed, it is possible that a somewhat different balance of dimensions is associated with successful outcome for programs of differing size. The most successful program in study two (ward G-2) deviated considerably from the average of the seven wards on the System Maintenance dimensions; its scores were more than 1.5 standard deviations above the mean on Order and Organization and Program Clarity, and it had the second highest score on Staff Control. Ward A-2, on the other hand, which had the highest dropout rate and the second lowest release rate, was considerably lower on all three System Maintenance dimensions. Thus there were large differences between the two ward programs on the System Maintenance dimensions, whereas the Treatment Program dimensions were essentially the same for the two wards, with the important exception of Practical Orientation. Figures 8.1 and 8.2 show that ward E-1, which had the highest community tenure rate in the first study, had substantially higher scores on Autonomy, Practical Orientation, and Personal Problem Orientation (i.e., three Treatment Program dimensions) than did the less successful ward H-1. However, these two wards were very similar on both the Relationship and the System Maintenance dimensions. The small wards exhibited greater ward-to-ward variation in the Treatment Program dimensions, whereas for the large wards, ward-to-ward variation was greater in the System Maintenance dimensions.

These comparisons are only suggestive, but they imply that there are certain overall differences in the manner in which large and small "successful" programs function. Well-operating programs may prepare their patients to cope with their immediate environment after release from the hospital in somewhat different ways: successful small wards are more likely to emphasize personal responsibility and the means by which to "make it" after release, coupled with a supportive and helpful environment during the patients' stay on the ward. Successful larger wards, on the other hand, may emphasize staff control and an ordered, regimented environment with no particular emphasis on autonomy—which may be just the kind of living conditions many patients must face once they leave the relative security of the hospital program.

It is particularly important that the present results corroborate those of previous studies in indicating that treatment environment may be at least as important as objective characteristics differentiating among programs, such as size and staffing and patient background characteristics. This conclusion is probably limited to situations in which these structural and patient background characteristics are within a certain range on all programs studied. In previous studies, Kellam at al. found no main effects related to patient-staff ratio and only one related to ward size, and Ellsworth et al. reported negative correlations between staffing and community tenure. Linn (1970) concluded that the presence of hospital policies and programs related more highly to turnover rates than did patient background characteristics. In our study, perceived treatment environment was more highly and consistently related to treatment outcome than were either ward size or staffing or patient background characteristics.

In conclusion, we can discern some relatively consistent findings across studies linking treatment environment and treatment outcome. Since different types of patients react differently to varied ward milieus, there must be important interaction effects between patient and ward milieu characteristics which at least partly determine treatment outcome. We have presented some interesting tentative results relating treatment environment and treatment outcome. More important, however, is our outline of a methodology that might be used profitably by other investigators in this area. The next logical step is to undertake national cooperative studies systematically assessing patient background and behavior, ward characteristics and policies, and treatment environment and treatment outcome. Systematic information about patients' relevant community milieus (i.e., living group or family setting, work situation, and characteristics of relevant social or task-oriented groups) must be included in the studies. In this way it may be possible to obtain more dependable information on the complex interactions among relevant patient, ward program, and community environment characteristics and different treatment outcome criteria.

REFERENCES

Cohen, J. and Struening, E. Opinions about mental illness: Hospital social atmosphere profiles and their relevance to effectiveness. *Journal of Consulting Psychology,* **28**: 291–298, 1964.

Ellsworth, R., Foster, L., Childers, B., Arthur, G., & Kroeker, D. Hospital and community adjustment as perceived by psychiatric patients, their families, and staff. *Journal of Consulting and Clinical Psychology Monographs,* **32**: 1–41, 1968.

Ellsworth, R., Maroney, R., Klett, W.,Gordon, H., & Gunn, R. Milieu characteristics of successful psychiatric treatment programs. *American Journal of Orthopsychiatry,* **41**: 427–441, 1971.

Gurel, L. Correlates of psychiatric hospital effectiveness. In Gurel, L. (Ed.) Intramural Report 64-5, *An assessment of psychiatric hospitals effectiveness,* VA Psychiatric Evaluation Project, Washington, D.C., 1964.

Kellam, S., Sheppard, G., Goldberg, A., Schooler, N. Berman, A., & Shmelzer, J., Ward atmosphere and outcome of treatment of acute schizophrenia. *Journal of Psychiatric Research,* **5**: 145–163, 1967.

Linn, L. State hospital environment and rates of patient discharge. *Archives of General Psychiatry,* **23**: 346–351, 1970.

Moos, R. & Schwartz, J., Treatment environment and treatment outcome. *Journal of Nervous and Mental Disease,* **154**: 264–275, 1972.

Spiegel, D. & Younger, J. Ward climate and community stay of psychiatric patients. *Journal of Consulting and Clinical Psychology*, **39**: 62–69, 1972.

Ullmann, L. *Institution and outcome: A comparative study of psychiatric hospitals*, Oxford, Pergamon Press, 1967.

Chapter Nine

DEVIANT PERCEPTIONS

There is an extensive literature on the various tendencies to respond deviantly, particularly to testing situations and paper-and-pencil questionnaires. Deviant responses have been regarded as particular kinds of response sets or biases. The literature on response sets is vast, and a number of kinds of response sets (e.g., acquiescence, evasiveness, social desirability, and denial) have been identified. Investigators have also studied such simple response biases as turning right instead of left when entering a museum or gallery and calling "heads" more often than "tails".

Berg (1955) was interested in the relation between deviant response patterns and personality. He believed that biased responses were general and that deviation in one area was associated with deviation in other areas. Berg noted that this hypothesis could be tested simply by identifying the common or modal responses to any suitable series of stimuli and predicting that subjects whose responses consistently go against these modal preferences will be deviant in the sense of exhibiting symptom patterns associated with abnormal states. He felt that the types of stimulus patterns used were largely irrelevant as long as they were sufficiently unstructured-
—that is, they bore the potential to bring out a deviant response set. In summaries of his work, Berg (1955, 1959) presents a number of studies supporting these notions.

The main thrust of Berg's deviation hypothesis is that deviant response tendencies are general across different kinds of item content and different kinds of perceptual and other experimental tests. In an important paper in this area, Sechrest and Jackson (1962) studied several alternative conceptual definitions of deviant behavior patterns, aiming to appraise their generality across diverse response classes. They took three approaches to the understanding of deviant response patterns: (1) a correlational approach, based on the assumptions that deviation is unidirectional and that subjects deviant on one measure will be consistently deviant in either a high or a low direction on other measures; (2) the identification of individuals deviant in any direction across a number of measures, based on the assumption that deviation may be bidirectional and that subjects deviantly high or low on one measure will be deviant in one direction *or* the other on additional measures; and (3) the study of those subjects on either extreme of a deviation measure, based on the assumption that individuals may be deviant by choosing deviant alternatives either more frequently *or* less frequently than most persons.

They utilized male and female college students in one group and female nursing students in a second group. The measures of deviancy were obtained from the subjects' responses to the Welsh Figure Preference Test, an Independence–Conformity Inventory, a Person Preference Test, and three Minnesota Multiphasic Personality Inventory (MMPI) subscales. The authors concluded that generality was quite limited even when the possibility that deviation may occur in either direction was taken into account. When the deviation measures were scored so that subjects could be classed as either atypically nondeviant or atypically deviant, significant relationships were obtained with reputational unconventionality and atypicality, suggesting that there may be a "normal" range of deviation and that individuals deviating in either direction from this normal range may be atypical. The results showed that deviant response tendencies were not a "general trait" as Berg had hypothesized; rather, it appeared that several types of deviant response tendencies could be identified.

These results are not surprising when viewed in the light of other research on the generality–specificity problem, that is, the problem of the consistency of different types of questionnaire responses and behavioral actions across a variety of settings. As briefly reviewed in Chapter 1, the variance accounted for by consistent differences among settings and by the interaction between setting characteristics and personal characteristics is usually as great or greater than the variance accounted for by consistent differences among persons. Basically this research corroborates exactly what Sechrest and Jackson concluded—namely, that the generality of deviant perceptions cannot be assumed and that it may be fruitful to think in terms of different types of deviant response tendencies.

Types of Deviant Response Tendencies

Four types of deviant response tendencies were investigated. The first measure was the extent to which the individual perceived his treatment milieu deviantly from the norm, regardless of direction. The second measure was the overall discrepancy between the individual's views of an ideal treatment milieu and the normative ideal conceptualizations on his ward. The general prediction was made that individuals who perceived their treatment milieus deviantly and/or who held deviant values would feel less satisfied, would like other patients less, would feel that they had less favorable opportunity to enhance their personal development, and would see themselves as taking fewer "positive' initiatives in the program.

The third deviancy measure was a directional deviancy score marking the extent to which an individual perceived the milieu as more positive or more negative than other people. This measure was utilized because of some intriguing findings, by investigators on psychiatric wards and in other environments, suggesting that individuals who see their environments more positively are actually more satisfied and do better in those environments. For example, Kish et al. (1971), utilizing the WAS, learned that patients who obtained high Internal scores on the Rotter I–E control Scale perceived their ward more positively on 8 of the 10 WAS subscales. The authors also found that the Internals were hospitalized for a shorter period and that they perceived themselves as taking more initiatives in the areas of Involvement, Support, Practical Orientation, and Staff Control. They note that the differences in perceptions may be realistic, since the Internal patient is seen by staff as having a greater potential for improvement and is thus treated in a more therapeutic fashion. Patients may perceive treatment milieus more positively when the milieus are in fact more positive for them.

In an interesting corroborative study, Ellsworth and Maroney (1972) attempted to determine whether patients who report positive ward attributes actually behave differently from those who report negative ones. Staff rated the behavior of 75 patients on a scale measuring the patients' cooperation, ability to communicate with staff, ability to plan realistically, and so on. A total score of cooperation–communication behavior was computed for each patient. Statistically significant correlations were found between patient behavior as rated by staff and the Perception of Ward (POW) scores of 75 patients. The patients who saw their program and experiences in more positive terms were rated by staff as being more cooperative and communicative than those who reported negative experiences.

In another study reported in the same article, Ellsworth and Maroney obtained POW scales at the time of release for patients who had been in the hospital at least 14 days and for whom data on later community adjustment were also available. Analyses of the relationships between perceptions of staff receptivitiy and outcome scores (adjusted for initial symptom severity) were made for different subgroups of patients. The findings indicated that patient perception of staff receptivity correlated positively with adjusted outcome scores for the following groups of patients: (a) patients who were single (never married), (b) patients whose relatives indicated they had "never" functioned adequately, (c) patients with high prehospitalization ratings on anger and agitation, (d) patients with high scores on prehospitalization employment, (e) patients whose relatives indicated they had "agreed" to come to the hospital, (f) patients with low prehospitalization ratings on confusion, and (g) patients with some college education.

The authors speculated that these subgroups of patients might experience better community adjustment if they were treated in a program high in staff receptivity. In an intriguing study testing this hypothesis they found that five of the seven specified patient subgroups had treatment outcomes in the predicted direction when treated in a program characterized as high in staff receptivity (as contrasted with a different program). It is important to note that differences in treatment effectiveness between the two programs for these patient cohorts were not accounted for by better overall treatment outcomes for one program. Thus the staff receptivity characteristics of a program may be differentially effective for particular patient subgroups, which apparently can be identified by careful analyses of their directional and deviancy scores.

In another study Herr (1965) was concerned with the question of whether students who achieved well academically perceive the environmental press of their high school differently from students who had poor records of academic achievement. Herr found that students categorized as high or middle achievers perceived more press for affiliation and dependence on others, assistance and protection, intense open emotional display, detached impersonal thinking, problem-solving analysis and theorizing, and so on. The low achieving students perceived more press for such characteristics as self-depreciation and self-evaluation, indifference or disregard for the feelings of others, direct or indirect aggression, and withholding friendship and support. These results suggest that students who see their high school environments more positively are also better achievers.

According to the findings just outlined, then, people who see their environments more positively are more satisfied with and perform better in those environments. Our third measure of directional deviancy was derived with the idea of replicating these findings.

The fourth score—the similarity between the individual's perception of the ward milieu and his view of an ideal milieu—is an individual real–ideal similarity score rather than a measurement of discrepancies from a norm. Substantial research in other areas indicates that real–ideal similarities are strongly related to various measures of adjustment. Initially, work was done on the relations between real–self and ideal–self perceptions, and the congruence between the two was used as a measure of adjustment and also as a measure of the outcome of individual psychotherapy (Rogers, 1951; Rogers and Dymond, 1954).

Pervin (1967a) studied college characteristics and student–college interaction using his Transactional Analysis of Personality and Environment (TAPE), an instrument based on the semantic differential. Students from 21 colleges rated several concepts on 52 different scales. These concepts were: my college, myself, students, faculty, administration, and ideal college. Ratings of satisfaction with different aspects of college life were also made. In general, discrepancies between student perceptions of themselves and of their college were related to dissatisfaction with college. Pervin also noted that the extent of this relationship varied considerably across schools: for example, correlation between the item "In terms of your own needs and desires, how satisfied are you with the academic aspects of your college?" and self–college discrepancy varied from a low of −.18 to a high of .65 in different colleges. Pervin (1967b) replicated these results in a further study and also reported that satisfaction with the environment did not simply reflect satisfaction with self. Pervin and Smith (1968) had 169 subjects rate the concepts of self, ideal–self, and my club on 52 adjective scales. Perceived self–club similarity was found to be related to ratings of satisfaction with the club environment. Thus satisfaction with the environment was not merely a reflection of satisfaction with the self.

In a final relevant study we utilized two samples of institutionalized delinquent males and tested the validity of the concept that satisfaction with one's environment represents an instance of person–environment fit (Trickett and Moos, 1972). Delinquents were asked to use a semantic differential technique in rating themselves and various reference groups (e.g., guards) in the institution. The similarity between self ratings and ratings of other groups was correlated with reported satisfaction about various aspects of the institution. Self-environment similarity was correlated with satisfaction with the environment, but only for specific relationships; that is, similarity to guards correlated with satisfaction with guards but not with satisfaction with the institution in general. Thus greater congruence between self conceptions and perceptions of real and ideal environments. is related to greater satisfaction with the environment.

Four Measures of Deviancy

Let us review the four measures of deviancy that were developed.

1.   Total Deviancy (real) is the absolute discrepancy between an individual's perception of the treatment milieu and the normative perception of his reference group (i.e., patients or staff).

2.   Total Deviancy (ideal) is the absolute discrepancy between an individual's views of an ideal treatment milieu and the normative ideal milieu conceptualizations of his reference group.

3.   Directional Deviancy reflects the extent to which an individual perceives his treatment milieu as more or less positive than his reference group. High scores on the first nine subscales and a low score on Staff Control were considered to be in the "more positive" direction.

4.   Real–Ideal Similarity is the squared difference summed over subscales between the individual's perception of his treatment milieu and his view of an ideal treatment milieu.

The 23 wards we studied in one state hospital as described in Chapter 7, provided the basic data. Patients and staff on these wards had taken Forms C and I of the WAS and had reported their general reactions to the ward. There were only moderate intercorrelations among the four Deviancy scores. For example, Total Deviancy (real) correlated positively (.31) with Total Deviancy (ideal) and negatively with both Real–Ideal Similarity (–.29) and Directional Deviancy (–.30) The highest correlation (.41) was between Directional Deviancy and Real–Ideal Similarity. The results indicate that these four Deviancy measures, although moderately correlated, assess somewhat different aspects of deviant perceptions.

Total Deviancy (Real and Ideal)

In the next set of analyses the real and ideal Total Deviancy scores were correlated (over patients, within each of the 23 wards) with the individual patient's reactions to the program. The number of cases varied somewhat from ward to ward but was usually between 35 and 65 patients. Table 9.1 shows the mean correlation, the number of within-ward correlations in the predicted direction ($N = 23$), and the number of significant within-ward correlations. In general, the results serve to confirm the predictions (except for anxiety), although the correlations are of only modest size.

Thus patients who see their program (either real or ideal) in a deviant manner also feel less satisfied, like the staff less, and feel they have fewer opportunities for personal development. Since there was some interward variability in the magnitude and in the direction of these relationships, a further analysis was carried out. The logic followed an analysis we had performed in an earlier study (Trickett and Moos, 1972). We gave the Correctional Institutions Environment Scale (CIES) to residents in two correctional units, to provide evidence on the similarities of the unit social environments. The aim was to replicate a relationship between self–environment similarity and satisfaction with the environment across two units. It thus seemed to be important to furnish some objective information regarding the actual similarity between the social climates of the two units. In that study the two units had almost identical CIES profiles, and the findings were generally replicated from one unit to the other.

The logic utilized in the work summarized in Figure 9.1 was analogous though somewhat different. There were six wards on which relatively high and consistently significant correlations were found between Total Deviancy (real) and the other variables. Almost all the relevant correlations were statistically significant on these six wards. Another group of seven wards had correlations that were generally in the right direction, but they were lower than those in the first group. In a third group of eight wards, the correlations between Total Deviancy and the relevant variables were mostly in the right direction, although very few were significant and some were in the reverse direction. Finally, there were two wards on which the correlations between Total Deviancy and general reactions were in the reverse direction; that is, they were consistently positive rather than negative.

Mean standard scores for the patient perceptions on each of these four groups of wards were calculated. Figure 9.1 compares the profiles for group

TABLE 9.1 RELATIONSHIPS BETWEEN TOTAL DEVIANCY SCORES AND PATIENT REACTIONS

| Patient Reactions | Deviancy Scores | | | | | |
| | Total Deviancy (Real) | | | Total Deviancy (Ideal) | | |
	Mean Correlation	Number in Predicted Direction (N = 23)	Number Signifi-cant (N = 23)	Mean Correlation	Number in Predicted Direction (N = 23)	Number Signifi-cant (N = 23)
Satisfaction	−.21	19	8	−.23	20	9
Like staff	−.19	16	7	−.15	20	4
Anxiety	.05	13	3	.10	15	3
Personal Development	−.17	17	5	−.21	17	6

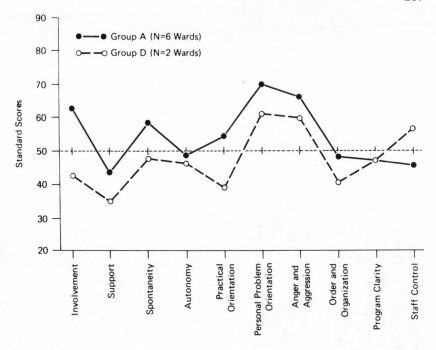

Figure 9.1 WAS Form C patient profiles for six wards in group A and two wards in group D.

A (the six wards on which the results were strongly in the predicted direction) and group D (the two wards on which the results were opposite to the predicted direction). The treatment milieus of the two groups of programs are dramatically different. The programs on which deviant patients were less satisfied have much higher scores on the Relationship dimensions of Involvement and Spontaneity and the Treatment Program dimensions of Practical Orientation and Personal Problem Orientation; in addition, they have a somewhat lower score on Staff Control. Thus the two groups of programs differ from each other on five of the 10 WAS dimensions. The treatment environments of the other two groups of programs fell between the two extreme groups on the same dimensions.

The results confirm our initial prediction—namely, that deviancy should be most substantially related to dissatisfaction on wards having the most active treatment programs. The wards in group A clearly have more active treatment programs than those in group D. Thus deviant perceptions of the environment may be related to such factors as greater individual

TABLE 9.2 RELATIONSHIPS BETWEEN DIRECTIONAL DEVIANCY AND REAL–IDEAL SIMILARITY SCORES AND PATIENT REACTIONS

Patient Reactions	Deviancy Scores					
	Directional Deviancy			Real–Ideal Similarity		
	Mean Correlation	Number in Predicted Direction ($N=23$)	Number Significant ($N=23$)	Mean Correlation	Number in Predicted Direction ($N=23$)	Number Significant ($N=23$)
Satisfaction	.39	23	19	-.29	22	14
Like staff	.35	21	19	-.21	20	8
Anxiety	-.25	18	11	.19	18	7
Personal Development	.38	22	17	-.28	21	15

satisfactions when the environment itself is particularly negative and/or undifferentiated. The characteristics of an environment are themselves critical moderator variables, affecting both the magnitude and the direction of various hypothesized relationships.

Directional Deviancy and Real–Ideal Similarity

Similar intraward correlations were calculated next for each of the 23 wards between the Directional Deviancy and the Real–Ideal Similarity scores and the patient's reactions to the program. Table 9.2 summarizes the results, which are more consistent and more striking than the results for the Total Deviancy scores. Table 9.2 indicates that patients who see their wards more positively feel more satisified, like the staff more, feel less anxious, and feel that the ward gives them a greater chance for personal development. For example, all 23 intraward correlations between Directional Deviancy and general satisfaction are in the right direction, and 19 of the 23 are statistically significant. The results for Real–Ideal Similarity are generally similar, although not quite as strong in magnitude. Since the data are so consistent over the 23 wards, we can also conclude that the relationships between these two scores and general reactions do not vary in different treatment environments, at least to the extent that the treatment environments of the 23 programs themselves varied.

Deviancy and Treatment Outcome

The correlations between deviancy, particularly Directional Deviancy, and more positive reactions to programs may simply indicate that certain patients answer a variety of items (i.e., about the treatment and about their reactions to it) more positively. It is also possible, as the results of Kish et al. suggest, that patients who see their milieu more positively are in fact functioning in a more active goal-directed treatment environment; that is, their Directional Deviancy may reflect accurate perceptions. If so, these patients should be more satisfied. Thus individuals who view their treatment program more positively might have better treatment outcomes at a follow-up interval. Fortunately we had some data that allowed us to make a partial test of this possibility.

As discussed in Chapter 5, two programs were assessed at three different intervals with the WAS. It was thus possible to calculate for each patient in these programs two of the deviancy scores—Total Deviancy (real) and Directional Deviancy. The patients also completed a variety of questionnaires while they were in the hospital; in addition, they were followed up at 6-month and 12- to 18-month intervals.

At the time of each follow-up, patients were asked a number of different questions. Information on eight of the questions was consistent enough within the two patient samples to permit analysis. The eight questions were:

1. In general, how are you getting along most of the time?
2. Most of the time, how is your attitude toward yourself and life in general?
3. In general, how are you getting along with other people?
4. How many friendships do you have (people who mean something to you beyond saying hello)?
5. How is your physical health most of the time?
6. How much tension are you having most of the time?
7. How much depression are you having most of the time?
8. Is drinking causing you any difficulty

Both Total and Directional Deviancy scores were obtained for the patients who had completed the WAS and on whom a variety of other questionnaire data as well as 6-month and final follow-up data were available. The deviancy scores were calculated for each individual patient against the mean scores for the test that had been administered while the patient was in the program. If a patient had taken the WAS twice, the first administration was used. Correlations were then calculated between the individual's Total Deviancy score and the eight follow-up variables, separately, for the 6-month and the final follow-up. There were 40 patients in each of the two programs who had complete data. The results for the experimental program at the 6-month follow-up reveal statistically significant relationships between Total deviancy and all eight follow-up variables (see Table 9.3). Patients who perceived the experimental program deviantly tended to feel more tense and depressed. They also complained of having fewer friends, of experiencing worse physical health and more drinking problems; in addition, they reported a poorer attitude toward self and poorer overall adjustment at the 6-month follow-up interval. Most of these relationships have disappeared at final follow-up, although there are still some negative correlations between Total Deviancy and overall adjustment.

TABLE 9.3   RELATIONSHIPS BETWEEN TOTAL DEVIANCY (REAL) AND FOLLOW-UP VARIABLES IN TWO PROGRAMS

Follow-up Variable	6-Month Follow-up		Final Follow-up	
	Experimental Program ($N = 40$)	Control Program ($N = 40$)	Experimental Program ($N = 40$)	Control Program ($N = 40$)
Overall Adjustment	−.36***	−.16	−.34**	.05
Positive Attitude Toward Self	−.31**	−.06	−.32**	.13
Getting Along Well With Others	−.35**	.30**	−.30**	−.09
High Number of Friends	−.29*	.07	−.16	.02
Physical Health	−.43***	.07	.09	.13
Tension	.27*	−.40***	.10	−.08
Depression	.31**	−.33**	.22	−.03
Drinking Problems	.39***	−.05	−.02	.15

*$p<.10$.
**$p<.05$.
***$p<.01$.

The results for the control program are quite different: specifically, there are few correlations between Total Deviancy and the eight follow-up variables. The three significant relationships appearing at the 6-month follow-up interval are reversed in direction from those in the experimental program. The patients who saw the control program deviantly complained of less tension and less depression and stated that they were getting along better with other people at the 6-month follow-up interval. None of the relationships between Total Deviancy and the follow-up variables was significant in the control program at the final follow-up interval.

The experimental program had a significantly more active, directed, and coherent treatment milieu than did the control program, particularly in the middle and later stages of the project (see Chapter 5). The results further bolster the point that the type of treatment milieu or environment in which an individual functions may operate as a "moderator" variable in the kinds of relationships found between, in this case, deviancy of environmental perceptions and treatment outcome. Patients who saw the experimental program deviantly (i.e., who presumably were not well integrated into the treatment milieu) tended to have a poorer treatment outcome as assessed at the 6-month follow-up interval. There was even some tendency for them to report worse treatment outcome at the final follow-up interval. The control program, on the other hand, disclosed few significant relationships between Total Deviancy and the follow-up variables, and those which did occur were reversed in direction. The patients who saw the control program deviantly did better on at least three of the eight variables at the 6-month follow-up interval.

The findings substantiate one of the well-known risks of directed structured treatment milieus—namely, patients who are not well integrated into such milieus have signficantly poorer outcomes than those who are well-integrated. If the treatment environment is highly structured, a patient must either fit into it (and then presumably perceive it rather accurately) or have a particularly difficult time, thus presumably poorer treatment outcome. It is seldom possible to adapt passively by inaction, or to "fade into the woodwork" in a program of this type. On the other hand, if a treatment milieu does not put specific premium on actively involving each patient in the program, it is possible to adapt by "opting out." In this situation, we would expect deviant perceptions to have little or no relationship to treatment outcome. Finally, insofar as the treatment milieu is disorganized, uninvolving, and unstructured, deviant perceptions may be adaptive and may relate positively to satisfaction and/or actual treatment outcome.

The second analysis related Directional Deviancy to the same eight follow-up variables. In this analysis each of the 10 WAS subscale scores was correlated with each of the follow-up variables for the 6-month and the final follow-up data. Overall, the results indicate that patients who saw the experimental program more positively had a better outcome at both 6-month and final follow-ups. For example, patients who experienced less tension at the 6-month follow-up interval saw the experimental program more positively on nine of the WAS subscales. Patients who complained of less depression at the 6-month follow-up interval saw the experimental program more positively on all 10 WAS dimensions. Patients who saw the control program more positively also tended to show a better treatment outcome at 6-month follow-up, but there was no such tendency at final follow-up. These results corroborate our earlier findings that patients who perceive their treatment milieus more positively actually tend to do better.

Since patient background variables in the two programs were very closely matched, the differences between the results on the two programs almost certainly bear no relation to differences in these variables. On the other hand, it is possible that "better" patients (i.e., those with less previous time in hospital, etc.) perceive their treatment milieus more positively and also state that they are doing well at follow-up. Moreover, it is possible that positive perceptions of treatment milieus are simply mediating variables between more positive patient background characteristics and more positive treatment outcome. This line of reasoning supports the notion discussed earlier that the treatment milieu is in fact more positive for patients whose predicted treatment outcome is more positive, among other things, because staff pay more attention to such patients. Alternative explanations for these results need to be tested out in future research. To some extent, however, treatment outcome may be at least partially predictable from perceptions of the treatment milieu.

INTEGRATION WITH PREVIOUS RESEARCH

The extent to which a patient perceives his treatment environment deviantly (and/or is deviant from the value norms held by other patients in the environment) is negatively related to the patient's reactions to his program and to his treatment outcome as assessed at follow-up. Basically, patients who see their treatment milieu deviantly are less satisfied, like the staff less, feel that what they are doing is less likely to enhance their abilities and their self-esteem, and feel that they are doing less well at 6-month follow-up. Whereas deviancy per se has mild negative consequences in most situations, the relationship between deviancy and reactions to the program and the treatment outcome varies as a function of the characteristics of the milieu. The social milieu is a "moderator" variable; deviancy must be viewed as an adaptive reaction in some milieus. Perhaps, then, experimental research does not generalize across settings precisely because the settings have important differential characteristics. Social climate indices may have utility both in selecting environments in which replication studies should be carried out and in providing explanations for the failure of certain relationships to be replicated in varying milieus.

We also found that individuals who perceived greater real–ideal milieu similarity were more satisfied with the milieu, liked the staff more, and felt less anxious and better able to develop their personal abilities. The strongest and most consistent finding is that people who view environments more positively do better in those environments. These results are corroborative of work described earlier in the chapter, (e.g., Ellsworth and Maroney, 1972; and Herr, 1965). Kish et al., concluded, as do we, that patients perceive treatment milieus positively when these milieus are positive for them.

Some additional literature provides further rationale for these findings. Rapoport (1960) has presented intriguing findings relating to value discrepancies. The staff he studied considered their values to be representative of "normal" society and viewed deviation from such values as evidence of personal pathology. Rapoport found that new patients had a range of values vis-a-vis the treatment ideology and that these could not be simply attributed to their psychopathology or their background. New patients whose values initially resembled those of the program and new patients who subsequently adopted the program's values adjusted better in the hospital and were considered to be more improved on discharge than were those with discrepant views. These results corroborate our own; however, Rapoport found that whereas congruent values were good predictors of success in the program, they were notably less successful predictors of good adjustment after discharge.

Many previous studies have indicated that nonconformity results in rejection from the group (e.g., Sherif and Cantril, 1947). Festinger, Schachter, and Back (1950) reported that group deviants received far fewer psychometric choices than did conformers. Schachter (1951), investigating the consequences of deviation from a group standard, learned that the group deviate was the most rejected individual, whereas people who took the "mode" position were least rejected. Individuals called "sliders" (they took a deviant position initially, but later changed toward the group norm) were in between, indicating the relevance of training people to be less deviant. Schachter also found that deviation resulted in receipt of more peripheral assignments in the role structure of the group (i.e., being on less influential committees) and that deviates were rejected more in high than in low cohesive groups. This supports our finding that the consequences of deviancy are related to the overall characteristics of the milieu.

Wood et al. (1966) found that inmates labeled "troublemakers" by correctional institution staff differed significantly from other inmates in the way they perceived their institution. These investigators assessed inmates' definitions of the institution in three separate areas: (1) as an opportunity structure, (2) as an authority structure, and (3) as a predictable environment in which future events are contingent on one's behavior. They found that inmates whose definitions were positive or favorable were the ones who adapted to the institution, cooperated with its constraints, and made productive use of its resources. Significantly, they also found that demographic life history and delinquency history variables did not differentiate among high and low "troublemaking" inmates.

Wood et al. point out that the results leave open the question of whether deviant perceptions arise during the course of the institutionalization or are brought to the institution by the inmate. This is relevant for the institutional staff in choosing an intervention strategy. If the inmate arrives at his perceptions mainly through his institutional experiences, personnel could concentrate on monitoring, regulating, or changing those experiences. If individuals have initial negative expectations, on the other hand, change efforts might best be concentrated in the early period of commitment, with heavy emphasis on countering unfavorable views by structuring and interpreting the setting in the most acceptable and meaningful way possible. Since an individual's adaptation is related to his perceptions of his milieu, it is in the interests of an institution to see that its resources and objectives are not misinterpreted.

Role Induction in Individual and Group Psychotherapy

Many investigators and clinicians have felt that providing systematic information about a new milieu or a new experience helps to socialize an individual and increases the probability of positive outcome. Anticipatory socialization experiences for patients or staff who have tendencies to perceive their environments deviantly might enhance their satisfaction with and functioning in the milieu. Work of this sort has been carried out in individual and group psychotherapy settings.

Orne and Wender (1968) suggested that some patients who lacked motivation for treatment might be capable of profiting from psychotherapy if they were taught what to expect—that is, if they understood the "rules of the game." They state that since inadequate socialization generally has negative effects, explicit anticipatory socialization procedures for individual psychotherapy patients should be beneficial. Hoehn-Saric et al. (1964) studied the effects on psychiatric outpatients of a pretreatment interview designed to clarify the patients' expectations of psychotherapy and to increase the congruence of their behavior with therapists' expectations of how psychiatric patients should act. Lennard and Bernstein (1960) have commented that dissymmetry of expectations between patients and therapists interferes with the therapeutic task and is an important reason for the premature termination of treatment often requested by patients who are less educated and whose cultural background differs from that of most therapists. Hoehn-Saric et al. utilized 40 patients; 20 were prepared for psychotherapy with a role induction interview; and 20 served as controls. The experimental group exhibited better therapy behavior than the control group on five different measures; also, they had a better attendance rate, were rated more favorably by therapists, and showed more favorable treatment outcome.

Sloane et al. (1970) attempted to distinguish between the effects of giving information and the hope-inducing suggestion of improvement. They studied four groups of neurotic patients who received different indoctrinations by a research psychiatrist. The first group was assigned to a psychotherapist without further explanation, whereas the second group was told that they would feel and function better after 4 months of psychotherapy. The third group had an anticipatory socialization interview that provided information but did not suggest that improvement would occur. The fourth group obtained information about psychotherapy and was told that they would feel and function better after 4 months of treatment. The patients who received an explanation about psychotherapy improved significantly more than those who did not. The suggestion that patients would feel better in 4 months had no effect on outcome. As a matter of fact, patients who received this suggestion were judged by therapists to be less likeable than those who did not. These findings indicate that giving information may be more important than holding out the expectation of improvement.

Yalom et al. (1967) have extended this procedure to preparing patients for group therapy. They found that an initial role induction interview strongly increased the extent of "here and now" interpersonal interaction and slightly increased the faith in group therapy of the oriented patients. They also pointed out that in laboratory groups increased clarity of goals and of the methods of goal attainment resulted in greater member attraction to the group, increased sympathy for group emotions, decreased hostility among members, increased motivation, increased member security, increased efficiency, and decreased member frustration. Ambiguous group member role expectations reduce group satisfaction and group productivity.

To our knowledge, no one has systematically experimented with giving information about treatment milieus to incoming patients or staff. The evidence from individual and group psychotherapy strongly indicates that this approach would be desirable. Modeling procedures might supplement direct information-giving techniques. Heller (1971) has observed that there have been a number of psychotherapy analog studies demonstrating that modeling procedures facilitate the discussion of personally revealing topics. Studies have revealed (a) that modeling procedures provide an effective means of teaching role behaviors, particularly when task instructions are ambiguous; (b) that modeling procedures can be useful in inducing realistic expectations of therapy, even for chronic psychotic patients, and (c) that modeling procedures may be most effective when the consequences of the model are either positive or neutral (as would generally be the case with psychiatric treatment).

In this connection, Vanderhoff (1969) investigated the effects of group counseling on low achieving students' perceptions of their college environment and on their grade point average. The logic was that the unsuccessful student may relate less well to the environment of the college than his more successful classmate and that counseling may help him to better understand his institution by providing him with a greater opportunity to achieve his educational goals. Analysis of item responses to CUES indicated that higher achieving students attributed less importance to belonging to the right club or group and felt that course work was less demanding and required less outside preparation than did lower achieving students. Higher achieving students had a better understanding of the opportunities provided by the institution. However, group counseling did not appear to be effective in altering the low achieving students' perception of their college environment.

The presentation of information about treatment milieus to prospective patients and/or staff might serve to reduce their discrepant perceptions and to enhance their treatment progress (or work adjustment), especially if the type of information and its manner of presentation are congruent with the individual's preferred coping styles. As discussed in Chapter 11, written program descriptions often give a somewhat inadequate or incomplete picture of the treatment milieu; thus they may exaggerate discrepant perceptions—exactly the reverse of the intended effect. There is a need for systematic investigation of different methods of writing and presenting program descriptions, as well as other methods for informing patients and staff about ongoing program characteristics. Accurate, well-presented information about the treatment milieu represents the first step in enhancing adjustment to the milieu and beneficial patient outcome.

REFERENCES

Berg, I. Response bias and personality: The deviation hypothesis. *Journal of Psychology*, **40**: 61–72, 1955.

Berg, I. The unimportance of test item content. In Bass, B. & Berg, I. (Eds.). *Objective approaches to personality assessment.* Van Nostrand—Reinhold, New York, 1959.

Ellsworth, R. & Maroney, R. Characteristics of psychiatric programs, and their effects on patients' adjustment. *Journal of Consulting and Clinical Psychology*, **39**: 436–447, 1972.

Festinger, L., Schachter, S., & Back, K. *Social pressures in informal groups: A study of housing community.* Harper & Row, New York, 1950.

Herr, E. Differential perceptions of "environmental press" by high school students. *Personnel and Guidance Journal*, **7**: 678–686, 1965.

Hoehn-Saric, R., Frank, J., Imber, S., Nash, E., Stone, A., & Battle, C. Systematic preparation of patients for psychotherapy. I. Effects on therapy behavior and outcome. *Journal of Psychiatric Research*, **2**: 267–281, 1964.

Kish, G., Solber, K., & Uecker, A. Locus of control as a factor influencing patients' perceptions of ward atmosphere. *Journal of Clinical Psychology*, **27**: 287–289, 1971.

Lennard, H. & Bernstein, A. *The anatomy of psychotherapy: Systems of communication and expectation.* Columbia University Press, New York, 1960.

Orne, M. & Wender, P. Anticipatory socialization for psychotherapy: Method and rationale. *American Journal of Psychiatry*, **124**: 1202–1212, 1968.

Pervin, L. A twenty-college study of student-college interaction using TAPE (Transactional Analysis of Personality and Environment): Rationale reliability and validity. *Journal of Educational Psychology*, **58**: 290–302, 1967a.

Pervin, L. Satisfaction and perceived self-environment similarity: A semantic differential study of student-college interaction. *Journal of Personality*, **35**: 624–633, 1967b.

Pervin, L. & Smith, S. Further test of the relationship between satisfaction and perceived self-environment similarity. *Perceptual and Motor Skills*, **26**: 835–838, 1968.

Rapoport, R. *Community as doctor.* Tavistock, London, 1960.

Rogers, C. *Client-centered therapy.* Houghton Mifflin, Boston, 1951.

Rogers, C. & Dymond, R. *Psychotherapy and personality change.* University of Chicago Press, Chicago, 1954.

Schachter, S. Deviation, rejection and communication. *Journal of Abnormal and Social Psychology*, **46**: 190–207, 1951.

Sechrest, L. & Jackson, D. The generality of deviant response tendencies. *Journal of Consulting Psychology*, **26**: 395–401, 1962.

Sherif, M. & Cantril, H. *The psychology of ego-involvements.* Wiley, New York, 1947.

Sloane, R., Cristol, A., Pepernik, M., & Staples, F. Role preparation and expectation of improvement in psychotherapy. *Journal of Nervous and Mental Disease*, **150**: 18–26, 1970.

Trickett, E. & Moos, R. Satisfaction with the correctional institution environment: An instance of perceived self-environment similarity. *Journal of Personality*, **40**: 75–88, 1972.

Vanderhoff, T. The effects of group counseling on low achieving students' perception of their college environment. Doctoral dissertation, Colorado State College, 1969.

Wood, B., Wilson, G., Jessor, R., & Gogan, J. Troublemaking behavior in a correctional institution: Relationship to inmates' definition of their situation. *American Journal of Orthopsychiatry*, **36**: 795–802, 1966.

Yalom, I., Houts, P., Newell, G., & Rand, K. Preparation of patients for group therapy. *Archives of General Psychiatry*, **17**: 416–427, 1967.

PART THREE

Community-Based Programs

Chapter Ten

THE SOCIAL CLIMATES OF COMMUNITY–BASED TREATMENT SETTINGS

This chapter describes the independent development of the Community-Oriented Programs Environment Scale (COPES), which is a scale directly parallel to the Ward Atmosphere Scale (WAS). The assumption that the immediate psychosocial environment is an important aspect of the overall treatment process is reflected in descriptions of community-based programs, as it was in descriptions of hospital-based programs. Extensive information about the history, funding, types of therapy, staffing, and patient characteristics of different programs can be obtained from accounts of Elm City Rehabilitation Center (Moses, 1969), of Woodley House (Doninger et al., 1963), of day hospitals in Great Britain (Farndale, 1961), of day–night services in the United States (Conwell et al., 1964), and of halfway houses (Glasscote et al., 1971, Keller and Alper, 1970).

Although a broad view of the treatment milieu can be inferred from published reports, there is clearly a need for more systematic methods for describing and comparing the actual social environments provided by different types of community-based psychiatric programs. In this regard, the excellent detailed descriptions of 11 halfway houses presented by Glasscote et al. (1971) include discussions of the origins of each house, the staff and staffing patterns, the characteristics of the residents, the physical facilities, and financial arrangements; in addition, the authors deal briefly with the actual treatment programs. A study indicating the extent to which the characteristics of the treatment environment are inferrable from such descriptions is presented in Chapter 11. Suffice it to say that although some program descriptions are better than others, it is difficult to accurately characterize different programs using these descriptions, partly because they lack completeness and comparability.

In a stimulating suggestion, Glasscote et al. (1971) call for studies to measure the "quality of life" of matched groups of former patients—some would be assigned to halfway houses, whereas others would be discharged early into more regular community living arrangements. Citing the rising level of expectations throughout society, they argue that one important criterion of the success of a community treatment program is its ability to provide the individual with a sense of satisfaction, well-being, and self-fulfullment. These authors concluded that halfway houses "offer a humane, compassionate, appropriate, warm, empathic environment which we believe is badly needed by a sizeable number of people who leave state hospitals to try to acquire the skills and confidence they need to live and work in the community" (p. 27). In reality, halfway houses vary considerably along the dimensions just listed; thus a standard assessment technique by which these and other community-based programs can be systematically compared should be extremely useful.

In an earlier survey Raush and Raush (1968) supplied very informative descriptive data on 40 halfway houses. They were quite aware of the significance of the social environments of these houses, stating that "the major impact of the halfway house on its residents very likely comes from the milieu it provides. . . . Environments do influence people . . . and if they do, possibly some environments are better than others for affecting a course of social adaptation to the ordinary requirements and opportunities of the community" (p. 160). They discuss the social structure, the value systems, the rules and rituals, the types of interactions, and the "resilience potential" of halfway houses. They also assert that a method by which to assess social environments in widely varying halfway house programs would be extremely useful.

Many others have directly or indirectly alluded to the importance of the social environment. For example, in describing the important characteristics of the Massachusetts Mental Health Center, Kramer (1962) emphasized that the environment had been rendered less authoritarian by altering the staff role from a traditional orientation. Wilder et al. (1968), in the description of Overing apartments, stress the high expectations which are held of the residents and identify the primary therapeutic agent at the apartments as an environment that encourages independence. Lamb et al. (1969), discussing the development of community mental health services in a county in California, indicate that the total social environment is assumed to be a key aspect of most therapeutic programs. Fairweather et al. (1969) give an account of an experimental halfway house program, noting the importance of establishing an environment that places increasing responsibilities on the residents. These authors discussed in some detail the socioeconomic environment of the community around their lodge; they also assessed some aspects of the social environments of their experimental community-based program and their control hospital-based program by systematically measuring group processes. They found that group processes could be characterized by three relatively independent dimensions which they labeled (1) group cohesiveness, (2) group performance, and (3) leadership and role delineation. Their techniques furnish one of the few examples of an attempt to assess and compare aspects of social group processes of hospital-based and community-based treatment programs.

Additional relevant work was carried out by Apte (1968) in a study of 25 halfway houses in England and Wales; these establishments aimed at providing an environment that facilitated residents' development, initiative, independence, self-esteem, and healthy interpersonal relationships. Apte wanted to measure the effectiveness of the various environments by using a 65-item scale that evaluated the degree of staff control of physical movement, privacy, and activities and social relationships within the house. He found a higher return rate to the community in permissive than in restrictive halfway houses. Since he was unable to use matched groups of patients, however, he could make no definite conclusions about the actual effects of the therapeutic milieu.

Two main factors led us to develop the Community-Oriented Programs Environment Scale (COPES) for assessing the psychosocial milieus of transitional community-based psychiatric treatment programs: (1) the consistent emphasis by theoreticians and researchers alike on the importance of the social environment and (2) the literature, briefly reviewed in Chapter 1, providing evidence of the critical role of situational and environmental factors in the determination of individual behavior. A technique that makes possible direct comparisons among different types of community-based programs (e.g., sheltered workshops, foster care homes, self-help programs) as well as between community-based and hospital-based programs seemed to us to have great potential utility. In addition, it offers the opportunity to attempt to replicate the general relationships found with the WAS (e.g., between treatment environment and treatment outcome) in a quite different set of treatment programs.

ASSESSING ACTUAL TREATMENT SETTINGS

Most of the items in the initial form of COPES were adapted from the WAS by patients and staff who had great familiarity with the characteristics of the social environments of various community programs, especially day hospitals and halfway houses. Additional items were formulated from program descriptions, interviews of patients and staff in various programs, and in other ways. The choice of items was again guided by the general concept of environmental press. For example, an emphasis on involvement is inferred from the following items: "Members* put a lot of energy into what they do around here" and "This is a lively place." An emphasis on Order and Organization is inferred from still other items: "Members here follow a regular schedule every day" and "Members' activities are carefully planned." Some of the items in the initial form were direct translations from similar items in the WAS, whereas other items were worded somewhat differently to obtain better item splits in community programs. As with the WAS, the COPES items are to be answered true if an individual believes they are generally characteristic of his program and false if he believes they are not generally characteristic of the program.

A resulting 130-item Form B of COPES was administered to members and staff in 21 community-oriented treatment programs, which were selected to obtain a broad range of program types. The programs chosen included nine day care centers, two coeducational residential centers, one men's and one women's residential program, two rehabilitation center programs, a community care home, a resident workshop, and two adolescent residential centers.

About half the houses tested were transitional residences for former mental patients, whereas the other half were designed to serve as an alternative to hospitalization. Some of these were residential and some were day care centers. Although most of the programs were open to men and women, three houses accepted only men and one took only women. Most of the members were able to function fairly normally and were at least eligible for full-time employment; one of the programs dealt with men having a chronic history of illness and was attached to a sheltered workshop. There

---

*No single adequate or generally acceptable term exists for identifying program participants. The words "patient," "resident," and "member" thus are used interchangeably here, although the designation "member" is somewhat preferable because it has no pejorative connotations.

was a very wide range of structure in the programs. The adolescent centers and the home for men were fairly structured and kept close control over their members, whereas many of the other programs allowed members the greatest possible amount of autonomy.

Tested in the 21 programs were 373 members and 203 staff. More than 80% of the members and essentially all the staff approached were both willing and able to take COPES adequately. Items were initially sorted by agreement among three independent judges into 12 rationally derived press subscales paralleling the 12 WAS subscales. The 10-subscale Form C of COPES was derived by using the following criteria.

1.   Each subscale should have acceptable internal consistency, and each item should correlate more highly with its own than with any other subscale. Two of the original 12 subscales were dropped because they did not meet these criteria. The original variety subscale had low item–subscale correlations and showed poor internal consistency, and most of the items in the original Affiliation subscale correlated as highly with other subscales (particularly Involvement) as they did with Affiliation. Only two items on Form C showed a correlation of less than .25 with their appropriate subscales in the member or the staff subsamples. More than 90% of the items for members and more than 95% for staff correlated above .30 with their appropriate subscales. Table 10.1 summarizes the internal consistencies for the 10 subscales, the average correlations between each item and its own subscale and the average correlations between each item and all the other subscales. Internal consistencies were calculated following Stern (1970), using Cronbach's α and average-within-program item variances. The results indicate that all the subscales have acceptable internal consistency and moderate to high average item–subscale correlations. In addition, the items correlate much more highly with their own than with other subscales.

2.   Insofar as possible, not more than 80% nor less than 20% of subjects should answer an item in one direction. This criterion was established to avoid items that were characteristic only of extreme programs. Ninety-five percent of the COPES Form C items had item splits between 20–80 for members or staff or both; that is, only 5% of the items showed an item split that was more extreme than 80–20 for both members and staff.

3.   There should be approximately the same number of items scored true as scored false within each subscale, to control for acquiescence response set.

TABLE 10.1   INTERNAL CONSISTENCIES AND AVERAGE ITEM-
-SUBSCALE CORRELATIONS FOR COPES FORM C SUBSCALES

Subscale	Internal Consistency		Average Item– Subscale Correlation		Average Item– Other Subscale Correlation	
	Members	Staff	Members	Staff	Members	Staff
Involvement	.79	.82	.48	.46	.16	.16
Support	.67	.64	.44	.42	.15	.14
Spontaneity	.63	.75	.43	.46	.16	.14
Autonomy	.62	.89	.38	.49	.11	.15
Practical Orientation	.64	.64	.44	.43	.12	.10
Personal Problem Orientation	.78	.84	.52	.50	.13	.16
Anger and Aggression	.82	.86	.51	.52	.10	.13
Order and Organization	.81	.87	.53	.53	.15	.15
Program Clarity	.68	.77	.45	.44	.15	.13
Staff Control	.67	.76	.40	.45	.10	.12
Mean	.79	.78	.41	.47	.13	.14

4.   Items should not correlate significantly with the Halo Response Set Scale, which assessed both positive and negative halo in program perceptions and was also given to members and staff.

The use of these four criteria resulted in the 10-subscale final Form C of COPES. Table 10.2 lists the subscales and gives brief definitions of each. The conceptualization of the dimensions is identical to that for the WAS. The Program Involvement, Support, and Spontaneity subscales measure *Relationship* dimensions. The next four subscales (Autonomy, Practical Orientation, Personal Problem Orientation, and Anger and Aggression) are the *Treatment Program* dimensions. The last three subscales (Order and Organization, Program Clarity, and Staff Control) are taken as assessing

TABLE 10.2   COPES SUBSCALE DEFINITIONS

1. *Involvement* measures how active members are in the day-to-day functioning of their program, (spending time constructively, being enthusiastic, doing things on their own initiative).
2. *Support* measures the extent to which members are encouraged to be helpful and supportive toward other members and how supportive staff are toward members.
3. *Spontaneity* measures the extent to which the program encourages members to act openly and to express their feelings openly.
4. *Autonomy* assesses how self-sufficient and independent members are encouraged to be in making decisions about their personal affairs (what they wear, where they go) and in their relationships with the staff.
5. *Practical Orientation* assesses the extent to which the member's environment orients him toward preparing himself for release from the program. Such things as training for new kinds of jobs, looking to the future, and setting and working toward goals are considered.
6. *Personal Problem Orientation* measures the extent to which members are encouraged to be concerned with their personal problems and feelings and to seek to understand them.
7. *Anger and Aggression* measures the extent to which a member is allowed and encouraged to argue with members and staff, to become openly angry, and to display other aggressive behavior.
8. *Order and Organization* measures the importance of order and organization in the program in terms of members (how do they look), staff (what they do to encourage order), and the house itself (how well it is kept).
9. *Program Clarity* measures the extent to which the member knows what to expect in the day-to-day routine of his program and the explicitness of the program rules and procedures.
10. *Staff Control* assesses the extent to which the staff use measures to keep members under necessary controls (e.g., in the formulation of rules, the scheduling of activities, and in the relationships between members and staff).

System Maintenance dimensions. The full-scale and its scoring key are given in Appendix B.

The next step was to obtain the 10 subscale scores for each subject. Means and standard deviations of all the subscale scores were calculated for each program, separately for members and staff. The results of one-way analyses of variance indicated that all 10 subscales significantly ($p < .01$ for all 10 subscales for members and for 9 of the 10 subscales for staff) differentiated among the 21 programs. Thus we had achieved the major purpose of this phase of the research—namely, to develop a scale whose dimensions would significantly discriminate among the average perceptions of members and the average perceptions of staff on different types of programs.

The 10 subscale scores were intercorrelated, separately for the 373 members and the 203 staff, to discover whether it might be fruitful to work with a smaller number of dimensions. The highest intercorrelation was exactly .50, and the only cluster of subscales that showed even moderate intercorrelations in both the member and the staff samples was composed of the Relationship dimensions of Involvement, Support, and Spontaneity (see Moos, 1974). The average correlation among the subscales was .23 for the member sample and .24 for the staff sample. Thus the 10 dimensions measure rather distinct although correlated characteristics of member and staff perceptions of community-based program treatment environments.

ASSESSING IDEAL TREATMENT SETTINGS

The 120 items (excluding the 10 response set scale items) of COPES Form B were reworded to allow members and staff to answer them in terms of the type of program they would ideally like to be on. The rationale for this form was identical to the rationale for the development of Form I of the WAS. We could find no previously available techniques that assessed the value orientations of members and staff regarding their program treatment environment. Again, Form I may be used in conjunction with Form C in order to identify specific areas in which members and/or staff feel that change should occur (for more details, see Chapter 11).

The current version of COPES Form I is directly parallel to Form C; that is, each of its items is parallel to one item in Form C. When filling out Form I, members and staff are instructed to answer each item as if they were describing an *ideal* program. Item–subscale correlations and internal consistencies were calculated for the 10 Form I subscales for a subsample of 15 programs. The average item–subscale correlations for the 10 subscales varied from .35 to .55; the subscale internal consistencies, which varied from a low of .70 for Program Clarity to a high of .88 for Personal Problem Orientation, were quite substantial for both the member and the staff samples. The results were very similar to those obtained earlier for Form I of the WAS.

AMERICAN COMMUNITY–ORIENTED PROGRAMS

The development of normative samples for COPES is in a more preliminary phase than that reported for the WAS. As with the hospital-based programs, however, an attempt was made to include a broad range of community-based programs, representing several alternatives to hospitalization. Thus far 54 programs have been surveyed. Both members and staff were tested in 32 of the programs, and only members were tested in the remaining 22 programs.

The 32 programs on which both members and staff were tested included 2 rehabilitation workshops, 2 partial hospitalization programs; 11 halfway houses and 17 day care centers. One of the workshops was oriented to physical and occupational rehabilitation; it employed physical and occupational therapists, part-time assistants, and nine part-time affiliated physicians who supervised the program, among other staff. The other workshop was a VA hospital program; it served patients with relatively chronic psychiatric problems and was staffed by two psychologists, a nurse, and clerical help. The two partial hospitalization programs were administered by state hospitals and allowed for hospitalization for either day care or night care only. The halfway houses included three adolescent homes, five homes for both men and women, two homes for men, and one for women. They varied in capacity of from 5 to 30 members. All were administered by professionally trained psychologists or psychiatric social workers whose role was to advise the live-in staff and to counsel the patients. Specifically designed to prepare their residents for living independently, these programs usually required members to leave the program after 6 months to a year.

The 17 day care programs tested included 4 VA centers with about 30 members each, 4 programs administered by general or psychiatric hospitals, 2 county programs, and 7 privately run programs with approximately 15 members each. All these programs were relatively highly staffed and offered concentrated direction in practical problem solving, improving social behavior, and self-care.

The additional 22 programs on which only members were tested included 20 community care foster homes for veterans, a patient-administered self-help program, and a small outpatient support group. As a rule, between four and seven veterans lived in the community care or foster homes, which were administered by a local VA hospital. There is a live-in foster parent, usually a woman, who handles cooking, supervises housekeeping, and helps plan occasional trips for the men. The homes are not meant to be treatment centers; rather, they provide a home setting for men who have had long-term hospitalization and who are able to function at a minimal level. A few of the men attend day care centers or local sheltered workshops, but most remain at home during the day. A team of social workers consult with foster parents on any behavior problems that arise and hold monthly meetings to help handle administrative matters. Because these homes are small, encouraging a family-type atmosphere, the foster parents were included in our testing as "members" rather than staff.

The patient-administered VA program, on an open ward on hospital grounds, was completely run by a patient council. All administrative and behavior problems were dealt with by this elected patient group. Prospective members were screened and chosen by the group as a whole. All members had to either work, go to school, or attend a day treatment center. The program was specifically designed to prepare men to live independently after a 6-month period. The outpatient support group was a group of six former patients who met twice a week in the evening to discuss their mutual problems. Although strictly speaking COPES does not apply to groups, this group was a specific source of encouragement and support for its members, who were all newly released from the hospital; moreover, we were interested in extending our techniques for the measurement of social environments to social and psychotherapeutic groups. Thus the overall range of programs included in the current American normative sample is quite broad, but the geographical representation is as yet relatively limited. Only seven programs outside California are included in the sample (one in Illinois, one in Massachusetts, one in Oklahoma, three in Pennsylvania, and one in Washington State. In this American normative sample we tested 778 members and 357 staff.

Figure 10.1 compares the mean scores for members and staff on the 32 programs on which both members and staff were tested. A comparison of the social environments of the 32 programs with staff and the 22 programs without staff is presented later. The actual means and standard deviations for members and staff appear in Moos (1974). The most important result indicated by Figure 10.1 is that there is much more agreement in the way members and staff in community-oriented programs see their programs than there is for patients and staff in inpatient ward programs. Members and staff in the community-oriented programs saw the average emphasis on the Relationship dimensions almost identically. This contrasts sharply with the results obtained for patients and staff on wards, where staff perceived

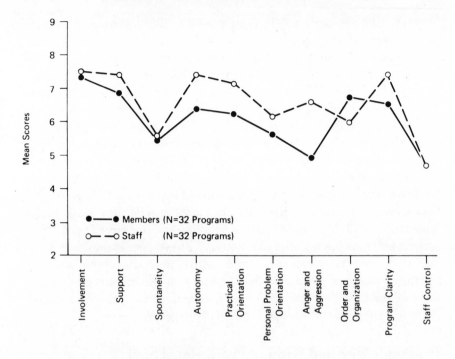

Figure 10.1 COPES Form C means for members and staff on 32 American programs.

considerably more emphasis on each of the three Relationship dimensions than did patients. The results for the four Treatment Program dimensions are generally similar for COPES and for the WAS. Staff on community-oriented programs see more emphasis on all four Treatment Program dimensions than do members, although the member–staff differences on Practical Orientation and Personal Problem Orientation are not as great as the patient–staff differences on these two dimensions. The discrepancies on Program Clarity and Staff Control between members and staff are somewhat less than those between patients and staff on ward-based programs.

The results suggest that the "two-subculture" notion is considerably less applicable to community-based than to hospital-based programs. Overall, members and staff perceive relatively similar emphases on the Relationship and System Maintenance dimensions, although the directions of the differences that do exist are consistent with those found on wards (i.e., staff consistently see treatment programs more positively than do members). Thus there is a relatively greater amount of integration and communication between members and staff in community-based programs than between patients and staff in hospital-based programs.

There are still some substantial differences between average member and average staff perceptions on certain specific items on the Treatment Program dimensions. For example, members answer true at least 25% more often on the following: "The staff tend to discourage criticism from members," "There is relatively little emphasis on making specific plans for leaving this program," "There is relatively little emphasis on teaching members solutions to practical problems," "The members rarely talk with each other about their personal problems," and "Members here rarely become angry." Items on which staff answered true at least 25% more often than members included, "Members are taught specific new skills in this program," "Staff here think it is a healthy thing to argue," and "Staff sometimes argue openly with each other." These item examples indicate that staff perceive a somewhat more active treatment orientation than members, most specifically in the emphases on leaving the program, on deriving solutions to practical problems, on making concrete plans, and on the sharing of personal feelings, particularly anger and aggression.

Programs With and Without Professional Staff

Since we sampled programs with and without professional staff, an informative comparison between the social environments of these two types of programs was possible. The background characteristics of both sets of patients were relatively similar, since in most cases a patient could just as easily have been placed in one type of program as in another. The major difference was that at least some professionally trained staff (psychiatrists, psychologists, and/or social workers) were directly affiliated with one set, whereas no professionally trained staff were affiliated with the other. The 22 programs without professionally trained staff were almost entirely community care homes ($N = 20$), as mentioned earlier. When answering the COPES, the men in the homes were instructed to consider the foster parents as staff. The other two programs included the patient-administered ward (the patients were to consider the patient leaders as staff), and the supportive former patient group (without staff).

We were primarily interested in how much the social environment, or perhaps the "quality of life," differed in programs with and without professional staff. Are patients living in community care homes actually experiencing a social milieu different from that of patients living and/or functioning in day care centers, resident workshops, rehabilitation

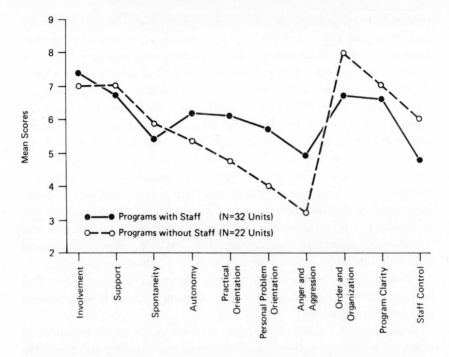

Figure 10.2 COPES Form C means for members on programs with and without professional staff.

programs, and so on? Figure 10.2 compares the social environments in these two types of programs.

We obtained results in three main areas: (a) Programs with and without professional staff do not differ in their emphasis on any of the three Relationship dimensions. (b) Programs with professional staff have much more emphasis on all four Treatment Program dimensions, particularly Personal Problem Orientation and Anger and Aggression, than do programs without staff. (c) Programs without professional staff place somewhat more emphasis on all three System Maintenance dimensions than do programs with staff. Thus professional staff make the greatest difference in the treatment program areas, which is essentially what we would expect, since they have primary interest and responsibility in organizing programs along these four salient dimensions. However, professional staff may not strongly influence the quality and intensity of the relationships among patients (at least as perceived by patients), and they may have some effect in diminishing the emphasis on system maintenance.

Since this comparison of programs with and without professional staff seemed to be quite important, the average proportion of true responses for each item was calculated for members in these two sets of programs. Members in the 22 programs without professional staff answered true significantly more often (the differences were 20% or greater for each item) to the following items on the three Relationship dimensions: "Members put a lot of energy into what they do around here," "Staff [i.e., foster parents] always compliment a member who does something well," "Members spontaneously set up their own activities here," "Members can generally do whatever they feel like here," "When members disagree with each other they keep it to themselves," "Very few things around here ever get people excited," and "Very few members ever volunteer around here." These items indicate that members in programs without professional staff are just as involved in the program but that there is some lack of excitement and initiative (volunteering), that members feel just as positively, if not more positively, about their foster parents as they do about professional staff, and that there is a somewhat greater atmosphere of freedom of action (but less explicit emphasis on the open expression of feelings) in the programs without professional staff.

Items on the Treatment Program dimensions on which members in programs without professional staff answered true significantly more often included "There is relatively little emphasis on teaching members solutions to practical problems," "There is relatively little discussion about exactly what members will be doing after they leave the program," "Members talk relatively little about their past," "Members are rarely asked personal questions by the staff," "The members rarely talk with each other about their personal problems," and "Members are rarely encouraged to discuss their personal problems here." Members on these programs were significantly more likely to answer false to the following items: "Members are taught specific new skills in this program" and "Members are expected to make detailed, specific plans for the future." Finally, on the Anger and Aggression subscale, there were differences of 20% or greater on seven of the nine items. In each case, members in programs without professional staff stated that there was less emphasis on this dimension.

The responses just cited reveal that professional staff have a very strong influence on the four Treatment Program dimensions. The foster parents in the community care homes engender very little "press" toward a practical job orientation, toward making plans for leaving the home, toward discussion and understanding of personal problems, or toward the open expression and sharing of feelings of anger. On the one hand, these results indicate that professional staff have an important and potentially beneficial influence in emphasizing autonomy, independence, and a practical orientation. On the other hand, a serious question can be raised about the benefits derived from professional staff's influence in strongly emphasizing the open expression of feelings (including angry feelings), since the members will experience very little performance press in these areas in the community environments in which they must later function, where psychiatrically oriented professional staff are seldom present. Staff in many psychiatric programs may be rewarding patients in specific behaviors that are not particularly functional in settings other than treatment programs. An important point to note here is that Involvement, Support and Spontaneity can be just as high on programs that do not specifically emphasize the open sharing of personal feelings.

Finally, on the System Maintenance dimensions, members in programs without professional staff answered true significantly more often to the following items: "The staff make sure that this place is always neat," "It is important to carefully follow the program rules here," "The staff make and enforce all the rules here," "If a member fights with another member he will get into real trouble with the staff," and "Members never quite know when they will be considered ready to leave this program." Items on which members in these programs answered false significantly more often included: "Things are sometimes very disorganized around here," "The day room or living room is often untidy," "This place usually looks a little messy," and "People are always changing their minds here." These items indicate that the foster parents in the community care homes emphasize neatness and orderliness to a somewhat greater extent than do regular professional staff. They are also seen as changing their minds less frequently and as being somewhat stricter. However, the men in these programs are not certain when they will be ready to leave the home. Since this decision is in part made by social workers who have close liaison with the home but do not live in it, this relative lack of clarity is understandable. In any case, individuals without specific professional training may emphasize order, clarity, and control as much or more than professionally trained staff.

These results, though preliminary, are quite intriguing and thought provoking. They indicate that the influence of professional staff in live-in programs is probably more limited than has been thought; that is, this influence is mainly related to the four Treatment Program dimensions. The strong emphasis on the Relationship dimensions in programs without professional staff is directly consistent with research in individual and group psychotherapy, which indicates that paraprofessional and other minimally trained staff can establish relationships that are no different in quality (e.g., accurate empathy, genuineness) from those established by highly trained professional staff (see, e.g., Truax and Carkhuff, 1967, Gruver, 1971). The results for the System Maintenance dimensions are not unexpected, since professional staff often specifically tend to deemphasize these variables because of their potentially constrictive influence.

Whether the major difference due to professional staff is more beneficial or more harmful is a moot point. An emphasis on autonomy and independence and on a practical problem-solving orientation is probably generally beneficial. An emphasis on the open expression of feelings, particularly angry feelings may or may not be beneficial, depending on the types of community situations to which the patient will be exposed and on the exact discriminations that he learns to make. It is obvious that the open expression of angry feelings, although potentially cathartic, may result in strong negative reinforcements in many community settings. Another implication of these results has to do with the training of foster parents and other nonprofessional staff. Such individuals can and should be specifically trained in methods for encouraging autonomy and a practical orientation, since they currently do not emphasize these dimensions which generally have beneficial effects on patients' personal growth.

In this connection it is important to note that members in programs with professional staff show greater real–ideal program discrepancies than do members on programs without professional staff. For example, the real–ideal discrepancies were greater for members in programs with professional staff for the Relationship dimensions of Involvement, Support, and Spontaneity and for the System Maintenance dimensions of Order and Organization and Program Clarity. Since it is unlikely that patients in these two types of programs initially had different views of ideal treatment milieus, this suggests the possibility that the presence of professional staff may increase members' dissatisfaction, at least as assessed by real–ideal program discrepancies. Patients in programs with professional staff wish to have more emphasis on Order and Organization and Program Clarity, presumably indicating that they would prefer the kinds of treatment milieus run by nonprofessional staff. On the other hand, members in programs without professional staff are dissatisfied with the lack of emphasis on Practical Orientation; thus perhaps there is validity in the suggestion that nonprofessional staff might be specifically trained in methods by which autonomy, independence, and a practical problem-solving orientation can be encouraged.

COPES American Form I Sample

Most of the programs tested with COPES Form C were also tested with the ideal program form. By the time the work with community-oriented programs was begun, our research on inpatient programs had convinced us that the measurement of value orientations of members and staff was important, particularly in relation to profile feedback and the implications for change that could be discussed with program participants. The COPES Form I was completed by members on 47 of the 54 programs also tested with the COPES Form C, and by staff on 26 of the 32 programs tested with Form C. A total of 618 members and 252 staff completed COPES Form I. The Form I norms are given in Moos (1974).

Figure 10.3 compares the members and staff on the 10 Form I subscales. The overall views of ideal treatment programs of members and staff are relatively similar, although staff again see an ideal milieu as having more emphasis on all three Relationship and on all four Treatment Program dimensions, whereas staff and members alike see it almost identically on the three System Maintenance dimensions. The general differences between members and staff on these community-based programs are very similar to those between patients and staff in hospital-based programs (see Figure 3.5). Staff seem to surpass members in wanting to make treatment programs more involved and cohesive and in wanting to increase greatly the treatment-oriented aspects of the program.

Some interesting findings emerge when the results in Figure 10.1 (COPES real form) are compared with those in Figure 10.3 (COPES ideal form). Members seem to be more satisfied with their programs than are staff. Although there are some real–ideal discrepancies for members on the Relationship dimensions (i.e., members wish to have somewhat greater emphasis on all three such dimensions), these discrepancies are much smaller than those for staff. Differences between real and ideal program environments, however, are relatively similar for members and staff on the four Treatment Program dimensions and on the System Maintenance dimensions of Program Clarity and Staff Control.

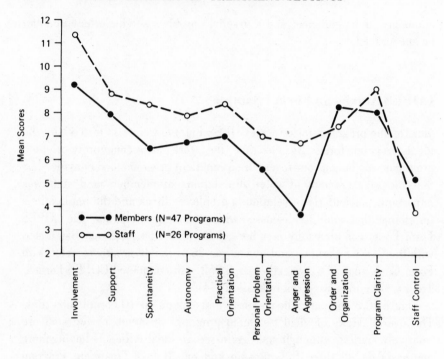

Figure 10.3   COPES form I means for members and staff on American programs.

BRITISH COMMUNITY–ORIENTED PROGRAMS

It was fortunately possible for us to collect a British reference group sample of 20 programs in collaboration with Paul Insel. The British sample included 2 psychiatric day hospitals and 18 halfway houses. The day hospitals, located at two major teaching hospitals in London, were characterized by high staff–patient ratios and mainly short-stay patients who could function at least to a limited extent in the community. One day hospital had 14 patients and 6 staff; the other had 21 patients and 12 staff.

Three of the halfway houses were administered by the Borough of London. There were between five and ten members in each of these houses, and each had three staff members. Specifically designed to help members deal with drug and/or alcohol problems, the programs usually required members to leave the establishment after one year.

The remaining 15 halfway houses were administered by a privately endowed foundation and were most interested in admitting members with a very high probability of successful rehabilitation. These houses are distributed across England, but most were in the south of England. They range in size from 4 residents and 1 staff member to 21 residents and 7 staff members. The treatment program they offer is aimed at providing a supportive environment with open expression of anger and aggression. They employ a semiprofessional staff and have an in-service training program that helps staff develop a therapeutic outlook, as opposed to a custodial orientation.

Residents in these programs are mostly young (mean ages are in the early 20s), and they are often admitted to the programs by court referrals. The programs encourage short-term stays from 6 to 12 months.

These programs can be characterized as active and energetic, with an emphasis on democratic processes in the living environment. For example, decisions that affect the lives of members of the house are voted on; each member and each of the staff receives one vote. The members are urged to exercise their rights, and they usually feel that their feelings and opinions are important in decision-making processes. The treatment program includes group therapy sessions once or twice a week in which members are encouraged to express feelings about themselves and the staff. These voluntary sessions are well attended and relatively successful in providing a pathway of communication between members and staff.

The 20 programs were all very small, and the total numbers of members and staff tested were only 209 and 74, respectively. COPES Form I was given to members and staff on 19 of the 20 programs, and 176 members and 55 staff completed the test. It should be noted that since the current British sample is *not* comparable to the current American sample, no conclusions about similarities or differences between American and British community-based programs can be based on these results. Of the 20 British programs, 17 were halfway houses of a particular type; all were relatively small, and the majority belonged to one highly structured organization.

Figure 10.4 graphs the COPES Form C data for members and staff in the 20 British programs. The actual means and standard deviations are given in Moos (1974). As with the British hospital sample, it appears that staff see more emphasis on all three Relationship and all four Treatment Program dimensions. The differences between members and staff are somewhat less on the System Maintenance dimensions, although staff perceive more emphasis on Program Clarity and less on Staff Control than do members. On the other hand, the shape of the overall profile is quite similar for members and staff. There is one rather striking feature about these profiles—namely, the highest mean score for both members and staff is on

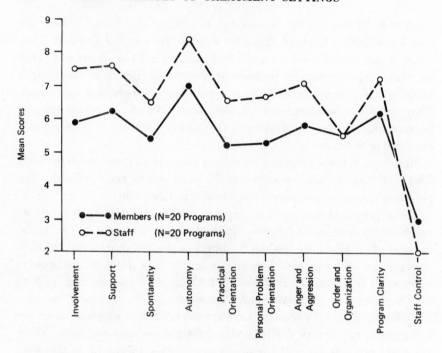

Figure 10.4   COPES Form C means for members and staff on 20 British programs.

Autonomy, whereas the lowest mean score for both is on Staff Control, indicating that the British programs very strongly emphasize patient self-reliance and independence.

Figure 10.5 presents the results for members and staff on the 19 programs that also completed COPES Form I. Members and staff conceive of ideal treatment programs in very similar ways. Staff wish to have somewhat more emphasis on the Relationship and the Treatment Program dimensions; as a rule, however, the differences are considerably less than those revealed on the American COPES Form I sample.

A comparison of the results appearing in Figures 10.4 and 10.5 indicates some substantial real–ideal discrepancies between members and staff, particularly on all three Relationship dimensions and on Practical Orientation and Program Clarity. Real-ideal discrepancies for the staff are relatively similar in that staff also wish much more emphasis on the dimensions of Involvement, Spontaneity, and Practical Orientation, whereas they are relatively satisfied with the emphasis on Autonomy and Staff Control.

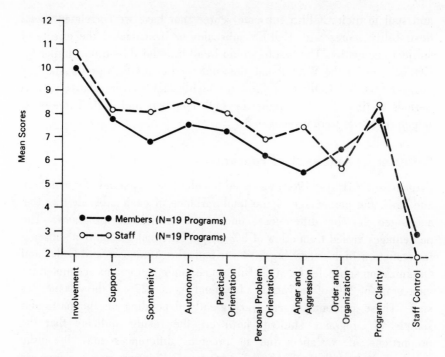

Figure 10.5   COPES Form I means for members and staff on 19 British programs.

TEST ADMINISTRATION AND TEST STATISTICS

Our experience in administering the COPES Form C and Form I has been very similar to that in utilizing the WAS. The COPES has been given as a paper-and-pencil questionnaire and with tape-recorded instructions and IBM answer sheets. We prefer the tape-recorded method of administration with the use of IBM answer sheets, because of the increased comparability of the instructions and the testing procedure across programs and subjects, and because the data-processing procedures involved are easier and less expensive. Issues of introducing the concepts of assessing program environment, of anonymity, of confidentiality, and so on are discussed in detail in Chapter 2; in these respects, the COPES resembles the WAS.

Since the WAS and the COPES are conceptually and methodologically parallel, and since most of the basic test statistic issues were very carefully investigated with the WAS, little of the groundwork was repeated with the COPES. We have not related the background characteristics of members and staff to their COPES subscale scores, nor have we correlated social desirability scores with COPES subscales or investigated the effects of subject anonymity. The results would in all likelihood be quite similar for COPES and for the WAS. Some data obtained on COPES profile stability suggest that the COPES profiles are highly stable over relatively short periods of time (2 to 6 months) for both members and staff. Three other important issues were investigated.

Differences Among the Programs

Estimated Ω^2 (Hays, 1963) was used to calculate, separately for members and staff, the percentage of the total variance of each subscale that was accounted for by differences among the initial 21 programs. The percentages varied from a low of 5% on the Practical Orientation subscale for staff to a high exceeding 50% on both the Autonomy and Order and Organization subscales for staff. Differences among programs accounted for an average of 20% of the variance for members and 27% of the variance for staff. These percentages can vary greatly depending on the particular sample of programs studied; however, the results indicate that the proportions of variance due to program differences may be quite substantial. As with the WAS, the proportions of interprogram variance are of similar magnitude to those usually accounted for by standard individual difference measures of personality.

Random Samples on Programs of Varying Sizes

The practical problem of the proportion of members and staff who need to answer COPES to obtain an adequate profile in a particular program was investigated by (1) taking 50% random samples of members and staff who actually completed COPES, (2) deriving separate profiles for these random samples, and (3) assessing the similarity of the profiles by utilizing the intraclass correlation (Haggard, 1958). The procedure followed was similar to that carried out on the WAS data as reported in Chapter 2.

The profile correlations were all quite high, indicating that it is not necessary to test all the members or staff in larger programs, particularly if an investigator is primarily concerned with a general assessment of the program environment. As a rule of thumb, an investigator needs to test only half the members on programs having 21 or more members and half the staff on programs having 11 or more staff. The mean intraclass correlation was .88 for the 7 programs with 21 or more members and .92 for the 3 programs with 11 or more staff. As expected, the results for COPES were very similar to those for the WAS. The random sample selected must of course be a sample of all members and staff currently in the program, not just of those members and staff who are willing to take the test. In any event, there were almost no refusals to participate in the community-oriented programs we tested. Thus the random samples of members and staff reported here are essentially random samples of all the members and staff in the programs under study.

COPES Form S (40-item Short Form)

As with the WAS, a 40-item Short Form of COPES was developed for use by investigators or program staff who wish to obtain a relatively rapid assessment of the treatment environment of a particular program. The procedure was identical to that used for deriving the Short Form of the WAS (4 items were chosen from each of the 10 COPES subscales, etc.). Means for the items selected were then calculated for the entire sample of 54 programs for members and 32 programs for staff. Standard scores were obtained for members and staff for each of the 21 programs used in the development of Form C. Intraclass profile correlations between the 10 COPES Form C and the 10 COPES Form S standard scores were then calculated for each program.

The results were extremely good for both members and staff. The intraclass correlations between Form C and Form S were above .75 for 19 of the 21 programs for members and 18 of the 21 programs for staff. The lowest profile correlations were .68 for members and .60 for staff. Thus utilizing Form S results in COPES program profiles highly similar to those obtained with the regular Form C. The 40 items included in the COPES Short Form are marked with an asterisk on the scoring key given in Appendix B. The Short Form means and standard deviations for members and staff for the American normative sample are presented in Moos (1974).

REFERENCES

Apte, R. *Halfway houses.* Bell & Sons, Ltd., London, 1968.

Conwell, M., Rosen, B., Hench, C. & Bahn, A. The first national survey of psychiatric day–night services. In Epps, R. & Hanes, L. (Eds.) *Day care of psychiatric patients.* Charles C. Thomas, Springfield, Ill., 1964.

Doniger, J., Rothwell, N. & Cohen, R. Case study of a halfway house. *Mental Hospitals,* **14**: 191–199, 1963.

Fairweather, G. Sanders, D., Cressler, D. & Maynard, H. *Community life for the mentally ill.* Aldine, Chicago, 1969.

Farndale, J. *The day hospital movement in Great Britain.* Pergamon Press, London, 1961.

Glasscote, R., Gudeman, J. & Elpers, R. *Halfway houses for the mentally ill.* Joint Information Service of the American Psychiatric Association, Washington, D.C., 1971.

Gruver, G. College students as therapeutic agents. *Psychological Bulletin,* **76**: 111–127, 1971.

Haggard, E. *Intraclass correlation and the analysis of variance.* Dryden, New York, 1958.

Hays, W. *Statistics for psychologists.* Holt, Rinehart & Winston, New York, 1963.

Keller, O. & Alper, B. *Halfway houses: Community-centered correction and treatment.* Heath-Lexington, Lexington, Mass. 1970.

Kramer, B. *Day hospital: A study of partial hospitalization in psychiatry,* Grune & Stratton, New York, 1962.

Lamb, R., Heath, D. & Downing, J. (Eds.). *Handbook of community mental health practice.* Jossey-Bass, San Francisco, 1969.

Moos, R. Assessment of the psychosocial environments of community-oriented psychiatric treatment programs. *Journal of Abnormal Psychology,* **79**: 9–18, 1972.

Moos, R. *Community-Oriented Programs Environment Scale Manual,* Consulting Psychologists Press, Palo Alto, Calif., 1974.

Moses, H. Halfway or more? *Rehabilitation Record,* **10**:35–37, 1969.

Raush, H. & Raush, C. *The halfway house movement: A search for sanity.* Appleton-Century-Crofts, New York, 1968.

Truax, C. & Carkhuff, R. *Toward effective counseling and psychotherapy: Training and practice.* Aldine, Chicago, 1967.

Wilder, J., Kessell, M., & Caulfield, S. Follow-up of a high expectations halfway house. *American Journal of Psychiatry,* **124**:103–109, 1968.

Chapter Eleven

THE CLINICAL
USE OF COPES:
FEEDBACK AND
SOCIAL CHANGE

Rudolf H. Moos and Jean Otto

Profile Interpretations and Feedback

Like the Ward Atmosphere Scale, COPES was designed not only as a multipurpose research tool (providing information about differences in member and staff perceptions of treatment milieus, allowing for the comparison of different programs, and comparing a program with itself over time), but also as an evaluative technique that would be useful to staff in participating programs.

As explained in the previous chapter, a wide variety of community-based treatment programs were tested with COPES. The diversity among COPES profiles was as great as it was among WAS profiles. Detailed examples of WAS profile interpretations were given in Chapter 4. Since the COPES and the WAS are directly parallel, only two additional examples are offered here.

An Adult Residential Center

Figure 11.1 shows the COPES profile for members and staff in program 113, a small residential center for men and women 16 years of age and over who are returning to the community after hospitalization, who might otherwise have to be hospitalized, or who are coming from a crisis situation.

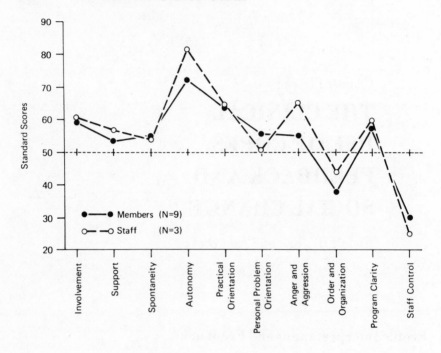

Figure 11.1   COPES Form C profiles for members and staff on program 113.

Members are involved in regular daytime activities and have responsibility for housework and cooking. Other than attending a management meeting and a group therapy meeting, they are encouraged to be as independent as possible. Rules and restrictions are kept to a minimum. The house is staffed by a resident manager, a part-time student manager, and a program director. The staff also consult with visiting social workers.

Members and staff showed high agreement on the characteristics of their treatment environment. Both groups agreed that the emphasis on the Relationship dimensions was slightly above average; indeed, eight of the nine members and all three of the staff agreed that members often did things together on weekends and that discussions in the house were very interesting. All members and staff felt that members were strongly encouraged to express their feelings (Spontaneity).

The Treatment Program dimensions were also adjudged similarly by members and staff, except that staff saw above-average emphasis on Aggression whereas members saw it as average. The emphasis on

Autonomy and Practical Orientation was thought to be somewhat above average, and encouragement of members to be concerned about their personal problems was perceived to be average. In the area of Autonomy, eight of the nine members and all three of the staff agreed that members were encouraged to take leadership and to be independent; everyone agreed that members had to demonstrate continual progress toward their goals and that members told one another about personal problems.

Members and staff were also in accord regarding the System Maintenance dimensions, with both groups saying that the emphasis on Order and Organization and Staff Control was somewhat below average and that on Program Clarity was somewhat above average. For example, two-thirds of the members and all staff agreed that things were sometimes disorganized; but all responded that members followed a regular schedule. None of the staff and only two of the members felt that the staff made and enforced all the rules.

Thus program 113 was characterized by moderately high emphasis on the Relationship dimensions and on facilitating independence and practical planning. The program did not strongly emphasize understanding personal problems, nor did it especially urge members to openly express their anger. The program rules and procedures were perceived to be clear and explicit, but there was little emphasis either on having a highly organized and structured program or on having staff control program decisions.

A Community Care Home

Figure 11.2 presents the COPES profile for program 108, which serves women and is located in a comfortable home in a city residential area, helping them to make the transition from hospital to community living. The women may go to work, school, or a day care center during the daytime. The house is managed by two women who act as house mothers to the residents and encourage the women to participate in community activities; two additional staff serve as administrative consultants on a part-time basis.

This profile illustrates a different type of treatment environment and also reveals greater disagreement among members and staff, particularly on the Relationship dimensions. Members rated Involvement and Spontaneity as about average, whereas staff saw the emphasis on these variables as well below average. For example, all four members felt that they put a lot of energy into what they did in the program, but all four staff members disagreed. Only one of the four members felt that members hid their

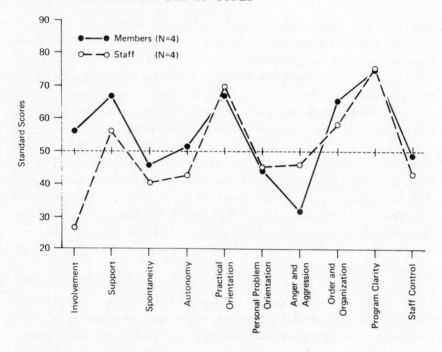

Figure 11.2   COPES Form C profiles for members and staff on program 108.

feelings from staff, but three of the four staff felt that this was true.
Members rated Support as very high, but staff saw it as only slightly above
average.

There was more agreement between members and staff on the Treatment
Program dimensions. Both felt that Practical Orientation was strongly
emphasized and that Autonomy and Personal Problem Orientation were
slightly below average. All members and staff agreed that members had to
demonstrate continued concrete progress toward their goals and that they
had to make specific plans for the future. Members and staff also agreed
that members were encouraged to be independent but that staff rarely gave
in to pressure from members. Both members and staff saw little emphasis
on Aggression; for example, they agreed that members rarely argued
openly.

Members and staff viewed the program as an orderly and organized one,
with clear rules and expectations. All members and staff agreed that
members knew the program rules and the consequences of breaking them.
Both groups felt there was above-average probability that staff would use

measures to keep members under necessary controls (e.g., both agreed that once a schedule was arranged for a member, she had to follow it).

The two profiles show how COPES may be a useful tool for identifying the significant aspects of a treatment program. The adult coed residential program, with few formal activities or rules, puts great emphasis on Autonomy and Independence. The members in this program were highly involved and felt free to communicate openly with one another. The home for women with a more chronic psychiatric history stressed Support and Practical Orientation and provided a moderate level of Staff Control. The wide range of differences among community-based treatment programs is further illustrated by noting that on most items at least 80% of the members in one or more programs responded in one direction, whereas at least 80% of the members in one or more other programs responded in the opposite direction; this was true for 10 of the 12 items on the Involvement subscale and for all 10 items on the Anger and Aggression subscale.

Staff Reactions to COPES Feedback

Feedback sessions in which staff were given the results of the COPES Form C and Form I questionnaires were held for all the programs tested. Feedback questionnaires were distributed in 10 of these programs to evaluate the accuracy and completeness of the profiles as the staff perceived them and to ascertain whether staff felt that the results had implications for specific changes in treatment methods, activities, or personal relationships in the program. The feedback questionnaire was identical to the one used in hospital-based programs (see Chapter 4).

The majority of staff felt that both the COPES Form C and Form I profiles portrayed the basic characteristics of their treatment milieu relatively accurately and completely. In the comments some staff indicated specific areas that they felt COPES did not cover. For example, one staff member mentioned that COPES did not evaluate the family-type life of the home. Another did not think the treatment program was validly rated because the home works in conjunction with other social agencies that provide group therapy and vocational training. Several staff members indicated that members' profiles were inaccurate because members had an inadequate understanding of the scale. For example, one said, "In general our members' judgment and perception is somewhat inaccurate since generally their judgment is lacking (or they would not be here)." A staff member at one home felt that the Practical Orientation items should reflect more of the "survival skills" they teach (e.g., cooking, cleaning, washing clothes). However, 82% of the staff who received feedback felt that important program changes were implied by the evaluation.

COPES allows staff to define more accurately the type of program they have, bringing to the task not only their own perceptions but also those of the members. A self-initiated analysis often results as discussion of the profile leads to interest in the differences and similarities of staff and member perceptions. Staff then begin to explore their own ideals as well as those of the members, relating these ideals to actual program performance. COPES serves as a concrete guideline for discussion. As a result of feedback, staff are often able to identify specific changes that might improve their program. This use of COPES as an analytic tool replicates the work done with the WAS described in Chapter 4. In both cases staff learn that research can be a nonthreatening process and, more important, that it can supply information that is easily understood and immediately applicable to their program (see Moos and Otto, 1972).

CHANGING SOCIAL ENVIRONMENTS

We developed methods of assessing social environments and made such assessments useful to participants through feedback because we wanted to facilitate planned change in social settings. Attempts at changing group environments began on a large scale with the development of human relations training in industrial settings, in which change generally is centered around improving employee morale and/or production procedures (Bavelas and Strauss, 1961; Beckhard, 1971; Mann, 1971).

Heller (1969) has developed a multidimensional "Group Feedback Analysis" approach to field research. The method is composed of three steps: (1) administration of traditional questionnaires which are subjected to standard statistical tests, (2) feedback of questionnaire results, and (3) content analysis. Content analysis comprises respondents' reviewing their thoughts on the subject under study. Heller used this technique with groups in 20 California companies. A battery of 22 questionnaires covering areas such as relative importance of managerial skills and use of different decision-making styles was administered. Each company received feedback of the test results and subsequently could focus on the areas of greatest individual interest. By comparing their company to other companies tested and noting differences between responses of an individual and of the group, each management sector was able to evaluate company policies and to clarify their thinking on company operations. Heller regards his technique primarily as an information-gathering device, but the inclusion of content analysis clearly lends itself to the facilitation of change.

Miles et al. (1971) identify the basic processes that result from feedback and content analysis such as Heller describes. Presentation of data leads to client inquiry of why certain results were obtained and to discussion of problems that were not the primary focus of the data collection. Client involvement at this level promotes acceptance of the data and creates a positive attitude toward using the data. Group meetings, which increase client responsibility for making changes, can lead to positive interactions between members of problem-solving groups as well as to clarification of issues and, through increased discussion of values, to the establishment of a useful conformity of norms based on reason. As practical group problems are being worked on and change effected, groups also learn how to interact more effectively, and this leads to "process" changes. The authors emphasize the usefulness of objective data from surveys, rather than subjective data as provided by human relations trainers, since surveys allow for a higher degree of involvement by clients in planning, collecting, analyzing, and interpreting data.

Changing the Milieu of an Adolescent Residential Center

To demonstrate how detailed feedback of COPES results can be useful in facilitating social change, we conducted a study in an adolescent residential center (Moos, 1973). The center was a coeducational home for teenagers referred from hospitals or the juvenile courts. The youngsters were diagnosed as having primarily mental or emotional difficulties; many also had drug problems and a history of school failure. With a capacity to serve 14 adolescents, the program has 4 live-in house managers and a director who is a research psychologist. Residents stay in the program for about 4 months and progress through as many step levels, each level having increasing responsibilities and privileges. Residents are rated weekly on a point system by other residents and staff. At these meetings progress is evaluated in such areas as personal care, money management, interpersonal relationships, and meeting step level expectations. There is a member government, and the members take responsibility for basic housekeeping and cooking. Most have a therapist outside the house.

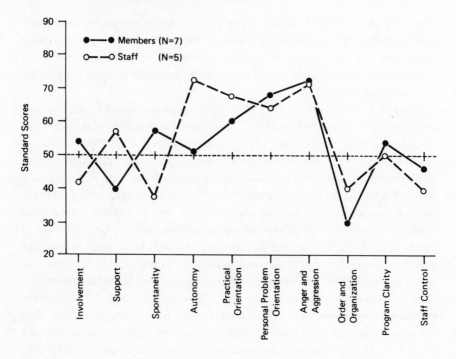

Figure 11.3   COPES Form C profiles for members and staff on program 104.

Initial Program Perceptions

Figure 11.3 plots the initial COPES Form C profiles for the residents and staff. Residents felt that the program strongly encouraged them to be spontaneous, to freely express their feelings (including angry feelings), and to be concerned with discussing and understanding their personal problems. For example, most residents felt that "Members are strongly encouraged to express themselves freely," that "Personal problems are openly talked about," and that "Staff encourage members to express their anger openly." The residents believed that there was slightly above-average emphasis on preparing them for release from the program; however they reported somewhat below-average emphasis on Support and Order and Organization. All the residents felt that "Things are sometimes very disorganized," and five agreed that "This place usually looks a little messy."

The residents and staff displayed some fairly large disagreements about

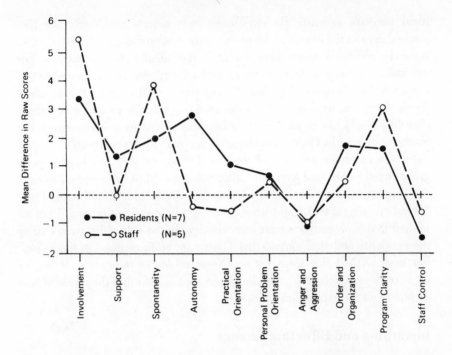

Figure 11.4 Real–ideal discrepancies as perceived by members and staff on program 104.

the characteristics of the program. For example, staff felt that the amount of emphasis on both Support and Autonomy was substantially above average, whereas the amount of emphasis on Involvement and Spontaneity was somewhat below average. For example, typical resident comments in the area of Spontaneity were "Members say anything they want to the staff" and "Members can generally do whatever they feel like"; most staff, however, felt these items were false. On the other hand, residents and staff agreed about the relative amount of emphasis on several of the other dimensions, most notably Personal Problem Orientation and Anger and Aggression.

Figure 11.4 compares the degrees of change the residents and staff would like to see in the program. The amount of change desired was calculated by subtracting the score the residents gave the actual program (Form C means) from the score they gave an ideal program (Form I subscale means). The same was done for staff. The profile shows the amount of increase or decrease needed in each area for the program to become an ideal program as currently envisioned by residents and staff. The line marked zero in the center of the profile indicates no change desired; that is, there is no discrepancy between real and ideal subscale means. For example, neither residents nor staff desired any change in the amount of emphasis on Personal Problem Orientation. Positive scores indicate a desire for increased emphasis in the area (e.g., residents and staff agreed that they would like to have fairly substantial increases in Involvement and Spontaneity and in Order and Organization and Program Clarity). Four of the seven residents and four of the five staff agreed that "It's hard to get a group together for card games or other activities," but none wished to have this feature in their ideal environment. All residents and staff agreed that "Members are careful about what they say when staff are around," but all wished that such cautions were unnecessary. In the area of Program Clarity the residents and staff agreed that "There are often changes in the rules," but most wished this were not so. Negative scores indicate a desire for decreased emphasis (e.g., residents and staff agreed that they wanted less emphasis on the expression of anger).

Instituting and Effecting Change

The profiles were discussed with residents and staff, and both groups showed an interest in systematically changing the program's social environment. One of the authors (Jean Otto) gave the feedback and met with residents and staff over a 4-month period. Several specific change attempts were made, and careful notes about all discussions and plans for change were kept. Following are some of the findings.

1.   There was a need to set up exciting involving special activities so that residents could really enjoy doing certain things together. Too much of the program structure involved problem-solving activities, and this had a dampening effect on the enthusiasm of residents and staff alike.

2.   Some staff felt that the residents wanted support for their acting-out behavior, whereas staff were anxious to discourage such behavior. A specific procedure by which residents could obtain peer support when they were having a personal problem was instituted. Any resident could call a "game" whenever they wished. All the other residents would then talk with the person about the problem he was having and would help him to seek a solution, or at least to feel better about the situation. For example, one girl called a "game" after she had had a very upsetting fight with her boyfriend.

The staff did not come to these games, which were usually held in the room of the person who was having the problem.

3.   Issues of Autonomy and Staff Control were important, especially since residents saw much less emphasis on Autonomy than did staff. The residents also indicated that they would ideally like much more emphasis on Autonomy. The main concern of staff was that residents often turned to them to make minor decisions that could have been made by the residents themselves; for example, residents often came to staff when they were sick and asked whether or not they should go to school. On the other hand, staff felt that residents entertained visions of having total freedom to do whatever they wanted to do without any concurrent responsibility.

Some of the specific changes initiated included the following.

1.   A position of crew-job chairman was started. One of the residents was made responsible for supervising the work around the house as it was assigned and checking the house every day to be sure that residents were doing their jobs adequately. This was initiated because there was some confusion over specific responsibilities for each job and also because the staff were assuming most of the burden of seeing that jobs were actually done.

2.   A position of food manager was established. The food manager was responsible for checking menus and for ascertaining whether the residents who were cooking dinner knew how to fix the meal and had all the supplies they needed.

3.   The resident coordinator position and sphere of responsibility was clarified. The coordinator who supervised both the crew-job chairman and the food manager, was given the authority to call resident group meetings whenever problems arose. In addition, he was placed on the screening committee, which decided about accepting new residents into the house. As might be expected in an adolescent residential center, Autonomy and Staff Control issues were quite complex and were discussed in detail.

The enumerated changes were also planned to have an effect on increasing Program Clarity. There was much discussion about this area in each of the resident–staff meetings, and several attempts were made to clarify expectations—for example, giving a resident the responsibility of teaching new residents their job obligations in the house, instituting a clearer structure in the process of individual goal setting, and establishing

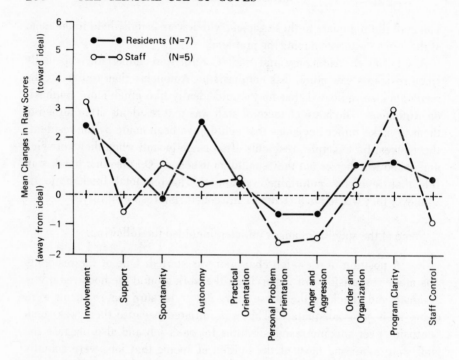

Figure 11.5 Mean changes in real–ideal discrepancies from the first to the second testing for members and staff on program 104.

a new rating procedure by which each resident rated the others on certain personal characteristics.

During the first two weeks of their stay, residents were required to keep a journal of their activities in and their reactions to the house. This journal was then used to help set personal goals. Originally new residents were simply told that they should think of specific operational goals for themselves, but they were given no clear way of figuring out what areas of personal behavior they should try to improve, nor how to go about the task. The journal was designed to help them focus on problem areas that others pointed out were problems for them. A procedure was also instituted whereby a new resident met with the director to go over his journal and set his goals.

COPES Forms C and I were given to residents and staff about 6 months after the initial testing. Figure 11.5 summarizes the mean changes in real–ideal program discrepancies from the first to the second testing. Points above the zero line indicate that residents and/or staff saw the program as closer to their ideal in the second testing, whereas points below the zero line indicate that the program appeared to be further away from their ideal in the second testing.

The residents generally felt that the treatment milieu was closer to their ideal in the second testing. The largest changes occurred in the Relationship dimension of Involvement and Support, the treatment Program dimension of Autonomy, and the System Maintainence Dimensions of Order and Organization and Program Clarity. In terms of Involvement and Support, for example, five of the seven members initially felt that the program had few social activities, but only two felt this to be true at the second testing. At the first testing only three members believed that members were given a great deal of individual attention, but at the second testing six reported that this was true. In terms of Autonomy, five members originally felt that there was no real membership government, but only two expressed this opinion at the second testing. Four of the seven members originally agreed that staff almost always acted on members' suggestions, but at the second testing all assented to this statement.

The staff also saw the program as closer to their ideal program at the second testing, particularly in the Relationship dimensions of Involvement and Spontaneity and in the System Maintenance dimension of Program Clarity. Like the residents, more staff agreed that the item "This program has very few social activities" was false at the second testing. In the area of Program Clarity, all staff originally felt that "Members never know when staff will ask to see them," whereas at the second testing none subscribed to this statement. Thus specific demonstrable changes occurred in each of the four major areas that had been extensively discussed in the house following the initial feedback sessions.

Importantly, both residents and staff felt that the program was further away from their ideal in the dimensions of Personal Problem Orientation and Anger and Aggression. This response is mainly attributable to a decision by residents and staff that they would ideally like less emphasis on these two areas. Thus we see that since views of ideal milieus may also change with feedback and discussion sessions, it is impossible to change a psychosocial environment toward a "static ideal." Feedback of information must be regarded as a dynamic, ongoing process that may result in continual changes in perceptions of ideal and actual social milieus. In addition, changes in conceptualizations of an ideal environment may follow changes in the actual environment.

Coping with Resistance to Change

In discussing resistance to program evaluation, Ellsworth (1973a) has cogently pointed out that "clinicians are not likely to cooperate in a process that might demonstrate their ineffectiveness" (p. 3). He found that staff were much more likely to accept feedback as accurate if it showed that they obtained above-average results with their patients. And he indicated that such feedback might or might not enable a ward team to increase its treatment effectiveness (1973b). Our experience, too, was that staff tend to react more positively to feedback when their WAS or COPES profiles show above-average scores (except on Staff Control!) and that they are more likely to question the validity of the scales when their profile scores are below average. This problem has not been too difficult to deal with because the profiles are simply summaries of the perceptions of the program participants and thus have a certain undeniable face validity. However, some resistance is usually encountered when a change in organizational procedures or goals is planned. Staff may complain that they are no longer sure of what is expected of them, that the change will be detrimental to the program, or that patients' disruptive behavior will increase. An understanding of this phenomenon will help a person who feels that change would be beneficial in dealing with such resistance.

Many of the studies on resistance to change within organizations have centered on the methods by which industrial settings adapt to technological change. Several key causes of resistance emerge from this literature. First, if the planned change requires basic revisions in the functions served by personnel, confusion over what is expected (i.e., role conflict) may lead to resistance (Wolfe and Snoek, 1964). Kahn et al. (1964) identify four sources of role conflict.

1. A person may receive conflicting directives (e.g., simultaneously to maintain authoritarian control of a unit and to be more sensitive to individual patients' problems).

2. Two different superiors may pressure a person to behave in different ways.

3. A person's role in one group may conflict with his role in another group. For example, the head staff member of a unit may be open to change when he represents the administrative point of view, but he may become opposed to change as he gains sensitivity to difficulties encountered by fellow staff on the unit.

4. Role conflict may result if the new demands made on a person require behavior not consistent with his needs and values (i.e., if his "personality" does not fit the new role).

Wolfe and Snoek maintain that two types of resistance can result from role conflict. The individual may become aggressive or hostile toward administration, openly opposing change, or he may withdraw from the group, creating resistance by his lack of participation.

Closely related to the problem of role conflict is the problem of resistance that develops because an issue is too ego-involving. When individuals have formed strong opinions about an issue, they often become personally committed to their ideas and are unwilling to change them. This is similar to role conflict in which the new role is in opposition to a person's values. For example, Freedman (1964) studied the effect of ego involvement on the ability of high school and college students to change opinions. The students were given a two-part concept-formation test. Half the group were told that the test was a measure of their personality and intelligence. These students were less able to change their original concepts (i.e., were much more committed to them), presumably because the concepts were a measure of themselves and thus highly ego-involving.

In one of Ellsworth's (1973a) investigations, administrators and clinicians expressed fears that their programs would be proved to be ineffective. These personnel seemed to be already committed to maintain their programs and were not open to evidence of unsuccessful outcome. In addition, Ellsworth sensed that administrators believed in their own competence to determine the best treatment for their clients and did not wish to have their decisions questioned. When personnel are made to feel that change is being initiated just because they are doing their job improperly or poorly, they react as to a personal threat and resist defensively.

A third source of resistance is observed when those toward whom change is directed do not clearly understand why change is being initiated, the methods that will be used to bring it about, or the effect it will have on them. Beer (1971) explains that resistance will be encountered when people do not have a clear image of organizational structure, policy, and goals, and when the need for change is not clearly articulated with these three related elements. Zander (1950) also demonstrates that an understanding of the form of change will help to alleviate unnecessary fears. Lippitt, Watson, and Westley (1958) hypothesize that such resistance is most often encountered early in the change process. In addition to being motivated to resist by fear and ignorance, people may also feel incapable of sucessfully achieving change; that is, they may be underesimating their own abilities.

Finally, change that ignores existing social relationships within the organization may foster resistance (Lawrence, 1969). Administrative staff must recognize that initiating change in one area may affect the types of relationships to which people have become accustomed. Relationships with other groups in the organization may also be changed. For example, if staff are used to working closely together and if they receive a great deal of support from close mutual relations, any move that might make them behave independently will be resisted. Likewise, an individual who has relatively high status with respect to his associates usually resists any move to diminish his power.

How can these types of resistance be dealt with effectively? One obvious but important point is that resistance must be openly confronted rather than suppressed. If resistance is stifled, its source cannot be uncovered and dealt with, and the difficulty of successfully initiating change will increase as pressure against it mounts.

Kahn et al. propose several ways of resolving problems of resistance created by role conflict or alterations in existing social relationships. First, if a change is made in one role, other interlinking roles should be altered in a direction that is supportive of the new role. Careful consideration must be given to informal relationships among people, as well as to more formally defined relationships (e.g., supervisor to subordinate). Briefly rotating people into other positions may help them to realize the need for change in their former behavior; such an approach may also help to teach them to behave in a more supportive way with respect to their associates. The authors also suggest that small, relatively independent groups should be the primary focus for change. In this way consistent relationships between people can be developed from the beginning. Mann and Neff (1961) indicate that observers might be used as change "catalysts," since outsiders are often more sensitive to developing role or relationship problems than are administrative staff. Lippitt et al. believe that those involved should be given a clear idea of how the establishment of new relationships or roles will allow needs to be met more satisfactorily.

Problems centered in a person's ego involvement with former attitudes or values seem to be handled best by direcing the individual's involvement toward the change process; that is, by increasing his participation in the process. Lewin (1952) suggested such an approach in his studies of group decision making. He showed that people resist change that does not conform to previously set group norms. However, if individuals perceive that the group norm has changed as a result of peer action, change will be supported. A classic study of the effect of participation on behavior based on Lewin's hypothesis was carried out by Coch and French (1948). They found that workers who participated in the change process had higher efficiency and a lower turnover rate than workers who did not. Changes should always be presented as a change in administrative policy or a group procedure; it is unadvisable to direct change in a personal manner toward an individual. Areas to which a group is less committed might be chosen as initial foci for a change.

It is best to face resistance created by lack of clarity early in the process, increasing the amount of communication between those directing the change and those subject to it. A momentum toward change is created when people have a clear image of the discrepancies between the current and the ideal organization. Participation in the process of change increases the individual's understanding of the objectives of the process. Besides understanding the process of change, those involved should know what the rewards will be for accomplishing it. Successful social change attempts must be planned and executed with as much detailed care, sensitivity, empathy to all perspectives, and luck as any successful therapeutic relationship. The most general rule we can formulate from our experience is: "The slower you start, the faster you finish."

The Process of Social Change

Our own methodology which is based on many of the foregoing considerations, includes four basic components. To begin, a systematic assessment of the social environment is made. Like methods used by Mann (1971) and Heller (1969), this step elicits specific information by which groups within an organization can be compared. Both member and staff perceptions are included in the analysis. Next, feedback is given to participating groups, with particular stress on real–ideal program differences. Feedback is a key element in most of the studies described previously. Primarily, this feedback is designed to provide information about elements in the program as it currently operates. With the WAS and COPES, however, the presentation of member and staff ideals adds a new dimension in program evaluation. Staff members can identify areas that do not measure up to their own stated values.

This analysis leads to the third step of process change—concrete planning of specific methods by which change can occur. For example, items responded to in opposite directions on the real and ideal forms aid members and staff in focusing on specific changes that might be made. Furthermore, since these modifications are based on the participants' own opinions and goals, as opposed to those of an outside observer, the chances of acceptance and cooperative implementation of changes are much greater.

Finally, a reassessment of the environment is made for the purpose of monitoring the results of the change. It is important to note that in fact the process does not end here. The follow-up assessment revealed the development of new problems both in our study and in Beckhard's investigation of the Vernon Company (1971). Members and staff reevaluate their ideals while attempting to reach them. As ideals change, people become dissatisfied with areas that were not of concern previously.

The four components just outlined carry certain underlying assumptions: (1) The social environment must be systematically defined and assessed to permit the occurrence of meaningful discussion and evaluation of attempts to institute social change. (2) All or as many as possible of the participants in a social system should be included in the various steps of planning and instituting change. (3) The individual motivations and goals of the participants must be taken into account in formulating both the directions and the methods for social change. (4) The systematic utilization of research results can itself have an adaptive value in directing, facilitating, and evaluating change.

The feedback and discussion sessions make practical applications out of ongoing research. By initially tying research to salient issues in a social system, individuals participating in the system can help design and cooperate in research that is both acceptable and relevant to their felt needs. This type of paradigm has been discussed by Menne (1967) and Heller (1969), and the latter has pointed out that the increasing complexity and subtlety of problems investigated in field research has put a strain on standard research techniques. The combination of feedback and discussion sessions with perceived environment data is an important mechanism in the acceptance and use of research, as well as a critical source of information and ideas about future relevant research. In this regard, easily administered assessment instruments such as the WAS and the COPES may be reasonable short-term information-gathering techniques for overburdened staff who lack extensive facilities or personnel for evaluation. Such techniques shed light on the congruence of the perceived environment from the perspectives of different groups and help articulate the relationship of the current environment to the overall goals of the social system.

Two considerations help identify the conditions under which this methodology is likely to be effective. First, it is probable that social change can best be facilitated by the methodology described when dealing with relatively small groups, in which most of the members interact directly with one another. As mentioned previously, the method then maximizes the involvement of each individual in the social setting, thus in the definition and facilitation of change. Second, if the method is to work, the dimensions on which changes are planned need to be under "local" control. Members and staff in community-oriented treatment programs can profitably discuss changing the degrees of emphasis on Involvement, Support, Autonomy, and Clarity because these variables are essentially under their control. As a rule, plans for effecting change in such other variables as the amount of money spent on each member per day or the staffing ratio must be handled somewhat differently.

This methodology is also directly linked to concepts of problem solving, coping, and adaptive behavior. Many theorists have discussed each individual's needs for involvement, for efficacy, and for the prediction and control of his own environment (e.g., White, 1959). The metholdology presented here is consonant with these important needs, which also include actively helping to mold one's social environment in desired directions. Its utilization may even help some individuals achieve a new competence— that of being able to change and control their own environments.

EVALUATING PROGRAM DESCRIPTIONS

The rapid proliferation of new types of psychiatric treatment programs has increased the need and demand for more accurate and complete program descriptions. Since the psychosocial or treatment environment is usually considered to be a key element in the therapeutic process, these descriptions should provide detailed information about this aspect of the program. Knowledge about a program's social milieu is important for prospective patients and staff, for referring and other community agencies, and for individuals interested in new developments in the field. Hamburg and Adams (1967) demonstrate that information seeking is a significant coping mechanism for people facing a new situation (e.g., high school students entering college, patients suffering from sudden, severe physical injuries, or parents facing the imminent death of a child). Both patients and staff might be better prepared to make use of community programs if they have a more complete understanding of what the program offers.

The program descriptions that have been written to fill these needs have depended primarily on observational techniques, supplemented by questionnaires reporting type of staffing, member characteristics, treatment techniques, and physical setting. Yet it is important to determine whether such published descriptions give an adequate picture of the treatment environment or social climate of a program. Jansen (1970) found that the descriptions of halfway houses by Raush and Raush (1968) did not seem to form an accurate picture of the programs she visited. Jansen says, "But on visiting such houses I was struck by the discrepancies between write-ups and actual practices. This may well be caused by the complexity of community living where the real transactions are hard to put one's finger on." In this connection, Speegle (1969) learned that the college environment as described in eight college catalogs was not congruent with students' perceptions of that environment as measured by the College Characteristics Index and that none of the catalogs he studied included descriptions of the informal social atmosphere of the college.

COPES was used to study the published descriptions of a sample of community programs to evaluate the information about the treatment milieu presented (Otto and Moos, 1973). Descriptions were found for five community programs for which COPES test results of members and staff were also available. Ten "naive" judges were given copies of these articles and were asked to complete a COPES questionnaire on the basis of the information appearing in the article. Comparing the results of the judges with those of members and staff in the program itself provided a measure of how accurately the treatment milieu of the program could be inferred from the article.

Judgments of the Five Programs

Four programs were described in *Halfway Houses for the Mentally Ill* (Glasscote et al., 1971; pp. 161–171). Program 115 is a coed residential center serving 19 people. The members, who are referred from a variety of other country programs (e.g., a crisis clinic, an outpatient service, and a day treatment center), must already be capable of handling their daily affairs, taking their own medications, and assisting with housework. Three meetings a week are held to discuss house problems, to assign work, and to develop social skills. The program is primarily designed to furnish a supportive environment in which members will be able to meet their goals. Program 117 (pp. 52–61) is a men's residence center, also serving a less than average chronic population. The men may attend a day hospital, work, attend school, or receive training at the State Department of Vocational Rehabilitation. The house provides a weekly group therapy session and some minimal recreational activities. Program 118 (pp. 49–63) is an adolescent residence center for boys who are referred from the courts or local state hospital. The boys attend public schools, but the program provides afternoon, evening, and weekend recreational activities. Frequent group and individual therapy sessions are held. Chronically ill men who have experienced several hospitalizations of 15 years or more are housed in program 119 (pp. 49–62). They learn basic life skills such as grooming, cooking, and housekeeping, and they are given jobs in a specially supervised workshop. The last program, described in *Partial Hospitalization for the Mentally Ill* (Glasscote et al., 1969; pp. 105–117) is program 116, a day treatment center. Program members must be sufficiently stable psychologically to participate in fairly high pressure group therapy meetings. Members are expected to use the program to develop their social skills and independence by building a therapeutic community at the center.

To determine whether the articles furnished enough information for judges to differentiate among programs on each of the subscales, a one-way analysis of variance was done for each of the COPES subscale scores. The judges perceived statistically significant differences among the five programs on nine of the subscales (all except Program Clarity). Thus the descriptions clearly gave different impressions of the programs' treatment milieus. Intraclass profile correlations of the judges' COPES profiles and the profiles of members and staff were calculated, thus permitting an assessment of the extent to which the judges' opinions agreed with those of the members and staff in the programs.

The judges' perceptions matched those of the members and staff for programs 116 and 117 relatively well. The intraclass correlations were .51 and .74 for program 116 and .70 and .71 for program 117. However, the degree of agreement was much lower for the coed residence (115), the home for chronic men (119), and the adolescent center (118). The intraclass correlations averaged .25 for judges and members and .22 for judges and staff for these three programs. This indicates that two of the reports provided more accurate information about the social milieu than did the other three, although in each program there were usually one or two areas in which judges agreed fairly well with members or staff.

Accurate and Inaccurate Descriptions

Program 116 showed good agreement between judges and actual program participants. Since the article was written from interviews with the staff and administrators of the program, it is understandable that judges shared staff perceptions somewhat more than members' perceptions. By relating specific items on individual subscales to information in the article, it is possible to see how judges could be so accurate in evaluating this program. In the area of Program Involvement, for example, judges agreed with both members and staff on 10 items. (The criterion for agreement was that at least 60% of judges, members, and/or staff had to answer the item in the same direction.) The items relate to how active members are in program activities and to the level of activities: "Members are pretty busy all of the time," "It's hard to get a group together for card games or other activities" (scored false), and "This program has very few social activities" (scored false).

The article explains that each member is assigned to one of four committees which are responsible for making home visits, contacting absentees, doing kitchen work, maintaining and furnishing the home used for the center, and organizing social activities. There are daily community meetings involving all participants, and twice a week each member takes part in smaller, patient-led group therapy meetings. In addition, there are special interest groups for adolescents, women, or individuals with related hobbies. The article explains that there is only one hour of free time a day. The listing of all these activities leaves the impression of a very active center with involved members.

Another area in which judges agreed closely with participants was Autonomy. The items on the Autonomy subscale refer to members being independent in decision making in the program: "Members are expected to take leadership here," "The staff almost always act on members' suggestions," and "Very few members have any responsibility for the program here" (scored false). The committees mentioned before are an indication of the responsibilities members are expected to assume, but there were also several sections in the article describing the high degree of patient Autonomy in the program.

The judges' scores strongly resembled those of the members and staff in one of the mens' residence programs (program 117), as well. In the area of Order and Organization, judges agreed with members on seven items and with staff on eight items. The article mentioned that the house is kept clean and that members are taught to be well groomed, and organized daytime activities were listed. In the area of Practical Orientation, measuring the emphasis on preparing for leaving the home and on learning practical skills, judges agreed with members on six items and with staff on eight items. The article explained that staff help members learn how to cook, shop, and groom, as well as how to interact socially. The program takes a life-management approach, stressing learning to handle everyday problems, rather than focusing on gaining insight into personal problems. The judges agreed with members and staff on four items relating to Autonomy (i.e., the degree of independence and leadership encouraged in members). The article briefly explained that the program's goal was to prepare the men for autonomous living. Although this article was only two pages long, it furnished enough specific information to allow the judges to make some quite accurate appraisals.

One of the programs for which the judges made the least accurate distinctions was the adolescent program (program 118). Whereas members and staff in the program agreed on 7 items in Support, 7 items in Autonomy, and 10 items in Personal Problem Orientation, the judges showed little or no agreement with members or staff in any of these areas. The article said that group therapy and feedback sessions are held but failed to describe what is discussed or how members are supported by these sessions. The article also explained that members who are "functioning" better are moved to an adjacent house and have more privileges, but these privileges were not defined. Regular meetings are held discussing members' progress, but again no details were given. Primarily the article discussed members' characteristics, background, eligibility, and common problems with drugs and family.

Judges agreed with members and staff on more items for articles that supplied detailed discussions of the program philosophy and specific information about member–staff interaction. The length of the description was not the determining factor in judges' accuracy. However, one program for which there was high agreement between judges and staff included several quotations from the program director and presented accounts of specific incidents at the center.

GUIDELINES FOR WRITING PROGRAM DESCRIPTIONS

Descriptions of treatment programs should serve to provide as accurate and complete a picture as possible of the essential characteristics of these programs. As indications that descriptions of milieus may not be fulfilling their functions as well as they should, we have Jansen's (1970) findings regarding the congruence between her impressions and published descriptions of halfway houses and Speegle's (1969) data on the congruence between college catalogs and students' perceptions of their colleges. Our own results are in accord with those of Jansen and Speegle, suggesting that there may be systematic distortions in program descriptions, at least for certain programs. There seem to be two major reasons for inaccurate program descriptions. First, important information is sometimes simply not included. Second, the description may be biased in overly positive directions because it is written by an individual who has responsibility for the program and thus wishes it to be seen in a positive light.

In terms of the issue of completeness, improved program descriptions should more adequately and systematically include information relevant to each of the major methods currently available for characterizing human environments. Six different types of dimensions have been commonly used to describe human milieus (see Chapter 1). Each of these six types is specifically relevant to descriptions of psychiatric treatment programs.

1.   Relevant *ecological* variables are those related to architectural and physical design. There is extensive evidence that the physical design characteristics of the location in which a treatment program is housed may have important attitudinal and behavioral consequences for program participants (e.g., Good et al., 1965; Proshansky et al.; Sommer, 1969). Specific information might include the number of different types of rooms available in the house, the size of these rooms, the number and size of different bedrooms, the type and layout of furniture in the living or common room, the types of pictures and wall decorations, and wall colors. This section of a program description probably does not need to be extensive, but some information about the physical settings in which a treatment program functions should help to provide a "feel" of the program.

2.   Some of the *behavior settings* that frequently occur in a treatment program (e.g., individual therapy, group therapy, community meetings) are often mentioned in program descriptions. However, the more informal

settings (e.g., free time, lunch time, picnics, recreational activities) may be extremely important in determining the treatment milieu, and these are usually inadequately or incompletely described. Since Barker (1968) and his colleagues have shown that the specific characteristics of behavior settings exert significant influences on the behavior and attitudes of their inhabitants, at least the settings that occur most frequently should be described.

3. *Organizational structure* dimensions are usually already included in program descriptions. The kinds of variables falling into this category include the size of the program (number of members), the member–staff ratio, the basic cost of the program, and the number of types of staff. These are all important aspects of treatment programs. Since these organizational structure variables do not bear particularly high correlations to perceived climate variables, however, it appears that they describe only one facet of a program. Organizational structure dimensions are necessary but not sufficient for describing treatment programs.

4. Information about the personal and background *characteristics of the milieu inhabitants* appears in most program descriptions, but the information is generally much more complete for members than for staff. Average age, chronicity level, diagnoses, length of stay in the program, and length of previous hospitalization are all commonly used variables that are of obvious importance in understanding the basic characteristics of the program. More information about the background characteristics of staff would be desirable.

The type of information included in these first four methods of characterizing treatment programs is fairly concrete and is usually readily obtainable. This information defines the basic physical characteristics of the program, the specific types of settings in which members and staff function, the overall organizational structure, and the background characteristics of members and staff. The more abstract elements or "feel" of the program, although somewhat less readily defined or measured, are certainly of at least equal importance. For example, program descriptions should systematically include information about the two final factors, as follows.

5. Investigators need data on the psychosocial characteristics and the social climate of the program. Methods such as the WAS and the COPES may be used to specify the psychosocial or perceived climate

characteristics of the treatment milieu. Even if it is difficult to administer the entire COPES to all members and staff, it may be possible, for a selected sample of members and/or staff to take the 40-item Short Form or for one or two outside observers to fill out the COPES on the basis of their observations of the program. Most treatment programs have frequent visitors and these individuals could fill out the COPES on the basis of their visit. At a minimum, program descriptions should attempt to describe systematically each of the dimensions included in the Relationship, Treatment Program, and System Maintenance areas. In this way a relatively complete description of the psychosocial milieu should be assured.

6.   Information is also required on the kinds of behaviors and attitudes that generally tend .to be reinforced (i.e., a functional or reinforcement analysis of the treatment program). Examples of relevant functional analyses of environments include the work on Environmental Force Units (EFU) by Schoggen (1963), Wolf's (1966) intriguing analysis of the specific conditions in the environment which reinforce the development of general intelligence and academic achievement, and Buehler et al.'s (1966) methods for identifying and measuring the social reinforcers occurring among inmates and staff in institutions for delinquent children.

Ideally, characterizations of treatment programs should use information relevant to all six types of dimensions identified for representing human milieus. Each method gives a somewhat different perspective on a program, and the use of all six should furnish relatively accurate and complete program descriptions. Aspects of program descriptions that are subject to individual perceptions (e.g., social climate) should make use of data-gathering methods that include a variety of individual perspectives, thus ensuring that specific biases are not overemphasized. Moreover, since members and staff may have varying views of program characteristics, both views should be included in program descriptions. Systematic inclusion of the views of an outside observer or interviewer would also be helpful. These considerations are more important in portions of program descriptions that attempt to provide information about reinforcement contingencies or the psychosocial treatment milieu. Accounts of specific illustrative incidents in the program might also give substance to these portions of program descriptions.

Many investigators have suggested that different institutions know much more about the individuals they are attempting to recruit or place than those individuals know about the institution. For example, colleges know more about the characteristics of entering students than entering students know about the colleges they plan to enter. As a rule, social workers and other program staff know far more about the characteristics of an individual patient than they do about the program or programs into which they wish to place him. Furthermore, the patient himself seldom knows much at all about the salient program characteristics. It may be that this imbalance of information is partly responsible for the extremely high rate of premature termination of treatment. Information about individual and group psychotherapy seems to be helpful to patients entering these treatment modalities. Similarly, patients should be assisted by prior knowledge about residential programs, especially those which are community-based (since they frequently include somewhat healthier individuals, who are usually able to participate in selecting a program).

Inclusion of the types of information suggested here should make program descriptions more complete and accurate and therefore more useful, not only to professionals with academic interests in developments in the field, but also to prospective staff considering working in a particular treatment program, and to social workers who need to make referral decisions. Finally, patients themselves would gain, especially the growing proportion of those who wish to take a more active part in choosing the treatment program that might be most beneficial to them.

REFERENCES

Barker, R. *Ecological psychology.* Stanford University Press, Stanford, Calif., 1968.

Bavelas, A. & Strauss, G. Group dynamics and intergroup relations. In Bennis, W., Benne, K., & Chin, R. (Eds.). *The planning of change.* Holt, Rinehart & Winston, New York, 1961.

Beckhard, R. Helping a group with planned change. In Hornstein, H., Bunker, B., Burke, W., Gindes, M., & Lewicki, R. (Eds.). *Social Intervention: A behavioral science approach.* Free Press, New York, 1971.

Beer, M. Organizational climate: A viewpoint from the change agent. Paper presented at American Psychological Association Convention, Washington, D.C., 1971.

Buehler, R., Patterson, G., & Furniss, J. The reinforcement of behavior in institutional settings. *Behavior Research and Therapy,* 4: 157–167, 1959.

Coch, L., & French, J. Overcoming resistance to change. *Human Relations,* 1: 512–532, 1948.

Ellsworth, R. Consumer feedback in measuring the effectiveness of mental health programs.

In Guttentag, M. & Struening, E. (Eds.). *Handbook of evaluation research*, to be published, 1973a.

Ellsworth, R. Feedback: Asset or liability in improving treatment effectiveness. *Journal of Consulting and Clinical Psychology*, **40**: 383–393, 1973b.

Fleishman, E. A leadership climate, human relations training, and supervisory behavior. *Personnel Psychology*, **6**: 205–222, 1953.

Freedman, J. Involvement, discrepancy, and change. *Journal of Abnormal and Social Psychology*, **69**: 290–295, 1964.

Glasscote, R., Glassman, S., Jepson, W., & Kraft, A. *Partial hospitalization for the mentally ill: A study of programs and problems.* American Psychiatric Association, Washington, D.C., 1969.

Glasscote, R., Gudeman, J., & Elpers, R. *Halfway houses for the mentally ill.* American Psychiatric Association, Washington, D.C., 1971.

Good, L., Siegel, S., & Bay, A. *Therapy by design.* Charles C. Thomas, Springfield, Ill., 1965.

Hamburg, D. & Adams, J. A perspective on coping behavior: Seeking and utilizing information in major transitions. *Archives of General Psychiatry*, **17**: 277–284, 1967.

Heller, F. Group feedback analysis: A method of field research. *Psychological Bulletin*, **72**: 108–117, 1969.

Jansen, E. The role of the halfway house in community mental health programs in the United Kingdom and America. *American Journal of Psychiatry*, **126**: 142–148, 1970.

Kahn, R., Wolfe, D., Quinn, R., & Snoek, J. *Organizational stress: Studies in role conflict and ambiguity.* Wiley, New York, 1964.

Lawrence, P. How to deal with resistance to change. *Harvard Business Review*, **47**: 4–12, 166–176, 1969.

Lewin, K. Group decision and social change. In Swanson, G., Newcomb, T., & Hartley, E. (Eds.). *Readings in social psychology.* Holt, Rinehart & Winston, New York, 1952.

Lippitt, R., Watson, J., & Westley, B. *Planned change.* Harcourt Brace Jovanovich, New York, 1958.

Mann, F. Studying and creating change. In Hornstein, H., Bunker, B., Burke, W., Gindes, M., & Lewicki, R. (Eds.). *Social Intervention: A behavioral science approach.* Free Press, New York, 1971.

Mann, F. & Neff, F. *Managing major change in organizations.* Foundation for Research on Human Behavior, Ann Arbor, Mich., 1961.

Menne, J. Techniques for evaluating the college environment. *Journal of Educational Measurement*, **4**: 219–225, 1967.

Miles, M., Hornstein, H., Calder, P., Callahan, D., & Schiavo, R. Data feedback: A rationale. In Hornstein, H., Bunker, B., Burke, W., Gindes, M., & Lewicki, R. (Eds.). *Social intervention: A behavioral science approach.* Free Press, New York, 1971.

Moos, R. Changing the social milieus of psychiatric treatment settings. *Journal of Applied Behavioral Science*, **9**: 575–593, 1973.

Moos, R. & Otto, J. The Community-Oriented Programs Environment Scale: A methodology for the facilitation and evaluation of social change. *Community Mental Health Journal,* **8:** 28–37, 1972.

Otto, J. & Moos, R. Evaluating descriptions of psychiatric treatment programs. *American Journal of Orthopsychiatry,* **43:** 401–410, 1973.

Proshansky, H., Ittelson, W., & Rivlin, L. (Eds.). *Environmental psychology: Man and his physical setting.* Holt, Rinehart & Winston, New York, 1970.

Raush, J. L. & Raush, C. L. *The halfway house movement: A search for sanity.* Appleton-Century-Crofts, New York, 1968.

Schoggen, P. Environmental forces in everyday lives of children. In Barker, R. (Ed). *The stream of behavior.* Appleton-Century-Crofts, New York, 1963.

Speegle, J. College catalogs: An investigation of the congruence of catalog descriptions of college environments with student perceptions of the same environment as revealed by the College Characteristics Index. Doctoral dissertation, Syracuse University, Suracuse, N.Y., 1969.

Sommer, R. *Personal space.* Prentice-Hall, Englewood Cliffs, N.J., 1969.

White, R. Motivation reconsidered: The concept of competence. *Psychological Review,* **66:** 297–333, 1959.

Wolf, R. The measurement of environments. In Anastasi, A. (Ed.). *Testing problems in perspective,* American Council on Education, Washington, D.C., 1966.

Wolfe, P. & Snoek, J. A study of tension and adjustment under role conflict. In Bennis, W., Schein, E., Berelow, P., & Steele, F. (Eds.). *Interpersonal dynamics.* Dorsey, Homewood, Ill., 1964.

Zander, A. Resistance to change: Its analysis and prevention. *Advanced Management,* **15:** 9–11, 1950.

Chapter Twelve

THE EFFECTS OF COMMUNITY–BASED TREATMENT PROGRAMS

This section deals with a replication and extension of the material discussed in Chapter 6 on the relation between the structural and organizational characteristics of programs and their treatment environments. In brief review, there are several alternative ways of representing psychiatric treatment and other types of institutional environments. Chapter 6 supplies data relating two structural characteristics of programs (size and staffing), a program policy characteristic (the amount of adult status allowed patients), and an average behavioral characteristic of the patients (disturbed behavior) to patient and staff perceptions of treatment milieus. The results indicated that significant relationships of moderate magnitude existed between these objective program characteristics and perceived treatment climate. Since the different ways of assessing program characteristics are only moderately interrelated, each provide unique information and each should be utilized in attempts to construct reasonably complete program descriptions. These findings are consistent with those arrived at by investigators studying other institutions, particularly colleges and universities. The general conclusion is that various descriptive methods are needed to provide accurate and complete characterizations of institutional environments; the various methods, moreover, are differentially relevant for different purposes (e.g., rapid objective description, attempts at changing the social milieu).

These considerations, in conjunction with our special interest in obtaining further information on the relationships among different ways of characterizing environments, led us to develop a Program Information Form (PIF). The PIF is based on logic similar to that used in the Ward Information Form, but it includes a substantially more extensive sampling of variables of potential utility in describing psychiatric treatment programs.

THE PROGRAM INFORMATION FORM (PIF)

The PIF was developed by identifying potential items from a variety of sources, including detailed interviews with program administrators and staff and reading of program descriptions already available in the literature. The PIF went through several revisions based mainly on feedback from program staff. The final version consists of 30 items grouped into six sections. Program staff are told that whereas COPES asks questions about the social climate of the program, the PIF is designed to elicit information about the program's physical, structural, and background characteristics. Let us now list the six sections of the PIF and examples of items in each section.

1. *The Origins and population* section asks about the type of center (live-in home, day center, workshop, etc.), the type of community area adjacent to the center (hospital grounds, urban residential, urban commercial, rural, etc.), the total number of rooms in the center, the length of time that the center has been in operation, the total capacity of the program, the number of members currently in the program, the sex and age distribution of the members, their education, their length of stay in the program, and so on.

2. *The staff* section includes questions on the total number of staff, the number of staff in different positions (e.g., resident manager, administrative supervisor, psychologist, or psychiatrist), the number of staff with college degrees, the age and sex distribution of the staff, and the average length of time each has been working in the program.

3. *The rules and decisions* section seeks information on the areas in which members make the final decisions (e.g., attendance or nonattendance at program activities, curfews, restrictions for breaking rules, discharge, work assignments, medication and on the use of different techniques of rule enforcement (staff or member criticism, house restriction or restriction to room, loss of privileges or points, etc.).

4. *The financial arrangements* section requests such information as

whether members pay a set fee, the monthly per member cost of operating the program, and the proportion of the cost usually met by members' fees.

5. *The work and jobs* section includes questions on the extent of members' participation in housekeeping and cooking duties and on the number of members who have paying jobs in regular work situations, are going to school or acquiring vocational training, and so on.

6. *The evaluation and discharge* section represents an attempt to learn about the frequency with which members' progress is evaluated, about the number of members who were discharged or who dropped out of the program in the previous 3 months, and about the community placement (return to family, foster home, independent living arrangement, etc.) of the discharged members.

Printed materials about the programs such as written rules or descriptions were also obtained whenever possible. The information on the PIF was elicited with a written questionnaire form supplemented either by personal interview or by telephone contact when necessary. Since the PIF was not developed until after some programs had already been tested with COPES, and since some of the questions were not relevant for all programs (this was particularly true of the community care homes), we had relatively complete PIF information on a subsample of only 16 programs. All PIF items were scored for each of these 16 programs, but the results indicated that there was little or no variation across the programs for approximately half the items. Fifteen items grouped into four different categories were selected for detailed analysis.

Structural Program Variables

The first set of dimensions characterizing programs are identified as structural variables. There were initially six variables in this category: (1) the number of rooms included in the center, (2) the total capacity of the program, (3) the number of members, (4) the staff–member ratio, (5) the monthly program cost per member, and (6) the number of years the program had been in operation. When intercorrelated over the 16 programs, these variables showed only moderate interrelationships, except for a correlation of .94 between total capacity of the program and number of current members. Thus the variable of total capacity was dropped from further analyses.

Table 12.1 lists the rank-order correlations between staff COPES Form C

TABLE 12.1 RANK–ORDER CORRELATIONS BETWEEN STAFF COPES FORM C SUBSCALES AND STRUCTURAL PROGRAM VARIABLES (N = 16 PROGRAMS)

COPES Subscales	Number of Members	Staff–Member Ratio	Monthly Cost	Years in Operation
Involvement	.02	.28	.32	−.54**
Support	−.32	.23	.53**	−.54**
Spontaneity	.08	−.07	.37	−.52**
Autonomy	−.34	.01	.14	−.33
Practical Orientation	−.72***	.34	−.36	.24
Personal Problem Orientation	−.23	.41*	.51**	−.58**
Anger and Aggression	−.11	.27	.20	−.76***
Order and Organization	−.33	−.08	−.43*	.32
Program Clarity	−.46*	.39	−.61***	.18
Staff Control	.45*	−.56**	−.51**	−.13

* $p < .10$.
** $p < .05$.
*** $p < .01$.

subscales and the structural program variables. Mean member and mean staff perceptions for each of the Form C subscales were first correlated over the 16 programs. There were significant correlations between member and staff perceptions for all 10 subscales, 6 of the 10 being significant at the .01 level. Thus Table 12.1 gives only correlations for mean staff perceptions. The variable of the total number of rooms in the center did not correlate significantly with any of the COPES subscales and is thus not shown.

The average number of members in the 16 programs was 26; the range was 6 to 43. The average staff–member ratio was 1–5, ranging from somewhat less than 1–2 in the most heavily staffed program to 1–16 in the most poorly staffed one. As expected, staff on larger programs see less emphasis on the Relationship dimension of Support and all Treatment Program dimensions, most notably Practical Orientation and Autonomy. Staff in the larger programs also see less emphasis on Order and Organization and Program Clarity and more emphasis on Staff Control. The results are mostly similar (but of course in the reverse direction) for staff–member ratio. These findings are generally congruent with those for wards (see Table 6.2), except that some of the current correlations are higher and that both Practical Orientation and Program Clarity are highly related to size and staffing. The Practical Orientation dimension is more salient in community-based programs than in hospital-based programs, which may account for the substantially greater emphasis on this dimension in smaller, better staffed programs.

When the monthly cost of the 16 programs was estimated, it ranged from $225 to $600 per member. These are not exact cost figures; rather, they are the costs as estimated by the individual responsible for the financial management of the program. As the cost of the program increases, the emphasis on the Relationships dimensions increases, as does the emphasis on Personal Problem Orientation. However, the emphasis on the System Maintenance dimensions lessens.

The last structural variable assessed was the number of years the program had been in operation. The 16 programs had been operating for an average of 6 years; the newest program had existed for less than a year and the oldest program for more than 15 years. This variable was not related to any of the other structural variables. Staff see less emphasis on the Relationship dimensions and on Personal Problem Orientation and Anger and Aggression in "older" programs. Since the number of years of program operation is related to the average ages of both residents and staff, the correlations in Table 12.1 are partly a function of these variables, as is discussed later.

The results indicate that there are some substantial relationships between treatment environment as perceived by staff (and also by members) and these structural program variables. On smaller, more highly staffed, more costly, and "younger" programs, as a rule, the emphasis on the Relationship and Treatment Program dimensions is higher, whereas the emphasis on the System Maintenance dimensions is lower. A substantial proportion of the variance in the treatment environments of the programs studied is accounted for by these four structural program variables.

Average Member Background Characteristics

In the next analysis, four background characteristics of members were related to staff perceptions of treatment environment. The four characteristics were: (1) mean age, which was 31.9 years (S. D. = 7.6); (2) mean education, which was 12.2 years 1 (S.D. = 1.6); (3) mean length of stay in the program, which was 3.4 months (S.D. = 1.4 months); and (4) proportion of members who either currently had jobs or were going to school or taking vocational training. On the average, 24% of the members fell into one of these categories; the variation across programs, however, was from 0 to 52%.

TABLE 12.2   RANK–ORDER CORRELATIONS BETWEEN STAFF COPES FORM C SUBSCALES AND MEMBERS' BACKGROUND CHARACTERISTICS ($N = 16$ PROGRAMS)

COPES Subscales	Mean Age	Mean Length of Stay	Proportion of Members Working or Going to School
Involvement	−.31	−.21	.27
Support	−.46*	−.56**	.12
Spontaneity	−.13	−.48**	.20
Autonomy	−.31	−.23	.51**
Practical Orientation	−.33	−.29	.51**
Personal Problem Orientation	−.63***	−.54**	.41*
Anger and Aggression	−.64***	−.40	.46*
Order and Organization	.22	.00	−.24
Program Clarity	−.10	−.22	.16
Staff Control	.41*	−.06	−.59**

```
  *   p < .10
 **   p < .05
***   p < .01
```

Table 12.2 presents the rank-order correlations between the staff COPES Form C subscales and three of the four member background characteristics. The correlations for mean education are not given because there were no significant relationships between this variable and treatment environment. The results indicate that as the mean age of the members increases, staff perceptions of the emphasis on all three Relationship dimensions (most notably Support) and on all four Treatment Program dimensions (most notably Personal Problem Orientation and Anger and Aggression) decreases, whereas their perception of the amount of emphasis on Staff Control increases. The correlations between mean length of members' stay and the COPES subscales were somewhat similar in that staff saw much less emphasis on Support, Spontaneity, and Personal Problem Orientation in programs in which the members stayed longer. Finally, the higher the proportion of program members who were working or going to school, the more emphasis staff perceived on all four Treatment Program dimensions and the less they reported on Staff Control. The correlation between mean member age and the proportion of members who were working or going to school was $-.52$; however, the mean length of members' stay was not correlated with either of the other background characteristics.

Thus there are substantial relationships between treatment environment and the three member background characteristics named. Essentially, emphasis on Relationship and Treatment Program dimensions increases as the members function better, whereas emphasis on System Maintenance dimensions, particularly Staff Control, decreases. It is important to note that staff perceptions were correlated with members' background characteristics; therefore, these relationships could not be mediated by the individual characteristics of the perceivers. Programs with older patients have less emphasis on Personal Problem Orientation and Anger and Aggression and more emphasis on Staff Control, but not simply because older patients may perceive these areas differently from younger patients—this conclusion is also corroborated by the general lack of relationships between individual perceptions of environments and individual background characteristics of perceivers, as briefly reviewed in Chapter 3.

Average Staff Background Characteristics

Three background characteristics of staff were assessed, as follows: (1) mean age of the staff, which was 36.8 years (S.D. $= 8.5$), (2) proportion of the staff with a college degree, and (3) proportion of female staff. Over all programs, 58% of the staff had a college degree. This percentage varied from 33% in one program to 100% in another. Approximately 41% of the staff in the 16 programs were female, the percentage range from 17 to 70%. There were no significant relationships between the proportion of female staff and treatment environment.

Mean staff age was strongly related to staff perceptions of program milieus. As the age of staff increases, the emphasis on all three Relationship dimensions (most notably Involvement) and on all four

Treatment Program dimensions (particularly Personal Problem Orientation and Anger and Aggression) decreases; however, the emphasis on all three System Maintenance dimensions (especially Order and Organization) increases. The actual correlations are quite substantial in magnitude. On the other hand, the correlations between the proportion of staff with a college degree and treatment environment were generally negligible. The only significant relationship was that Autonomy increased as the proportion of staff with a college degree rose.

There was a slight but nonsignificant negative correlation ($r = -.22$) between the two staff background variables just mentioned. However, the mean age of staff correlated .71 with the mean age of members, and these variables correlated .48 and .54, respectively, with the number of years the program had been in operation. Thus there is an "age" dimension that strongly differentiates among the 16 programs in this sample. The programs that have been in operation the longest have the oldest members and the oldest staff. Since patients are usually placed into different programs, it is unlikely that a significant self-selection factor is involved; nevertheless, there is certainly a program selection factor in so far as staff attempt to pick new patients who will "fit" with patients already in the program.

Staff usually have a reasonable amount of choice over which program they wish to work in; more importantly still, they often can influence the decision-making input with respect to which new staff are hired. Thus both self-selection and program-selection factors must operate to maximize the degree of age similarity between members and staff.

Figure 12.1 graphically illustrates the findings by comparing staff perceptions for the six programs in which staff mean age was less than 30 with the seven programs in which staff mean age was greater than 40. The mean ages of the members in these two groups of programs were similarly discrepant. Staff in "younger" programs see more emphasis in the areas of Involvement, Spontaneity, Personal Problem Orientation, Anger and Aggression, and (to a lesser extent) Autonomy, whereas they see less emphasis on Order and Organization, Program Clarity, and (to a lesser extent) Staff Control. Some of these differences are very large in magnitude—the scores on Anger and Aggression are almost 4 mean raw score points apart, whereas the scores for both Personal Problem Orientation and Order and Organization differ by almost 3 mean raw score points. Members showed almost identical differences, but they were not quite as large as those for staff.

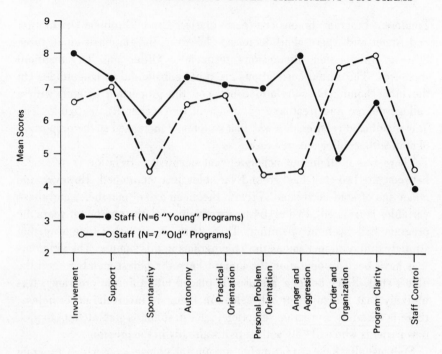

Figure 12.1   COPES Form C staff perceptions on "young" (N = 6) versus "old" (N = 7) programs.

Program Policy Variables

The fourth category of dimensions to be assessed consisted of program policy variables. Only the following two variables differentiated among the 16 programs included in our analysis: (1) the number of areas in which the members made final decisions and (2) the frequency with which members' progress was formally evaluated. The first variable was significantly correlated (positively) only with the Treatment Program dimension of Autonomy. The frequency of formal evaluations correlated significantly negatively with Autonomy and Practical Orientation and significantly positively with Staff Control.

In summary, relationships have been presented involving treatment environment and selected structural dimensions, members' background characteristics, staff background characteristics, and program policy variables. The results are preliminary, since only 16 programs were included; it appears, however, that perceived treatment environment bears relatively substantial relationships to the more objective characteristics, which also differentiate among programs. In general, the Relationship dimensions are emphasized more heavily in smaller programs with larger staff–member ratios, higher monthly costs per member, and younger members and staff.

The same programs place much more emphasis on the Treatment Program dimensions of Personal Problem Orientation and Anger and Aggression. All four Treatment Program dimensions are more strongly emphasized in programs that have a greater proportion of patients who are either working or going to school. Programs in which a greater proportion of staff have a college degree and in which members are allowed to make more decisions for themselves put more emphasis on Autonomy, whereas programs in which formal evaluations occur frequently insist less on Autonomy. Finally, programs in which staff are older have substantially more emphasis on all three System Maintenance dimensions, whereas more expensive programs place substantially less emphasis on the same dimensions. Otherwise, the clearest relationships are with Staff Control, which is higher on larger programs and on programs having a greater frequency of formal evaluations, and lower on programs having higher staff–member ratios and a higher proportion of working members.

The most striking results concern the high correlations between the number of years a program has been in operation and the average age of the members and the staff. The treatment environments of "younger" programs are very different from those of "older" programs. The data strongly substantiate the importance of developing a variety of measures by which to assess program characteristics. They also raise the intriguing possibility that members and staff somehow select or are selected by programs in which they are likely to be similar to the other participants. This notion encouraged us to develop some indices of program homogeneity and to relate these indices to treatment environment (see Chapter 13).

TREATMENT ENVIRONMENT AND SATISFACTION

A study done with COPES attempted to replicate the relationships between treatment environment, satisfaction, and personal development as found in hospital-based programs. For 13 of the programs tested with COPES, we administered a slightly modified version of the questionnaire assessing overall reactions to the program (see Chapter 7). There were six questions asking members to rate their general satisfaction with the program, how much they liked the members and staff in the program, how anxious they felt, and how they rated their experiences in the program as having provided a chance to test their abilities and to increase their self-confidence. Eleven questions were answered on 5-point scales. Rank-order correlations were calculated over the 13 programs between the COPES subscales and the members' reactions to the programs. General satisfaction and liking for members were again combined, as were the abilities and self-confidence items, because of their high intercorrelations.

The three Relationship dimensions were highly correlated with general satisfaction, liking for staff, and personal development (e.g., $r = .56, .57$, and $.81$, respectively, for Involvement). There were fewer relationships between these variables and either the Treatment Program or the System Maintenance dimensions, although the extent of emphasis on Personal Problem Orientation was significantly related to general satisfaction ($r = .79$), the emphasis on Order and Organization was significantly related to liking for staff ($r = .64$) and to personal development ($r = .51$), the emphasis on Program Clarity was positively related to personal development ($r = .50$), and finally the emphasis on Staff Control was negatively related to anxiety ($r = -.50$).

Broadly speaking, the foregoing results replicate those found for the WAS as summarized in Table 7.5, certain exceptions not withstanding. The clearest replication is for the Relationship dimensions, on which the results are essentially identical in hospital-based and community-based programs. Thus the finding that Involvement, Support, and Spontaneity are positively related to satisfaction, liking for staff, and hopefulness about expected treatment progress is clearly replicated. The "negative" finding that anxiety is not related to the emphasis on the Relationship dimensions also generalizes from hospital-based to community-based programs.

The results for the dimensions of Autonomy, Personal Problem Orientation, and Order and Organization were basically replicated in the two samples, although some of the relationships are not quite as strong in the community-based programs. Finally, the results for the dimensions of Practical Orientation, Program Clarity, and Staff Control were somewhat different in the current sample. Partly because of a restricted range of Practical Orientation scores in the 13 programs under consideration, no relationships appeared between Practical Orientation and any of the members' reactions. The results for the dimensions of Program Clarity and Staff Control are particularly intriguing when it is recalled that Stern conceives of the System Maintenance dimensions as catabolic. In this sample, Program Clarity was positively related to personal development and Staff Control was negatively related to anxiety. Thus both dimensions had some positive effects, at least in terms of members' reactions.

The strongest relationships between treatment environment and general reactions to the program occur for the Relationship Dimensions. When these dimensions are emphasized by staff, morale is generally high, members feel more satisfied, like one another and the staff more, and are more hopeful about treatment. As a rule, emphases on the Treatment Program dimensions of Autonomy, Practical Orientation, and Personal Problem Orientation are positively related to these member reactions. There is not a single example of a negative correlation between the emphasis on these three Treatment Program dimensions and any of the three above-mentioned reactions to treatment programs. The extent of emphasis on Anger and Aggression is generally not related to patient reactions to treatment programs. Finally, the relationships between treatment environment and reactions to programs are least clear and consistent for the System Maintenance dimensions, although Order and Organization and Program Clarity tend to be positively related to satisfaction, liking for staff, and personal development. The results for Staff Control, although not directly inconsistent, were not replicated. Staff Control, which was negatively related to patient satisfaction, liking for staff, and personal development in the ward studies, was negatively related to member anxiety in the community program studies.

DEVIANT PERCEPTIONS

An attempt was made to replicate the relationships between deviant perceptions and patients' reactions to their treatment programs, as described in Chapter 9. Since the 13 programs studied were all relatively small (total $N = 146$ members), it was not possible to calculate within-program correlations. The first two deviancy scores—Total Deviancy (real) and Total Deviancy (ideal)—were not utilized because our previous results had indicated that the correlates of these deviance scores were partly mediated by the characteristics of the social environment. However, since our previous results had also suggested that the relationships between Directional Deviancy and Real–Ideal Discrepancy and reactions to the treatment environment were highly consistent over the 23 wards we studied, correlations were calculated between these two deviancy scores and member reactions to their programs across all 13 programs. The results indicated (a) that Directional Deviancy was significantly positively correlated with general satisfaction ($r = .38$), liking for staff ($r = .23$), and personal development ($r = .27$), whereas (b) Real–Ideal Discrepancy was significantly negatively correlated with these three variables and significantly positively correlated with anxiety (average $r = .20$). These results, even to the point of the highly similar magnitude of the relationships, are essentially identical to those found in hospital-based programs, as discussed in Chapter 9 (see especially Table 9.3).

Thus as individual patients and staff perceive their treatment milieus more positively, they feel more satisfied, like the staff more, and feel more hopeful about the personal benefits obtainable from the treatment milieu. As the discrepancy between an individual's perceptions of the environment and his views of an ideal environment increases, that individual feels less satisfied, likes the staff less, feels less hopeful about the program, and exhibits more anxiety. Although these relationships are relatively small in magnitude (none accounted for more than approximately 15% of the variance in satisfaction scores), the consistency of their direction in both hospital-based and community-based programs is indeed suggestive. From the data, it appears that the systematic use of methods by which patients could learn about the normative perceptions and values in their environments might prove helpful, especially to the individuals who see their treatment most negatively.

DEVIANT EXPECTATIONS

The results on the correlates of deviant perceptions encouraged us to do additional work on the initial expectations of patients entering new treatment programs. There has been a substantial amount of research indicating that the effects of initial expectations may be crucial in determining various significant outcomes, as reviewed by Rosenthal (1968) and Rosenthal and Jacobson (1968). In Goldstein's (1962) review of this area, focusing particularly on psychotherapy, it is pointed out that both initial expectancies and the later confirmation or nonconfirmation of expectancies are important. According to the evidence thus far, the degree of mutuality or compatibility of patient and therapist role expectations seems to be critical.

We used COPES to assess the effect of the expectations of newly admitted members in four community-based treatment programs. We wanted to test the hypothesis that prospective members would make better use of a treatment program if their expectations of the social climate matched more closely those of actual program participants. For example, new patients who are better informed about a program (i.e., who are more realistic in their expectations of it) may have a better attendance rate, and so on.

COPES Form E (Expectations), which was derived from and is directly parallel to Form C, measures prospective members' expectations of the social climate of the program they are about to enter (see Moos, 1974).

COPES Expectation Forms were given to all patients who were accepted in four different programs for which COPES Form C scores were also available. Patients completed the form either before they actually began attending the program or within 48 hours of admission.

The four programs studied included a patient-run ward in a VA hospital, two day care centers, and a day hospital. The principal goal of the program on the patient-administered ward is to develop autonomy in its members. A patient council makes major policy decisions, leads small group discussion about unit problems, handles disciplinary matters, and supervises maintenance of the ward. The patients meet weekly as a group to decide about admission of prospective members and to discuss unit activities. A director, who acts primarily as a consultant to the men, handles serious disciplinary matters. The men are allowed free passes on evenings and weekends.

The two day care programs administered by the VA operate on a token-economy system. Men earn points for attendance at classes in social behavior and basic academic or life skills, such as math or cooking, and the points can be spent on recreational activities, coffee, and similar items. The main treatment goal of the two programs is to aid members in solving practical, day-to-day problems. Both programs operate on a quarterly basis.

The day hospital provides intensive group discussions for its members. Members are expected to set specific goals for themselves, such as reducing asocial and antisocial behavior, solving family problems, or obtaining employment. An attendance schedule is set up for each member, depending on need. Some members are required to attend daily; others may attend only once a week.

As mentioned previously, new members entering the programs were given the COPES Expectation Form. Staff members in each program rated new members as "good" (i.e., having attended regularly, participated well, and having made reasonably good use of the program) or as "poor" (i.e., having been frequently absent and having made minimal or no use of the program). The patients who could not easily be placed into one of these categories are not included in this analysis. Of the 94 Expectation Forms collected, the forms of 47 patients rated "good" and 26 patients rated "poor" are used here. The patients who remained in the program for 1 to 2 months were given COPES Form C.

Thus there were four sets of scores available for comparison: (1) The Expectation subscale scores of patients rated "good," (2) the Expectation subscale scores of patients rated "poor," (3) the COPES Form C scores of members in the program at the beginning of the study, and (4) the COPES From C scores of "good" patients who remained in the program for 1 to 2 months.

First the COPES Expectation scores of all "good" and "poor" patients were compared. The expectations of patients who later did poorly in the program were substantially higher on 7 of the 10 COPES subscales than were the expectations of those who later did well. The "poor" patients expected that there would be greater member involvement in program activities (Involvement), that they would receive considerably more staff encouragement and support (Support), and that they would be freer to openly express their feelings (Spontaneity). The same results were found for three Treatment Program dimensions; specifically, patients who utilized the program poorly had had more positive initial expectations in the areas of Autonomy, Practical Orientation, and Personal Problem Orientation than patients who utilized the program well. Finally, "poor" patients had expected greater Program Clarity than the "good" patients. The two groups had had similar expectations on the remaining COPES subscales.

Further comparisons indicated that the "good" patients in all four programs tended to change their perceptions of the program between the time they entered it and the period 1 or 2 months after admission. In two programs the overall congruence of the "good" patients and the members showed no appreciable change (although the initial accuracy of new members' expectations was relatively high for these programs), whereas in the other two programs patients' perceptions matched those of the members more closely at the second than at the first testing. Thus when initial expectations are moderately discrepant from actual program characteristics, these perceptions tend to change, becoming more accurate with experience in the program.

This evidence of the importance of initial expectations, with the evidence reviewed earlier on the generally negative effects of deviant perceptions, indicates that information-giving procedures may be helpful in enhancing early patient and staff adaptations to treatment milieus. The expectations regarding the social climate held by prospective members who later do well in a treatment program differ from those of prospective members who later do poorly. The expectations of those who do well are more realistic whereas those who do poorly have unrealistically high hopes. This is particularly true in those areas in which participating program members feel that the program has average or below-average emphasis.

The need for more comprehensive preparation of patients for entrance into treatment programs is suggested by this and other investigations into individual and group psychotherapy (see review in Chapter 9). Our study on published descriptions of treatment programs (see Chapter 11) indicated that these descriptions alone may not supply accurate or complete information about the treatment environment. The evidence summarized on role induction interviews and anticipatory socialization in individual and group psychotherapy supports the idea that a similar procedure in preparing patients for milieu treatment would be useful. Research on the utility of a "socialization interview" with newly admitted members is currently underway in two community programs.

THE EFFECTS OF STAFF ROLE

A number of studies have focused on the differences in such variables as attitudes, beliefs, and participation rates of staff members of different professional backgrounds and roles (e.g., psychiatrist, nurse, aide or technician, psychologist, social worker, student). For example, Lorei (1970) studied staff in 12 VA hospitals who rated the importance of 16 possible outcomes of decisions to release or retain psychiatric patients. Comparison of the outcome profiles of eight occupational groups showed small but significant differences in profile shapes and larger differences in profile levels. The groups differed most in their opinions regarding the importance of indigency, idleness, and family complaints about release. Nursing assistants differed most frequently from other groups. In another study, Lorei and Cohen (1970) found that the degree of difference among occupations within hospitals and their ratings of the relative importance of outcomes bore a high positive correlation with hospital size.

In earlier work in this area, Cohen and Struening (1963) determined profiles for 19 occupational groups on the Opinions about Mental Illness (OMI) Scale. They found, for example, that activity therapists, physicians, and nurses were low on authoritarianism; that aides were high on authoritarianism and social restrictiveness and low on benevolence; and that psychologists and social workers were very low on authoritarianism and social restrictiveness and high on mental hygiene ideology and interpersonal etiology.

Cohen and Struening were particularly impressed by the size of the discrepancies in attitude among staff groups. They argued that mental health professionals present to the patient a social stimulus differing greatly from that of the clerical, technician, nurse, and psychiatric aide staff. "These findings," they concluded "document the frictions between personnel groups in the hospital, a kind of cold class war of forces having disparate views about the nature of the human material entrusted by society to their care (pg. 122)."

Psychiatrists and aides were far apart; nurses tended to be in between and somewhat closer to the psychiatrists than to the aides, but quite distant from both. This structuring was primarily due to differences in authoritarianism and social restrictiveness. Cohen and Struening believe that the considerable increase in authoritarian–restrictive ideology as one goes down the occupational hierarchy is at least partly attributable to the social and educational class differences among these professional role groups. The authors also point out that the differences may be related to the allocation of responsibility among the three groups; that is, the aide may be the most coercive of the three because he bears the immediate responsibility for maintaining order and security. They suggest that the permissiveness of the psychiatrist (and of the psychologist and social worker), no matter how theoretically effective, may simply be "painfully nonfunctional for the aide or even the nonspecialist nurse (pg. 122)."

This literature on staff role differences aroused our interest in the extent to which staff of different roles do in fact perceive their treatment milieus differently. We obtained some data on the role position of staff members who filled out the COPES and the WAS. Thus it was possible to compare the perceptions of staff of different roles on the *same* programs. In our initial sample we used 21 programs on which one or more psychiatrists ($N = 36$), nurses ($N = 63$), and aides ($N = 102$) had completed the WAS.

These three groups perceive their treatment milieus similarly, although there are some differences. As with other data on staff role, the differences between psychiatrists and aides are greatest, but this is not true for all subscales. Psychiatrists see somewhat more emphasis on Involvement and Support and somewhat less on Spontaneity than do either nurses or aides. Psychiatrists also see greater emphasis on all four Treatment Program dimensions, but particularly on Practical Orientation and Personal Problem Orientation. Finally, on the System Maintenance dimensions, it is the aides who perceive the most emphasis on Order and Organization, Program Clarity, and Staff Control. The magnitude of the differences varies between 1 and 2 mean raw score points. These differences were generally replicated in a study of 20 additional programs which also had at least one psychiatrist, one nurse, and one aide. Thus there are relatively consistent overall differences in perceptions of the treatment milieu by representatives of these three staff role groups.

Relevant comparisons were also made for four more groups: psychologists ($N = 33$), social workers ($N = 30$), psychiatric residents ($N = 33$), and nursing students and other trainees ($N = 69$). Separate comparisons were established between the perceptions of each of these four groups and the perceptions of all the other staff in their programs. Social workers perceived less emphasis on all three Relationship dimensions and more emphasis on Staff Control than did the other staff in their programs. Perhaps surprisingly, there were essentially no differences between the perceptions of nursing students and other trainees and those of the rest of the staff, with the single exception that nursing students reported more emphasis on Order and Organization. Psychiatric residents saw their wards relatively similarly to other staff, except that they noted less emphasis on all three Relationship dimensions, especially Spontaneity.

These results were generally replicated in a second sample; however, the results for psychologists were inconsistent in the two samples. In the first sample psychologists perceived more emphasis on Involvement and Support and on all four treatment Program dimensions, also reporting less emphasis on Staff Control than the other staff on their wards. The results were directly opposite in the second sample. Thus a further analysis was made of the wards included in the two discrepant samples. The first sample consisted of 27 wards on which there were psychologists; 16 were located in state hospitals and none was located in university and teaching hospitals. In the second sample of 25 wards, however, only 3 were in state hospitals whereas 13 were in VA hospitals and 7 were in university and teaching hospitals. Thus the differences in the relative perceptions of psychologists and other staff appears to be related to the importance of the role occupied by the psychologist on the ward.

Psychologists usually have highly responsible roles on wards in VA hospitals. This was particularly true of the wards we studied, since our contacts were often made with the aid of the hospital psychology department. When psychologists have responsible roles, they tend to see the ward more positively than the rest of the staff. However, when psychologists have peripheral or ancillary roles, as is usually the case in state hospitals, they are apt to see the ward milieu more negatively. Thus the general conclusion linking patient–staff differences and staff role differences is that the more responsible the role position of the perceiver, the more positive his perception of the environment.

Staff role differences were generally similar, although much larger on British programs. There were fewer data available on staff role in the British sample, but it was possible to compare registrars ($N = 15$), nurses ($N = 52$), and aides ($N = 19$) on 14 wards. The registrars saw their programs much more positively than the nurses on all three Relationship and all four Treatment Program dimensions, and the nurses in turn saw the programs more positively than the aides. In the British system the registrar and the senior registrar are physicians; these individuals, particularly the latter, have the most responsible positions and make most of the important decisions about patients and day-to-day program policies. The differences that appeared on some subscales were of the magnitude of 2 to 3 mean raw score points.

Data collected on the relationship between staff role and COPES subscale scores essentially supported the findings just enumerated—that is organizational staff (administrators, psychiatrists, program directors, etc.) tended to see their treatment programs more positively than did nurses, aides, clerical helpers, and other ancillary staff. Taken together, the results suggest that staff who have greater administrative responsibility for a treatment program perceive that program more positively than do other staff. This is directly consistent with our earlier findings that staff generally view treatment programs more positively than do patients. The finding held true for hospital-based and community-based programs both in the American and British samples. Related evidence is also available from a variety of other environments; for example, correctional staff perceive the environments of correctional institutions more positively than do inmates (Wenk and Moos, 1972), teachers perceive the climates of their classrooms more positively than do their students (Trickett and Moos, 1973), supervisors perceive work group climates more positively than the employees they supervise (Friedlander and Greenberg, 1971), and administrators perceive university environments more positively than do faculty, whereas faculty perceive them more positively than do students (Peterson et al., 1970).

We have demonstrated that disagreements among staff of varying role orientations regarding the characteristics of the treatment environment may be relatively substantial. These differences must give rise to some of the intrastaff strains and problems that have been described by a variety of investigators (e.g., Caudill 1958). The use of feedback of information about outsiders' perceptions of the treatment environment, utilizing such scales as the WAS and the COPES, can serve to identify and presumably to reduce areas of intrastaff disagreement. The most important implications of these results are (a) that regular outside evaluations of the functioning of treatment programs are likely to be beneficial to staff and patients and (b) that sources of information about the characteristics of treatment programs (e.g., brochures) should not be compiled solely by program administrators and directors. These individuals may present an excessively positive picture of the treatment milieu, engendering positive expectations in prospective patients; such unrealistically high hopes, in turn, result in disappointment and negative reactions to the program, inadequate utilization of the program, poor attendance, and high dropout rates.

REFERENCES

Caudill, W. *The psychiatric hospital as a small society.* Harvard University Press, Cambridge, Mass., 1958.

Cohen, J. & Struening, F. Opinions about mental illness: Mental hospital occupational profiles and profile clusters. *Psychological Reports,* **12:** 111–124, 1963.

Friedlander, F. & Greenberg, S. Effect of job attitudes, training and organization climate on performance of the hard-core unemployed *Journal of Applied Psychology,* **55:** 295–387, 1971.

Goldstein, A. *Therapist–patient expectancies in psychotherapy.* Pergamon Press, New York, 1962.

Lorei, T. Staff ratings of the relative importance of the consequences of release from or retention in a psychiatric hospital. *Journal of Consulting and Clinical Psychology,* **34:** 48–55, 1970.

Lorei, T. & Cohen, J. Hospital and occupation group differences in opinion about the release or retention of psychiatric patients. *Journal of Clinical Psychology,* **26:** 223–229, 1970.

Moos, R. *Community-Oriented Programs Environment Scale Manual,* Consulting Psychologists Press, Palo Alto, Calif., 1974.

Peterson, R., Centra, J., Hartnett, R. & Linn, R. Institutional Functioning Inventory. Preliminary technical manual. Educational Testing Service, Princeton, N.J., 1970.

Rosenthal, R. *Experimenter effects in behavioral research.* Appleton-Century-Crofts, New York, 1968.

Rosenthal, R. & Jacobson, L. *Pygmalion in the classroom.* Holt, Rinehart & Winston, New York, 1968.

Trickett, E. & Moos, R. The social environment of junior high and high school classrooms. *Journal of Educational Psychology,* **65:**93–102, 1973.

Wenk, E. & Moos, R. Social climates in prisons. *Journal of Research in Crime and Delinquency,* **9:** 134–148, 1972.

Chapter Thirteen

HOMOGENEITY
AND CONGRUENCE

Program Homogeneity

The results presented in Chapter 12 on the high degree of age matching in treatment programs encouraged us to study various aspects of program homogeneity and its correlates. The degree of relative homogeneity or diversity that is appropriate for characterizing groups and institutions has received attention in a variety of contexts (e.g., Yalom, 1970). Three fairly recent research examples utilizing the concept of homogeneity illustrate some approaches.

Peterson et al. (1970) included a Human Diversity subscale in their Institutional Functioning Inventory (IFI). They defined Human Diversity as the degree to which the faculty and student body are heterogeneous in their backgrounds and present attitudes. A high score indicates that the college is viewed as having attracted students and faculty of diverse ethnic and social backgrounds, political and religious attitudes, and personal tastes and styles. A low score suggests that the campus community is relatively homogeneous in terms of faculty and student backgrounds and beliefs. The items on the Human Diversity subscale include "There are provisions by which some number of educationally disadvantaged students may be admitted to the institution without meeting the normal entrance requirements," "This institution deliberately seeks to admit a student body in which a variety of attitudes and values will be present," "One of the methods used to influence the flavor of the college is to try to select students with fairly similar personality traits" (scored negatively), and "A wide variety of religious backgrounds and beliefs are represented among the faculty."

The IFI subscale that assesses perceived Human Diversity may or may not be related to more objective measures of this variable. Some relationships between the subscale and other measures of university environments are cited by Peterson et al; for example, Human Diversity correlates positively with number of books in the library, proportion of faculty with doctorates, enrollment, and average faculty compensation. It is also positively related to student radicalism. Colleges and universities in which Human Diversity is high also have lower CUES Scores on Practicality and higher CUES Scores on Awareness. A wide range of attitudes among individuals should correlate with personal and political commitments (CUES Awareness), which in turn should be related to protest over social issues. It is important to note that although Human Diversity is a perceived climate dimension, administrators, faculty and students show extremely high agreement across universities in their relative perceptions of it.

Astin's (1962) work represents a different approach to the assessment of the characteristic of institutional homogeneity. As discussed in Chapter 6, the Environmental Assessment Technique (EAT) identifies six orientations in the student body as defined by the proportion of students majoring in different fields. The six orientations are as follows: (1) realistic (agriculture, forestry, and engineering, etc.), (2) intellectual (natural science, mathematics, philosophy, etc.), (3) social (education, nursing, sociology, etc.), (4) conventional (accounting, business, economics, etc.), (5) enterprising (public administration, political science, foreign service, etc.), and (6) artistic (art, music, journalism, foreign languages, etc.). Astin defined the Homogeneity of the Environment as the difference between the most frequent and the least frequent personal orientations at the college. He reasoned that a college dominated by one orientation should receive a high score on homogeneity, whereas it should have a low homogeneity score if the major fields of the students were distributed fairly evenly among the six orientations.

Astin identified a factor on which his Homogeneity of the Environment score had a high factor loading (.69). He found that more homogeneous environments had a higher realistic orientation, whereas institutions with more heterogeneous environments had higher artistic and enterprising orientations. Not too surprisingly, he also learned that more homogeneous institutions offered a smaller variety of courses and that they had smaller libraries. The Homogeneity of the Environment dimension was identified as one of the six principal dimensions along which higher educational institutions could be characterized. The homogeneity factor was correlated with the five CUES subscales in a sample of 61 schools (reported by Pace, 1969), and the results indicated that Homogeneity was significantly negatively related to CUES Practicality (although the correlation was relatively low: $-.32$). Homogeneity was not significantly related to the other four CUES dimensions. Thus the Homogeneity dimension may be relatively distinct and separate insofar as it is not highly related to other types of dimensions also characterizing the environments of institutions of higher education.

In a somewhat different approach, Lansing et al. (1970) examined the compatibility of neighbors and the homogeneity of neighborhoods in a study of planned residential environments. Gans (1968, Chapter 12) has stressed the importance of resident characteristics without specifically defining the terms homogeneity and heterogeneity. He states that little is known about which characteristics must be shared before people feel themselves to be compatible with others. The most and least important background characteristics, behavior patterns, and interests are not specifically known.

Lansing et al. argue that it is possible to determine for each microneighborhood what proportion of the residents have the same age, family income, education, attitudes about the neighborhood, and so on. The higher the proportion of residents who are coded the same for a given variable, the greater the neighborhood homogeneity with respect to that variable. For example, if four of five respondents report the "same" family income, then the proportion of .80 is assigned to all five respondents to indicate the level of income homogeneity present in the neighborhood. In Lansing's study, the prediction was that respondents in neighborhoods with high levels of homogeneity would be more likely to judge their neighbors as compatible (i.e., "friendly" or "similar"). The authors selected three types of variables for assessing neighborhood homogeneity:

1.   Demographic and socioeconomic variables (e.g., age of male heads of households, age of wives, education of male heads of households, education of wives, family income, year moved into present home, race).

2.   Neighborhood attitudes, rated on such dimensions as noisy–quiet, poorly kept up–well kept up, pleasant–unpleasant, good place–poor place, and attractive–unattractive.

3.   Other attitudes, such as overall satisfaction with the community.

Lansing et al. were somewhat surprised by the results arrived at by correlating the respondents' ratings of their neighbors as friendly or similar with measures of the socioeconomic and demographic homogeneity in the neighborhood. Most of the correlations were opposite to the predicted direction; that is, living in a neighborhood where characteristics of the type just listed were homogeneous did not lead the respondents to perceive neighbors as friendly or similar. One interesting finding was that male respondents were more likely to judge neighbors as "friendly" if the neighborhood was racially heterogeneous. The correlations were all quite low, and the authors concluded that "none of the measures of socioeconomic and demographic homogeneity considered here show consistently strong relationship to either perceived friendliness or similarity" (p. 125). However, when consensus (homogeneity) exists among neighbors about the qualities of the residential environment, the neighbors themselves are more positively evaluated. Thus attitude or perception factors may indeed be most important for compatibility. Lansing et al. also found that the perception of neighbors as compatible (i.e., friendly, similar) is very highly associated with satisfaction with the neighborhood.

We have taken three dissimilar methods of assessing (1) human diversity, (2) the homogeneity of higher educational institutions, and (3) microneighborhood compatibility to illustrate recent empirical work in this area. The importance of the issue of program homogeneity and the related problem of person–environment congruence resulted in our experimenting with two somewhat different empirical approaches utilizing two samples of community-based treatment programs.

16 Community-Based Programs

Three indices of program heterogeneity were obtained from the information contained in the PIF: (1) the age range of members, (2) the range of education of the members, and (3) the range of length of stay of the members. It is important to note that the three measures of dispersion (or heterogeneity) were not correlated with the average scores on the corresponding variable; age range, for example, was not related to mean age. Thus the effects of age range are not attributable to the effects of the mean age differences among the programs, and so on. On the other hand the three measures were themselves highly positively related; illustratively, the correlation between the age range and education range of the members was .59. The three measures listed were correlated with staff perception of treatment environments in the 16 programs, with the following results:

1. Staff saw more emphasis on the Relationship dimensions, particularly Involvement and Support, in more heterogeneous programs. Some of the relationships were substantial; for example, staff perceptions of Involvement and Support correlated .57 and .60, respectively, with members' age range.

2. Staff saw much less emphasis on Autonomy and on Practical Orientation in more heterogeneous programs.

3. Staff reported much more emphasis on Staff Control in more heterogeneous programs, their perceptions of Staff Control correlated .67 with the range of members' length of stay. Thus as program heterogeneity increases, staff perceive greater emphasis on the Relationship dimensions and on Staff Control, but less emphasis on Autonomy and Practical Orientation.

These results are of course preliminary, since they are based on a small number of programs and on only three indices of member heterogeneity. Nevertheless, two aspects of the results are quite intriguing. First, heterogeneity indices were generally unrelated to other salient program characteristics, but they were significantly related to each other. Such indices, therefore, may represent a quite separate dimension along which treatment programs and other environments should be characterized. This corroborates Astin's findings in educational environments. Second, program heterogeneity may have differential effects on different indices of treatment environment—for example, increased emphasis on Relationship dimensions accompanied by decreased emphasis on certain treatment program dimensions suggests that both positive and negative effects may be related to program heterogeneity.

12 Community Care Homes

A study was carried out on 12 of the community care homes briefly described in Chapter 10. These homes represent a unique group for study because size, staffing, and monthly cost per person are almost identical in all cases. Thus differences in the treatment milieus of the homes are not attributable to these factors. Background information was obtained from hospital and/or program records on each of the patients currently living in the home.

We computed two heterogeneity scores from this information. *The Background Heterogeneity Score* was calculated by rank ordering (over the 12 homes) the standard deviations for age and education and the number of occupational categories represented in the house. These three rank orders were then combined into one score, which was the background heterogeneity score. *The Chronicity Heterogeneity Score* was obtained by rank ordering the standard deviations for the total number of months in the hospital, the total number of hospitalizations, and the length of the most recent hospitalization and rank–ordering the sum of these three variables. The resulting score was the program chronicity heterogeneity score.

The two heterogeneity scores were correlated, over the 12 homes, with the resident COPES Form C subscales. The results indicated (1) that the Background Heterogeneity Score was not related to any of the treatment environment dimensions and (2) that the Chronicity Heterogeneity Score was significantly negatively related to resident perceptions of the emphasis on the Relationship dimensions of Involvement and Spontaneity, the Treatment Program dimensions of Personal Problem Orientation and Anger and Aggression, and the System Maintenance dimension of Program Clarity. Thus the greater the Chronicity Heterogeneity Score, the less emphasis in the home on the five dimensions named. Further analyses revealed that the Chronicity Heterogeneity Score was significantly positively related to the length of the last previous hospitalization, a variable which itself correlated with a number of treatment environment dimensions. Since, therefore, chronicity heterogeneity was not independent of chronicity, we cannot state with certainty whether it had any effects over and above those exerted by chronicity itself.

PERCEPTION AND VALUE CONGRUENCE

The findings relating to program heterogeneity and to "background matching," at least in terms of age, led us to identify other indices of program congruence. It appears that the average perception and value congruence in treatment programs is considerably greater than the hypothesis of random selection leads us to expect. When the WAS and the COPES are utilized as measures of program congruence, the effects of self-selection and program-selection are necessarily confounded with changes in perceptions and values that occur subsequent to functioning in a particular treatment milieu. Thus although there is evidence that a relatively high degree of program congruence exists, the reasons for such congruence cannot be specified without longitudinal studies in which patients and staff are followed from the time they enter a program.

TABLE 13.1   MEAN INTRACLASS PROFILE CORRELATIONS FOR THREE SAMPLES OF PROGRAMS

	Mean Intraclass Correlations		
	16 Community-Based Programs	18 British Community Programs	23 State Hospital Programs
Patient–Staff (Real)	.57	.65	.35
Patient–Staff (Ideal)	.76	.78	.56
Patient (Real vs. Ideal)	.45	.33	.70
Staff (Real vs. Ideal)	.42	.64	.32

Our results are quite intriguing when viewed in the light of program perception and value congruence. Table 13.1 presents mean profile similarity scores (intraclass correlations) for three samples of programs. Four profile similarity scores were calculated: (1) agreement between patients and staff with respect to the actual treatment milieu, (2) agreement between patients and staff with respect to an ideal treatment milieu, (3) real–ideal treatment milieu similarity for patients, and (4) real–ideal treatment milieu similarity for staff. The samples are the group of 16 community-based programs discussed earlier, the group of 18 British community-based programs described in Chapter 10, and the 23 state hospital wards described in Chapter 7.

Average patient–staff congruence with regard to perception of the environment is substantial for both samples of community-based programs, and it is moderate in the state hospital sample. Although patient–staff agreement varies widely from program to program, there is, on the average, much greater agreement than we would expect to obtain by chance. The extent of agreement might be utilized as a measure of the development of a program culture. Perhaps a more surprising finding is the relatively high degree of patient–staff value congruence exhibited in all three samples. The average value congruence is extremely high in both samples of community-based programs and quite substantial in the state hospital programs. Programs differ considerably in their extent of value congruence, but again the average congruence is much greater than we would expect to obtain by chance.

It is likely that at least two processes contribute to this high degree of perception and value congruence. First, patients and staff simply learn about the characteristics of their treatment milieus, and perceptual congruence develops out of a shared reality of events. A certain amount of value congruence must also come about through discussions of shared value orientations and through mutual attraction and similarity influences directed toward increasing congruence.

Second, there is probably a strong tendency for patients and staff who share neither the perceptions of the treatment milieu nor the dominant value orientations to leave the program. Although this aspect has not been systematically studied, Chapter 8 presented data on the astonishing proportion of patients who drop out of treatment programs. Similar evidence exists for individual and group psychotherapy in which many patients leave treatment under circumstances other than that of mutual consent between patient and therapist (e.g., Yalom, 1966). Even less information is available about the reasons for staff turnover, which is usually quite high, and it seems reasonable to suppose that it would be related at least partly to disagreements about real or ideal treatment environments.

The results presented in Table 13.1 for real–ideal congruence are somewhat more variable over the three samples. On the average, real–ideal congruence is greater than chance; however, it is of only moderate magnitude for the patients in the two community-based program samples. We find that such congruence is substantial for the patients in the state hospital sample because these patients have much lower expectations of what an ideal treatment milieu could be like. On the other hand, there is some general "socialization" for professional staff with regard to the characteristics of ideal treatment milieus; thus the staff on the 23 state hospital wards show only very moderate real–ideal congruence.

The results indicate that there is a third process, in addition to the two just suggested, which increases real–ideal congruence at least for patients. As actual treatment milieus change, expectations about ideal treatment milieus also change. Individuals who are functioning in somewhat "negative" environments, not quite realizing that their surroundings can be substantially changed, often have negative and undifferentiated expectations of what an ideal milieu might be like. As the milieu changes, expectations of improvement are aroused, and concepts of ideal milieus also change. The situation is somewhat different for staff, at least for professional staff who already have an overall model or image of the ideal treatment milieu.

One additional method of assessing real–ideal congruence was utilized. Rank-order correlations were calculated between mean real and mean ideal subscale scores, separately for patients and staff in each of the three samples. Positive relationships indicate that as the actual emphasis on a particular environmental dimension increases, the specified ideal amount of emphasis on that dimension also increases. For example, the correlation over the 16 community-based programs between the amount of emphasis that patients perceived on Personal Problem Orientation and the amount of emphasis they ideally wished to have on this dimension was .63. Apparently, then, patients in programs that put greater emphasis on Personal Problem Orientation ideally wish even more emphasis on this dimension.

In the first sample of 16 community-based programs, 8 of the 10 real–ideal subscale correlations for patients were positive (5 were statistically significant) and 9 of the 10 real–ideal correlations for staff were positive (5 were statistically significant). Essentially similar results were found for the 18 British programs, in which the correlations were also predominantly positive, about half being statistically significant. In the sample of 23 state hospital programs, 9 of the 10 real–ideal correlations for patients were positive (8 were statistically significant), whereas all 10 real–ideal correlations for staff were positive (7 were statistically significant).

Thus we can point to a strong tendency for patients and staff to ideally want a relatively high degree of emphasis on dimensions that are already being strongly emphasized. To put it another way, if one program has a higher degree of emphasis than another on Spontaneity or Personal Problem Orientation or Staff Control, both patients and staff in that program will usually wish to ideally have more emphasis on Spontaneity or Personal Problem Orientation or Staff Control than patients and staff in the other program. We have already noted that at least three mechanisms may be operating to cause these results. In any case, it is clear that patient and staff perception and value congruence are considerably greater than would be expected based on the hypothesis of random matching. Insofar as this observation is valid, treatment programs may be said to have differential and characteristic cultures.

The extent of overall patient–staff and real–ideal congruence varies substantially from program to program. In some programs the relevant intraclass profile correlations are greater than .90 (see, e.g., the profile for ward 205 in Chapter 4), whereas in others they are essentially zero, indicating a total lack of perception or value congruence. The existence of such discrepancies led us to become interested in the correlates of these congruence indices.

Our hypothesis was that patient–staff and real–ideal congruence would be positively related to patient morale, to patient liking for staff, and to perceived opportunities for personal development. Data were available from our study (see Chapter 7) of 23 programs in one state hospital. The relevant intraclass profile correlations for the 23 programs were themselves correlated with the mean patients' reactions to the programs. Patient–staff congruence about the actual milieu and patient real–ideal congruence were significantly positively related to patient general satisfaction, liking for staff, and perceived opportunities for personal development. Patient–staff ideal milieu congruence was positively related to general satisfaction and liking for staff, and staff real–ideal congruence was positively related to patient satisfaction and perceived personal development. Basically, the results on real–ideal congruence were replicated for both members and staff in the sample of 13 community-based programs discussed in Chapter 12. The results on member–staff perception and value congruence were not replicated because there was too little variation in these two congruence indices in the latter sample of programs.

HOMOGENEITY AND CONGRUENCE IN TREATMENT SETTINGS

Patient and Staff Values

There are very few experimental studies of changes in patient and staff values in treatment milieus, although this problem has been extensively discussed. As mentioned in Chapter 1, Almond developed a scale for the assessment of patient values and studied changes in these values during hospitalization in a short-term milieu therapy setting (Almond et al., 1969). Utilizing questionnaire and case study techniques, the investigators found that the majority of patients changed toward the prescribed value system of the ward community. The changes persisted through the time of discharge from the unit. Such increased patient–staff value congruence occurred most strongly on a factor scale assessing values of social openness and involvement. Even though value change in other dimensions was less clear, the authors concluded that there is a "meaningful and compelling process of acculturation for study ward patients from the moment of admission until and perhaps beyond discharge" (p. 350). These patient value changes are related to "role playing" influences, and the authors emphasize that patients occupy a specific role for weeks or months within the "protected walls of the ward." Almond et al. state that strong pressures in many programs produce a split between patient and staff cultures; the social system of the milieu they studied however, seemed to create compelling counterpressures toward the expected patient role.

In later work (Almond, 1971), three distinct patterns of value or attitude change were identified. Some patients entered the program with values similar to those of staff (preconverts), whereas others had initially discrepant values but changed over time in the direction of the staff (unit converts). There was also a small group of patients whose values stayed discrepant or became even more discrepant from the staff (rejectors and renegers). This series of studies substantiates the notion that there are strong "congruence-enhancing" influences in some therapeutic milieus.

Astrachan et al. (1969) present a very interesting study on the experimental introduction of values into a ward milieu. They were concerned with the conditions under which psychiatric patients adopt the values held by staff and how deeply such values take root. They introduced a value that was noncongruent but neutral to the preexisting value system of the ward setting and accentuated other values already present in the system. These experimental procedures were designed to measure how far, staff and patients would modify their behavior in line with the behavior of the research staff who emphasized the values in an indirect manner (i.e., by example rather than by precept). For example, an attempt was made to change the manner of addressing patients during meetings. Specifically, patients were generally spoken to by their first names, and the research staff, to a very limited extent, introduced the practice of using patients' family names. The procedure worked mainly for patients who were older or who had important current or past positions or affiliations outside the hospital (e.g., a noted professor!).

In another experiment on the same ward the investigators introduced the two congruent values of work (that it is important for patients to return to their functional work role) and planning (that it is important for patients to plan their activities and lives and that explicit focusing on planning should go on throughout a patient's hospital career). When the research staff emphasized a value for certain patients, the rest of the staff also tended to stress that value for the same patients in the same meeting. Generalization, however, was very limited. In discussing these findings, the authors indicate that longer value induction time periods and more explicit direct focus on values might have produced more marked effects. From our perspective, the results strongly support the notion that value change can and does occur among patients and staff in ward milieus, even when the measure of value change is behavioral. Taken together, the studies provide direct evidence supporting the hypothesis that patient–staff value congruence generally increases with experience in the treatment milieu.

Compatibility and Congruence

Meltzoff and Kornreich (1970) have briefly discussed the evidence of increased patient–therapist similarity as a consequence of psychotherapy. Relevant studies in individual psychotherapy include that by Schrier (1953), who used rating scales of patient and therapist personality characteristics in short-term therapy and presented support for the hypothesis that the patient modifies his perceptions of himself in the direction of his therapist's self-rating. In an intriguing study, Sheehan (1953) investigated Rorschach changes during psychotherapy to determine whether (and if so, how much) patients' personality shifts tended to become more like their therapists'. Of the 21 college student patients, 17 shifted toward the therapist. Sheehan's finding that two groups who shifted in nearly opposite directions each shifted toward their respective therapists suggests that the shifts were linked to the specific therapists. The patients who were rated by their therapists as most improved showed greater shifts toward the therapist.

Farson (1961) studied the changes in client–therapist self-description congruence during therapy and found that an individual client's self-descriptions did not become more congruent with his therapist's self-descriptions. On the other hand, the degree of overall congruence between the clients and therapists as a group increased at both terminal and follow-up intervals. The congruence was with therapists as a class rather than as individuals. Doubtless the same effect occurs in certain treatment programs; that is, patient and staff congruence increases as a function of treatment experience.

In somewhat controversial work, Rosenthal (1955) studied the relationship between patient improvement in psychotherapy and changes in moral values in the direction of the therapist. At the beginning and at the end of treatment; he administered a Moral Values Q-Sort dealing with the areas of sex, aggression, and authority. Ratings of patient improvement correlated significantly positively with change in the direction of moral values of the therapist. Specifically, the patients who were unimproved or worse tended to move away from the therapist's value system. Spohn (1960) has demonstrated that congruence of social values is one of the determinants of therapists' clinical judgments about patients. Parloff, Iflund, and Goldstein (1960), comparing two schizophrenic patients, found that after 8 months the successful patient was significantly closer to the therapist's values than was the unsuccessful one.

Thus there is evidence that the personality and values of patients may shift with psychotherapy in the direction of those of the therapist, particularly when treatment outcome is successful. Given the right treatment milieu, it seems likely that many patients would perceive the milieu similarly to staff and would tend also to adopt staff value orientations with regard to preferred treatment milieus.

In relevant work on community-based programs, Fleisher and Kuldau (1972) studied the relation between compatibility and stability in eight foster home care groups. According to the Fundamental Interpersonal Relations Orientation (FIRO-B) Scale measures of group compatibility, more men dropped out from groups that were incompatible in the area of control than from groups that were compatible in this area. It also developed that the groups became more compatible in the areas of control and affection after the dissonant individuals had departed. In addition, high individual incompatibility scores in the area of affection correlated significantly with short length of stay for the men who departed, that is, men who were most incompatible with the group in the area of affection stayed for the shortest period of time. On the average, men who departed were less compatible with their groups in the area of affection than those who remained. These findings further support the notion that individuals who are incompatible with groups tend to leave those groups. Moreover, individuals who are least compatible probably leave the soonest. This "dropout" effect produces an increase in the overall homogeneity or congruence of the group.

Correlates of Congruence

There is extensive evidence indicating that congruence of individual perceptions in different milieus increases interpersonal attraction and compatibility, thus probably empathy, helping behavior, and positive outcomes. All the research in this area cannot be summarized here. Overviews of some relevant literature in personality theory and social psychology are given by Maddi (1968) and Newcomb (1961). Maddi presents an extremely interesting review of consistency models of personality wherein similarities and discrepancies are noted between the cognitive and/or arousal states of the individual and information impinging on him from his environment. From this point of view, discrepancies between the individual and the environment produce discomfort, anxiety, and/or a motivation to act in a way that will reduce the discrepancy (Maddi, 1968; see especially Chapter 4).

Newcomb (1961) has marshaled data suggesting that similarity of social background, values, and presumably perceptions determines attraction and compatibility. He found that interpersonal attraction among college men who were living in the same house varied with the total number of issues about which individuals were in agreement. General agreement with respect to the importance of values and with respect to attraction to other peers was particularly important in the formation and maintenance of friendship dyads.

Whitehorn and Betz (Betz, 1960) demonstrated that psychotherapists (labeled type A) who obtained high success rates with hospitalized schizophrenics differed from therapists (type B) who obtained low improvement rates. However, McNair, Callahan, and Lorr (1962) found that psychiatric outpatients treated by type B therapists improved significantly more than patients of type A therapists. They suggest that type B therapists may do better with outpatients because they have more interests in common with them (e.g., more similar life backgrounds and/or more familiarity with patients' daily living problems). McNair et al. suggest that a "similarity" interpretation might also account for the greater success that the type A therapists had with schizophrenic inpatients in the Whitehorn and Betz studies.

Tuma and Gustaad (1957) reported a positive relationship between client–counselor personality similarity and client learning in counseling sessions, and Heine and Trosman (1960) found a positive correlation between similarity of patient and therapist expectations and the duration of individual therapy. Carson and Heine (1962) hypothesized that success in psychotherapy depends on the ability of the therapist to achieve an optimum balance between empathy and objectivity; therefore, the relationship between patient–therapist personality similarity and therapeutic success might be curvilinear. They derived an MMPI index of personality similarity for patient–therapist pairs and obtained support for their theory. Their findings paralleled those of Fiedler (1958), who concluded from his work with task groups that group effectiveness is related in curvilinear fashion to the psychological distance of the group leader.

In two related studies, Mendelsohn and Geller (1963, 1965) found that client–counselor similarity in Myers-Briggs Type Indicator (MBTI) scores was related to greater length of counseling contact, presumably reflecting more commitment to counseling on the part of both client and counselor as a function of increasing personality similarity. They also found that the evaluation and comfort–rapport attitudes toward the counseling experience of freshmen at a counseling center (but not nonfreshmen) were related to client–counselor similarity. Mendelsohn and Geller concluded that these results were consistent with the findings that personality similarity leads to greater attraction in brief contacts.

A number of studies on patient–therapist compatibility have utilized the FIRO-B Scale, which measures three interpersonal needs: Inclusion, Control, and Affection (Inclusion and Affection fit into our Relationship category, whereas Control falls into our System Maintenance category). Schutz (1958) presents a variety of methods for using these subscale scores to obtain compatibility indices between individuals. Sapolsky (1960) utilized FIRO-B and found that subjects' responses to the influence exerted by their experimenter differed in accordance with the compatibility existing between subject and experimenter. In a second study Sapolsky (1965) confirmed the hypothesis that the greater the compatibility between patient and doctor, the more the patient would (a) experience similarity existing between himself and his doctor, (b) believe that the doctor felt himself similar to him, and/or (c) perceive himself as being understood by his doctor. Sapolsky also reported that the degree of patient–doctor compatibility was positively correlated with the outcome of inpatient treatment. He concluded that this relationship was probably due to the differential effect of the compatibility variable on the way the doctor was perceived by the patient.

Subsequent studies have stirred up considerable controversy in this area, much as with the research on Type A and type B therapists. For example, Mendelsohn and Rankin (1969) found that client–counselor compatibility as measured by the FIRO-B Scale was related to clients' perceptions of the relationship and their evaluations of the counselor and the usefulness of counseling. However, compatibility was a poor predictor for male clients but an excellent one for females. They also noted differences in different need areas; for example, compatibility in the Control need area was related positively to outcome; rather surprisingly, however compatibility in the Inclusion and Affection need areas was related negatively to outcome. In this connection, Carson and Heine have suggested that high similarity of personality can lead to therapist overidentification with a patient and his problems. In a final study, Gassner (1970) found that high compatibility-matched patients (utilizing FIRO-B) had a significantly more favorable view of their therapists after 3 and 11 weeks of interaction. However, therapists did not prefer relating to their high-compatibility patients (as opposed to the low-compatibility individuals). No differences in the amount of behavioral change were found in the high- and low-compatibility groups, although the change measures were obtained after only 3 weeks of treatment. Gassner concluded that high levels of patient–therapist interpersonal attraction can be promoted by compatibility matching procedures.

Some work has focused on the effects of value similarity between clients and counselors. Interestingly, Burdock, Cheek, and Zubin (1960) noted a relation between psychoanalytic candidates' success in training and similarity with their supervisors' interest patterns as measured by the Strong Vocational Interest Blank. They suggested that trained analysts may be equating criteria for the well-adjusted personality with their own interests or value systems.

Welkowitz, Cohen, and Ortmeyer (1967) demonstrated that patients who were rated as most improved by their therapists were closer to the therapists in values than the patients who were rated as least improved. They also reported that values tend to move toward similarity in ongoing therapist–patient dyads. Thus we have support for the notion that individual value systems move toward greater similarity with dominant values in the environment. Other relevant studies in the area are reviewed by Meltzoff and Kornreich (1970, pp. 311–327). Research relating interpersonal similarity and attraction is also discussed by Goldstein, Heller, and Sechrest (1966) and Goldstein (1971). The results generally indicate that similarity of attitudes and perceptions increases interpersonal attraction.

Similar findings have been reported for social and task-oriented groups and for psychotherapy groups. For example, Schutz (1958) reviews evidence on the relation between dyad compatibility and preference for continued personal contact. He cites supportive studies predicting roommate travel companion, and house manager choices from compatibility scores. Hutcherson (1963) determined compatibility separately on the FIRO-B need dimensions for 8 male junior high school teachers and more than 700 of their students. He found that academic achievement was positively related to compatibility in the area of Control but not with regard to Inclusion or Affection. When Smelser (1958) compared compatible and incompatible groups formed by means of California Psychological Inventory (CPI) dominance scale scores and varied role assignments, he learned that the compatible groups were more productive on a specially designed train-running task. Moos and Speisman (1962) also successfully predicted the productivity of specially constructed compatible and incompatible dyads utilizing the FIRO-B, the CPI dominance scale, and the Leary Interpersonal Check List.

In work on group composition and group cohesiveness, Yalom (1970) studied 40 outpatients shortly before they began therapy in 5 newly formed therapy groups. The FIRO-B was administered, and the interpersonal compatibility of each member vis-à-vis each other member of his group was calculated. Yalom and Rand (in Yalom, 1970) then correlated individual and group compatibility scores with individual and total group cohesiveness scores obtained at the sixth and twelfth group meetings. The FIRO-B group compatibility correlated significantly with group cohesiveness, and any two group members who showed mutual extreme incompatibility were significantly less satisfied with the group. Yalom and Rand also reported a connection between low compatibility and the tendency to drop out of group therapy.

Finally, there is a body of literature investigating the effects of need and personality complementarity in mate selection and the stability of marriage (e.g., Winch, Ktsanes, and Ktsanes, 1955; Cattell and Nesselroade, 1967). Reviewing this area, Hicks and Platt (1970) have concluded that there are positive relationship between marital happiness and   (a) husband–wife similarities in socioeconomic status, age, and religion; (b) congruence of husband's self-concept with that held of him by his wife, and (c) the general compatibility of role expectation and role performance.

Thus the results of research carried out in individual therapy and other dyadic relationships, in social, task-oriented, and therapeutic groups, and in families and marital couples, are supportive of the notion that interpersonal compatibility relates positively to similarity of perception, interpersonal attraction, and individual or group productivity criteria.

HOMOGENEITY AND CONGRUENCE IN EDUCATIONAL SETTINGS

Substantial relevant work has been performed in colleges and universities. Studying three types of residential communities (freshman living units, upper-division living units, and living units in which freshmen and upperclassmen were mixed), Beal and Williams (1968) found that whereas freshmen in the mixed class housing situation were more satisfied with their college experience, upper-division women seemed to be more satisfied in the "segregated" living situation.

DeCoster (1967) assigned groups of high-ability students so that they formed 50% concentrations in certain residence halls. Control groups of students were randomly assigned to other residence halls. The high-ability students living in close proximity in the homogeneously assigned residence halls surpassed the scattered high-ability students in academic success and also perceived their living quarters as being more desirable. The concentrated high-ability students reported that their living units were conducive to study, that informal talk sessions had educational value, that they were influenced by fellow residents to do better in their studies, and that their fellow residents were considerate and respectful of others. On the other hand, there was some evidence that this concentration of high-ability students may have had negative effects on the academic achievement of the less talented students in the same residence.

In a study furnishing direct behavioral evidence (change of major) of a press toward congruence, Brown (1968) manipulated the environmental press of college living situations by placing students with similar academic majors on certain floors of residence halls. Freshmen room assignments were arranged so that the ratio of science students to humanities students was 4–1 on two floors of a residence hall, whereas the ratio of humanities students to science students was 4–1 on two other floors. A significantly greater proportion of the "minority" groups changed their majors to fields similar to those composing the majority groups on their residence hall floor. In addition, significantly more of the minority group students expressed dissatisfaction with residence hall life.

Astin (1964) found that the traits identified in members of entering freshmen classes are highly related to certain characteristics of the college. For example, the more able students, the more highly motivated students, and the more scientifically inclined students were most likely to enroll in affluent institutions. These students also tended to enroll in colleges with intellectual environments but not in colleges with social environments. Private, nonsectarian institutions seemed to recruit student bodies with greater potential for academic, scientific, artistic, and social achievement than did other types of schools. The author believed that "by some combination of circumstances, institutions seem to enroll students whose past achievements and educational and vocational plans are remarkably suited to the curricular offerings of the institutions" (p. 286). Astin tentatively attributes this effect to a combination of self-selection and college-selection factors.

In further work corroborating the results obtained by Brown (1968), Astin (1965) mounted a 4-year longitudinal study to investigate the effects of various college characteristics on the career choices of 3538 exceptionally able boys. Some support appeared for the hypothesis that the student's career choice comes to conform more and more to the dominant or modal career choice in his college environment. This was true even though a student's career choice at graduation from college was affected far more by his characteristics as an entering freshman than by the characteristics of his college environment. A student's chance of eventually pursuing a particular type of career is enhanced somewhat if he attends a college in which a relatively high proportion of other students are planning careers of that type.

Other studies have demonstrated that a "fit" or "congruence" exists between the average level of the specific needs of students and the particular environmental pressures. For example, Stern (1970) found that 28 of the 30 correlations between average scores on the matching Activities Index (AI) and College Characteristics Index (CCI) scales were positive. In Stern's interpretation this indicates that students who have a specific need attend institutions with appropriate press. Chickering examined student and college characteristics in 13 small colleges and also uncovered evidence of congruence between student personality and college environment (Chickering et al., 1969). Students with the most conservative religious beliefs chose colleges strongly supportive of such beliefs. Within this group, the most altruistic students went to church-related colleges at which service was emphasized. Students scoring highest on measures of intellectual interest selected colleges that varied most sharply from the traditional pattern. Students who were most reluctant to express their impulses in conscious thought or overt action were likely to attend schools characterized by numerous regulations and close supervision. Other relevant studies are cited in Feldman and Newcomb (1969); who reached the general conclusions that "the evidence thus gathered reveals a tendency for students incongruent with the specific college to be more dissatisfied with their experiences at the college and to be more likely to consider leaving and actually to leave" (p. 293).

There is also a large body of evidence indicating that students within friendship groups at college (both dyads and larger groups) tend to be similar with respect to various attributes, especially values, attitudes, and interests. To some extent this similarity is an outcome of students' initial selection of one another as friends. It has been repeatedly demonstrated that actual and perceived similarity of attributes can be related to initial attraction among college students in experimental settings and to actual friendship formation in natural settings. The mutual influences of friends on one another must act in part to increase their similarity beyond that produced by initial selection. However, Feldman and Newcomb (1969) point out that very little is known about the relative contributions of selection and ongoing normative influence on the homogeneity of college friendship groups. Newcomb (1961) found that the selection and reselection of friends played a more important role in producing similarity among friends than did value or attitude change. Further work needs to be done in various milieus on distinguishing between the effects of mutual selection and reselection (initial similarity) and mutual influence once the individual is in the setting (change toward greater similarity).

In summary, our own evidence and the evidence of other investigators indicate that the press toward program congruence or homogeneity is fairly strong. Among the reasons for the occurrence of homogeneity are the following: initial self-selection, initial program selection, dropout and reselection by individuals and programs, and actual changes that take place in individuals as they function within particular environments having dominant orientations. Although more research is required, investigators might feasibly consider selecting patients and staff for treatment programs on the basis of their background or value congruence with other individuals already in those programs. Various types of homogeneous and heterogeneous programs should be created and their differential effects on both patients and staff studied.

REFERENCES

Almond, R., Keniston, K., & Boltax, S. Patient value change in milieu therapy. *Archives of General Psychiatry*, **20**: 339–351, 1969.

Almond, R. The therapeutic community. *Scientific American*, **224**: 34–42, 1971.

Astin, A. An. Empirical characterization of higher educational institutions. *Journal of Educational Psychology*, **53**: 224–235, 1962.

Astin, A. Distribution of students among higher educational institutions. *Journal of Educational Psychology*, **55**: 276–287, 1964.

Astin, A. Effect of different college environments on the vocational choices of high aptitude students. *Journal of Counseling Psychology*, **12**: 28–34, 1965.

Astrachan, B., Harrow, M., & Flynn, H. The experimental introduction of values into a psychiatric setting. *Comprehensive Psychiatry*, **10**: 181–189, 1969.

Beal, P. & Willaims, D. An experiment with mixed class housing assignments at the University of Oregon, Student Housing Research (ACUHO Research and Information Committee), 1968.

Betz, B. Experiences in research in psychotherapy with schizophrenic patients. In Strupp, H. & Luborsky, L. (Eds.). *Research in psychotherapy*. American Psychological Association, Washington, D.C., 1962, pp. 41–60.

Brown R. Manipulation of the environmental press in a college residence hall. *Personnel and Guidance Journal*, **46**: 555–560, 1968.

Burdock, E., Cheek, F., & Zubin, J. Predicting success in psychoanalytic training. In Hoch, P. & Zubin, J. (Eds.). *Current approaches to psychoanalysis*. Grune & Stratton, New York, 1960; pp. 176–191.

Carson, R. & Heine, R. Similarity and success in therapeutic dyads: A reevaluation. *Journal of Consulting Psychology*, **30**: 458, 1962.

Cattell, R. & Nesselroade, J. Likeness and completeness theories examined by sixteen personality factor measures on stably and unstably married couples. *Journal of Personality and Social Psychology*, **4**: 351–361, 1967.

Chickering, A., McDowell, J., & Campagna, D. Institutional differences and student development. *Journal of Educational Psychology*, **60**: 315–326, 1969.

DeCoster, D. Housing assignments for high ability students. *Journal of College Student Personnel*, **7**: 10–22, 1966.

Farson, R. Introjection in the psychotherapeutic relationship. *Journal of Counseling Psychology*, **9**: 337–342, 1961.

Feldman, K. & Newcomb, T. *The impact of college on students*. Jossey-Bass, San Francisco, 1969.

Fiedler, F. Interpersonal perception and group effectiveness. In Tagiuri, R. & Petrullo, L. (Eds.). *Person perception and interpersonal behavior*. Stanford University Press, Stanford, Calif., 1958.

Fleisher, B. & Kuldau, J. Compatibility and stability in home care groups. *Social Psychiatry*, **7**: 11–17, 1972.

Gans, H. *People and plans.* Basic Books, New York, 1968.

Gassner, S. Relationship between patient–therapist compatibility and treatment effectiveness. *Journal of Consulting and Clinical Psychology,* **34:** 408–414, 1970.

Goldstein, A. *Psychotherapeutic attraction.* Pergamon Press, New York, 1971.

Goldstein, A., Heller, K., & Sechrest, L. *Psychotherapy and the psychology of behavior change.* Wiley, New York, 1966.

Hicks, M. & Platt, M. Marital happiness and stability: A review of the research in the sixties. *Journal of Marriage and the Family,* **32:** 553–574, 1970.

Hutcherson, D. Relationships among teacher–pupil compatibility, social studies grades, and selected factors. Doctoral dissertation, University of California, Berkeley, 1963.

Lansing, J., Marans, R., & Zehner, R. *Planned residential environments.* Institute for Social Research, Ann Arbor, Mich., 1970.

Maddi, S. *Personality theories: A comparative analysis.* Dorsey, Homewood, Ill. 1968.

McNair, D., Callahan, D., & Lorr, M. Therapist "type" and patient response to psychotherapy. *Journal of Consulting Psychology,* **26:** 425–429, 1962.

Meltzoff, J. & Kornreich, M. *Research in psychotherapy.* Atherton, New York, 1970.

Mendelsohn, G. & Geller, M. Effects of counselor–client similarity on the outcome of counseling. *Journal of Counseling Psychology,* **10:** 71–77, 1963.

Mendelsohn, G. & Geller, M. Structure of client attitudes toward counseling and their relation to client–counselor similarity. *Journal of Consulting Psychology,* **29:** 63–72, 1965.

Mendelsohn, G. & Rankin, N. Client–counselor compatibility and the outcome of counseling. *Journal of Abnormal Psychology,* **74:** 157–163, 1969.

Moos, R. & Speisman, J. Group compatibility and productivity. *Journal of Abnormal and Social Psychology,* **64:** 190–196, 1962.

Newcomb, T. *The acquaintance process.* Holt, Rinehart & Winston, New York, 1961.

Pace, R. *College and University Environment Scale,* Technical manual, 2nd ed. Educational Testing Service, Princeton, N.J., 1969.

Parloff, M., Iflund, B., & Goldstein, N. Communication of "therapy values" between therapist and schizophrenic patients. *Journal of Nervous and Mental Disease,* **130:** 193–199, 1960.

Peterson, R., Centra, J., Hartnett, R. & Linn, R. Institutional Functioning Inventory: Preliminary technical manual. Educational Testing Service, Princeton, N.J., 1970.

Rosenthal, D. Changes in some moral values following psychotherapy. *Journal of Consulting Psychology,* **19:** 431–436, 1955.

Sapolsky, A. Effect of interpersonal relationships upon verbal conditioning. *Journal of Abnormal and Social Psychology,* **60:** 241–246, 1960.

Sapolsky, A. Relationship between patient–doctor compatibility, mutual perception, and outcome of treatment. *Journal of Abnormal Psychology,* **70:** 70–76, 1965.

Schrier, H. The significance of identification in therapy. *American Journal of Orthopsychiatry,* **23:** 585–604, 1953.

Schutz, W. *FIRO: A three-dimensional theory of interpersonal behavior*. Holt, Rinehart & Winston, New York, 1958.

Sheehan, J. Rorschach changes during psychotherapy in relation to personality of the therapist. *American Psychologist*, **8**: 434–435, 1953.

Smelser, W. Dominance in cooperative problem-solving interactions. Ph.D. dissertation, University of California, 1958.

Spohn, H. The influence of social values upon the clinical judgements of psychotherapists. In Peatman, J. & Hartley, E. (Eds.). *Festschrift for Gardner Murphy*. Harper & Row New York, 1960.

Stern, G. *People in context: measuring person environment congruence in education and industry*. Wiley, New York, 1970.

Tuma, A. & Gustaad, J. The effects of client and counselor personality characteristics on client learning in counseling. *Journal of Counseling Psychology*, **4**: 136–141, 1957.

Welkowitz, J., Cohen, J., & Ortmeyer, D. Value system similarity: Investigation of patient–therapist dyads. *Journal of Consulting Psychology*, **31**: 48–55, 1967.

Winch, R., Ktsanes, T., & Ktsanes, V. Empirical elaboration of the theory of complementary needs in mate selection. *Journal of Abnormal and Social Psychology*, **51**: 508–513, 1955.

Yalom, I. *The theory and practice of group psychotherapy*. Basic Books, New York, 1970.

PART FOUR

Retrospect and Prospect

Chapter Fourteen

UNDERLYING
PATTERNS OF TREATMENT
SETTING

This chapter summarizes the empirical work and discusses implications for individual clinical practice of self-initiated change in treatment settings; also examined are new types of research designs for more comprehensive comparisons and evaluations ·of psychiatric and other "treatment" programs. We briefly present our work in the Social Ecology Laboratory in other types of social environments, including correctional institutions, military training companies, university student living groups, and junior high and high school classrooms, amplifying our theory that the underlying patterns of all these environments are similar. Finally, we consider the relevance of our work for comparing and evaluating treatment programs and for studying a variety of social environments along broadly commensurate dimensions.

OVERVIEW OF RESULTS

Our work was conceived as an integration of several lines of investigation. Initially most influential was research indicating that the variability of individual behavior from one environment to another is apt to be quite substantial. We found that patients' behavior in treatment settings often differs markedly from their behavior in out-of-hospital community settings. Thus the common assumption that adjustment in the treatment milieu is highly related to adjustment in the community is not correct. Second, both naturalistic descriptive studies and comparative program evaluations emphasized the importance of distinctive treatment milieus in accounting for beneficial treatment outcome, thereby pointing to the necessity of measuring and comparing these milieus. We noted that physicians, anthropologists, social scientists, and novelists have described psychiatric hospitals and programs, reaching various conclusions about their effectiveness. All agreed, however, that the immediate psychosocial environment in which patients function has a crucial impact on treatment outcome. This and other work convinced us of the necessity of developing systematic ways of assessing and comparing treatment milieus.

THE PSYCHOMETRICS OF PERCEIVED CLIMATE SCALES

We developed techniques to measure the social climates of hospital-based and community-based psychiatric treatment programs by asking patients and staff individually about the usual patterns of behavior in their program. We were compelled by the logic that behavior is shaped and directed by the environment as subjectively perceived by the people in it. In addition, we wanted to be able to measure people and their environments along similar or commensurate dimensions.

We then developed the Ward Atmosphere Scale (WAS) to assess the social climates of hospital-based treatment programs and the Community-Oriented Programs Environment Scale (COPES) to assess the treatment milieus of community-based programs. We collected data from more than 200 hospital programs in the United States, Canada, and the United Kingdom, and from 75 community programs in the United States and the United Kingdom. The psychometric data presented in Chapters 2 and 10 indicated that (1) the WAS and the COPES subscales have adequate internal consistency and test–retest reliabilities, (2) the subscales significantly discriminate among treatment programs, and (3) the 10 subscales on each test are only moderately interrelated. We also found that the treatment environment of programs that have a consistent treatment philosophy is extremely high over long periods of time (e.g., 2- to 3-year intervals). The treatment environment may remain stable even though there has been complete turnover in the patient population. We found that patient and staff perceptions of treatment milieus are only minimally related either to the respondents' personal background characteristics or to their tendency to answer items about themselves in socially desirable directions. The role position of an individual in an environment (e.g., patient or staff) seems to affect his perception of that environment much more than do his background characterisitcs.

Most important, both the WAS and the COPES subscales fall into three basic categories. The Involvement, Support, and Spontaneity subscales measure Relationship dimensions. The next four subscales—Autonomy, Practical Orientation, Personal Problem Orientation, and Anger and Aggression—assess Personal Development or Treatment Program dimensions and the Order and Organization, Program Clarity, and Staff Control subscales serve to evaluate System Maintenance dimensions. The relevance of this conceptualization for other social environments is discussed later in this chapter.

We developed 40-item Short Forms of both the WAS and the COPES for use by investigators or program staff who wish to obtain a relatively rapid assessment of a program's treatment environment. The short forms are especially useful in following changes in a program over time. We also briefly presented the development of versions of scales by which goals and value orientations (Ideal Forms) and and initial expectations (Expectation Forms) of patients and staff could be assessed. These forms are useful for a variety of research purposes, as discussed in Chapters 2, 9, and 12.

THE DIVERSITY OF TREATMENT PROGRAMS

The range of currently existing treatment programs is great. Some strongly emphasize the understanding of personal feelings and the open expression of anger, playing down as much as possible Order and Organization and Staff Control. Other programs put heavy stress on patient independence and autonomy and a task-related bahavioral planning orientation, being only moderately concerned with Clarity and Control. There were some examples of almost every conceivable type of treatment program. We found two university and teaching hospital programs with strikingly similar structural and patient background characteristics but strikingly different WAS profiles. We obtained results in a state hospital program indicating that the social milieu may be quite active and cohesive even when the program serves very difficult patients living in a relatively poor situation in a hospital with restrictive overall rules and regulations. From other results it appears that small relatively well staffed programs may have quite negative social environments, whereas large poorly staffed programs may have clear, coherent, and structured treatment milieus. The WAS and the COPES provide standard, relatively objective ways for systematically assessing and comparing treatment programs, and this is one of the major uses of the instruments.

Staff on the whole present a significantly more positive picture of treatment programs than do patients. The differences between patients and staff are much greater in hospital than in community programs. Compared with patients, staff in hospital programs see much more emphasis on each of the Relationship and Treatment Program dimensions but less emphasis on Staff Control. Patients and staff in community programs report relatively similar emphases on the Relationship and System Maintenance dimensions, but staff consistently perceive more emphasis on the Treatment Program dimensions. These results indicate that the "two-subculture" phenomenon is much more applicable to hospital than to community programs. To put it another way, patients and staff in community programs surpass their counterparts in hospital programs by communicating much more accurately and fully with each other and by being more cohesive and integrated. British staff also perceive their treatment programs significantly more positively than do British patients.

In our cross-cultural comparison of British and American hospital programs, American patients and staff appeared to perceive significantly more emphasis on the Relationship dimension of Involvement, the Treatment Program dimensions of Autonomy, Practical Orientation, and Personal Problem Orientation, and the System Maintenance dimension of Staff Control. We interpreted this finding as being consistent with our own impression and with general cultural stereotypes—that is, British staff leave their patients more "to their own devices" than do American staff.

We presented several program evaluation and program change studies indicating that the WAS and the COPES are sensitive to treatment environment changes as perceived by both patients and staff. Each of three program change studies revealed greater emphasis on the Relationship dimensions, signifying better patient and staff morale, more helpfulness and supportiveness, and greater personal openness and expressivity. Personal relationships in a program seem to improve regardless of the specific changes instituted. Changes in the Treatment Program dimensions are more directly related to the type of change introduced. Thus one study found relatively large increases in Personal Problem Orientation and Anger and Aggression in a program in which staff received group therapy training.

Another study revealed substantial increases in Autonomy and Practical Orientation when a token-economy program was instituted. On the other hand, not all attempts are sufficient to bring about large changes; in one investigation, for example, relatively little change resulted from a resocialization training program in a chronic backward of a state hospital. Our data indicate that the specific characteristics of treatment programs and policies, rather than hospital administration rules and regulations per se, are of most critical importance in determining the actual treatment milieu.

THE CLINICAL RELEVANCE OF RESEARCH: SOCIAL CHANGE

We presented three demonstration studies in which the treatment milieus of three psychiatric programs were successfully changed. One study was carried out in a small, heavily staffed university hospital program. The WAS served as a teaching device for program staff, and after intensive discussion of real–ideal program discrepancies, attempts were made to formulate specific change goals. A relatively large overall change in the social milieu of this university program demonstrated that assessment and intensive staff discussion could function as a stimulus for positive change. In the second study performed in psychiatric unit of a general hospital, the staff decided to use the WAS to describe the program and to identify ways in which it could help create a more beneficial treatment milieu. The results showed that significant changes occurred in the program and that both patients and staff perceived the milieu as being closer to an Ideal milieu after the feedback and change processes had been completed.

The third study was conducted in an adolescent residential center. Several change attempts were made over a 4-month period (e.g., rules and expectations were clarified, residents were given new and responsible positions in the program). Both residents and staff felt that the treatment milieu was generally closer to their ideal in the second than in the first testing. Significantly, both residents and staff also felt that the program was further from their ideal in the dimensions of Personal Problem Orientation and Anger and Aggression. This shift occurred mainly because residents and staff decided that they ideally wished less emphasis on the two areas named, illustrating that views of ideal environments can also be changed with feedback and discussion sessions. A psychosocial environment cannot be changed toward a "static ideal"; instead, feedback of information must be thought of as a dynamic, ongoing process that produces continuous change in real and ideal social milieus. Changes in values about ideal environments may follow changes in the actual environment.

Several conclusions emerge from the three studies just described.

1.   Systematic information about program perceptions aids staff in articulating their concerns.

2.   Some staff who infrequently verbalize their opinions are able to formulate salient issues in terms of WAS and COPES feebdback.

3.   Change attempts may have temporary negative effects, particularly decreased Program Clarity as perceived by patients. To avoid increased patient confusion, staff must explain to patients as fully as possible the overall plan for policy changes.

4.   Program changes may take place within a generally consistent treatment ideology; that is, a program can institute a series of carefully thought-out and graduated changes while still retaining its essential overall direction. However, it may be difficult to stop change once it has been initiated.

5.   Values may be changed by the actual practices in the treatment milieu. Thus a patient or staff member who functions in an environment that strongly emphasizes Autonomy and Spontaneity may end up valuing these dimensions more highly both in and out of hospital.

6.   Feedback and discussion sessions constitute a practical application of ongoing teaching and research.

Easily administered assessment techniques such as the WAS and the COPES are reasonable short-term information-gathering techniques for busy staff lacking extensive facilities of personnel for evaluation. The administration and analysis of these scales is a useful service that a hospital or university psychology department can provide to treatment programs. In addition, as indicated previously, we feel that feedback and discussion about the treatment environment of a program helps give ongoing research a practical application. Research can be tied to salient issues in a social system, thus allowing individuals participating in that system to collaborate actively in research that concerns them. These techniques are an important mechanism in the acceptance and use of research, as well as a critical source of information and ideas about future relevant research.

THE EFFECTS OF TREATMENT MILIEUS

Size and Staffing

Our results show that programs of smaller size and/or higher staffing tend to have more emphasis on Relationship and Treatment Program dimensions (particularly Personal Problem Orientation and Anger and Aggression) and less emphasis on Staff Control. Increased size and/or decreased staffing creates pressures toward a more rigid structure, increases staff need to control and manage, and decreases the degree of patient independence and responsibility and the amount of support and involvement staff are able to give patients. Greater size and less staffing are also related to fewer spontaneous relationships among patients and between patients and staff, as well as to diminished emphasis on understanding patients' personal problems and openly handling their angry feelings. Large size may create organizational pressures toward custodial rather than treatment operations. The custodial atmosphere may itself create "unreceptive" behavior, which justifies the need for futher regimentation. Thus large size may initiate a "vicious circle" that reinforces System Maintenance staff behaviors, especially Staff Control.

Sometimes the usual negative concomitants of large size and poor staffing can be ameliorated by changing certain aspects of the social and organizational environment. We found examples of active, coherent treatment milieus in large, relatively well-staffed programs and in small, relatively poorly staffed programs. The negative effects of large hospitals may be partially alleviated by a unit system in which the hospital is functionally divided into smaller sections. Dividing a large treatment unit into patient-staff treatment teams and/or other smaller groups may also enhance communication and cohesion.

We learned that patients' values about ideal programs may be affected by the staff–patient ratio and that staff values about ideal programs may be affected by patient behavior. Patients on more poorly staffed programs ideally want much more emphasis on Relationship and System Maintenance dimensions, whereas staff who work in programs on which patients are unusually aggressive and disruptive ideally want less emphasis on Spontaneity, Autonomy, and Practical Orientation, but more on Staff Control. Thus staff behavior influences patients' values regarding ideal programs, whereas patient behavior affects staff values regarding ideal programs.

We sampled community programs with and without professional staff and were thus able to compare their social environments. We were primarily interested in the extent to which the social environment or perhaps the "quality of life" differed in these programs. The programs did not differ in emphasis on the three Relationship dimensions, but programs with professional staff put much heavier stress on all four Treatment Program dimensions, particularly Personal Problem Orientation and Anger and Aggression. Programs without professional staff had more emphasis on the three System Maintenance dimensions. Thus professional staff make the greatest difference in the Treatment Program areas. They do not seem to strongly influence the quality and intensity of the relationships among patients, and they have some effect in diminishing the emphasis on System Maintenance.

These results are thought-provoking, since they suggest that the influence of professional staff in live-in community programs may be more limited than has been thought—that is, such influence may occur mainly with respect to the four Treatment Program dimensions. Research in individual and group psychotherapy indicates that paraprofessional and other minimally trained staff can establish relationships that do not differ in quality from those established by highly trained professional staff. These results are consistent with our finding that the Relationship dimensions are as strongly emphasized in programs without professional staff as in programs with such staff. The results for the System Maintenance dimensions are not unexpected, since professional staff often deemphasize these variables because of their presumed constrictive influence.

Whether the influence of professional staff is more beneficial or more harmful is a moot point. Emphases on Autonomy and Independence and on a practical problem-solving orientation are probably beneficial. An emphasis on the open expression of feelings, particularly angry feelings, may or may not be beneficial, depending on the types of community situations to which the patient will be exposed and on the exactness of the discriminations he learns to make. It is obvious that the open expression of angry feelings, although potentially cathartic, may produce strong negative reinforcements in many community settings. An implication of these results has to do with the training of foster parents and other nonprofessional staff. These individuals can and should be specifically trained in methods by which to emphasize Autonomy and a Practical Orientation, since these dimensions have beneficial effects on patients' personal growth.

Morale and Coping Styles

Our studies on hospital and community programs indicated that when Relationship and Treatment Program dimensions (except for Anger and Aggression) are emphasized, morale is generally high, patients feel more satisfied in the program, like one another and the staff more, and are more hopeful about treatment. Emphasis on Staff Control is generally negatively related to each of these variables. Also, patients engaged in less helping behavior in programs emphasizing Anger and Aggression. This suggests that some programs with active treatment milieus encouraging the open expression of anger may make patients more uncomfortable, thereby causing a decrease in helping behavior. These results give some indication of the variables mediating between treatment environment and treatment outcome. For example, patient-perceived Practical Orientation was related to release rate in two independent studies of treatment outcome. Practical Orientation was also related to patient helping behavior in the areas of friendship and enhancement of self-esteem and to staff helping behavior in the areas of friendship and directive teaching. These helping activities must in part be related to the rapid turnover rate in programs with a high emphasis on Practical Orientation.

Relationship dimensions assume critical importance in individual and group psychotherapy, in social and task-oriented groups, and in industrial and educational environments. These dimensions appear to have similar effects across different types of institutions. Much less is known about the differential effects of the Personal Development and System Maintenance dimensions, since they have not been as generally utilized in studies of group and institutional effects. It has been hypothesized that Relationship and Personal Development dimensions are anabolic (i.e., growth enhancing), whereas System Maintenance dimensions are catabolic (i.e., growth inhibiting). The justification for this statement remains to be evaluated. The clearest conclusion is that satisfying human relationships in all environments studied to date facilitate personal growth and development and are in this sense anabolic. However, the effects of Personal Development and System Maintenance dimensions merit further study. We feel that all three types of dimensions should be included in future systematic assessments of social environments.

Treatment Outcome

We developed three perceived climate indices linking three objective measures of treatment outcome to treatment environments. Programs with high dropout rates tend to have few social activities, little emphasis on involving patients in the program, and somewhat poor planning of patients' activities. Patients in such programs do not interact much with one another, and they have a good deal of free time with little or no guidance. Staff discourage criticism from patients and are unwilling to act on patients' suggestions. Patients tend to gripe about or criticize the staff, perhaps because the program is seen (by both patients and staff) as poorly organized. Programs with high dropout rates are rather unfriendly; patients do not really feel comfortable or at ease, and staff seem to be somewhat unhappy with the environment and with one another.

Programs with high release rates typically emphasize making plans for leaving the hospital (and having concrete plans before leaving) and training patients for new kinds of jobs. There is a fair amount of Staff Control, but staff are personally interested in the patients and tell them when they are making progress. There is relatively little emphasis on expressiveness; for example, patients rarely argue with one another, and they keep their disagreements to themselves. Neither patients nor staff see much Support in such programs. Even though the programs are practical and "unexpressive," their members regard them with a certain pride and involvement.

Programs that keep patients out in the community the longest emphasize the free and open expression of feelings, particularly angry feelings. Staff think it is a healthy thing to argue, are seen arguing among themselves, and sometimes start arguments in group meetings. Patients are expected to share their personal problems and feelings with one another and with staff. This emphasis on personal problems and the open expression of anger occurs within a context that also emphasizes Autonomy and Independence, a Practical Orientation, Order and Organization, and a reasonable degree of Staff Control. For example, patients are transferred from the program if they do not obey the rules, but they are treated with respect by the staff and are encouraged to be independent.

Our results corroborate those of previous studies in indicating that treatment environment may be as important as such objective characteristics differentiating among programs as size and staffing and patient background variables. In our studies, perceived treatment environment was more highly and consistently related to treatment outcome than were either program size and staffing or patient background characteristics. National cooperative studies systematically assessing patient background and behavior, program characteristics and policies, and treatment environment and treatment outcome are the next logical step in this area. Systematically acquired information about patients' relevant community settings must be included in these studies. In this way it should be possible to obtain more dependable information on the complex interactions among relevant patient, treatment program, and community environment characteristics and different treatment outcome criteria.

DEVIANT PERCEPTIONS AND EXPECTATIONS

Our results indicated that patients who see their treatment milieu deviantly are less satisfied, like the staff less, feel that what they are doing is less likely to enhance their abilities and their self-esteem, and actually do somewhat more poorly than other patients, at 6-month follow-up. Most important, the relationship between deviancy and reactions to the program and to treatment outcome varies as a function of the characteristics of the milieu. The social environment is a "moderator" variable, and deviancy must be viewed as an adaptive reaction in some environments. Research findings may not generalize across settings precisely because the settings have important differential characteristics. Thus social climate indices may have utility both in selecting environments in which replication studies should be carried out and in explaining why certain relationships are not replicated in varying milieus.

According to the results of our study of expectations, the effects of deviant expectations also depend on the characteristics of the program's social milieu. When the milieu is generally negative and inconsistent, patients with unrealistically positive expectations do poorly and are more likely to drop out of treatment prematurely. When the milieu is generally active, positive, and coherent, however, unrealistically high expectations do not have the same negative effects.

Prior information about treatment programs can enhance the accuracy of patients' expectations, thus reducing the incidence of patient maladaptation and dropout. Work in individual and group psychotherapy has shown that providing systematic information about the therapy helps to socialize an individual and increases the probability of positive outcome.

Anticipatory socialization experiences for patients or staff who have tendencies to perceive their environments deviantly might enhance such individuals' satisfaction with and functioning in their treatment milieu. The presentation of information about treatment milieus to prospective patients and/or staff might serve to reduce their discrepant perceptions and expectations and to improve their treatment progress, especially if the information and its manner of presentation are congruent with the individual's preferred coping styles.

In this connection, we point out that the rapid proliferation of new types of psychiatric treatment programs has increased the need and the demand for more accurate and complete program descriptions. Many people feel that published program descriptions do not give an adequate picture or "feel" of the treatment environment or social climate of a treatment program. Our study corroborated this opinion. Ideally, descriptions of treatment programs should use information relevant to the six major methods by which human milieus have been characterized (see Chapter 1). Each of these methods gives a somewhat different perspective on a program, and the use of all six can furnish relatively accurate and complete program descriptions. Better program descriptions should be of use to prospective staff considering working in a new treatment program, to social workers who make referral decisions, and to patients who wish to take a more active part in choosing their own program.

PROGRAM HOMOGENEITY AND CONGRUENCE

Our results demonstrate that the average perception and value congruence in treatment programs is considerably greater than the hypothesis of random patient selection would lead us to expect. When the WAS and the COPES are used as measures of program congruence, the effects of self-selection and program selection are necessarily confounded with changes in perceptions and values that occur subsequent to functioning in a given treatment milieu. The exact mechanisms by which the relatively high degree of program congruence occurs can be clarified only through longitudinal studies that follow patients and staff from the time they enter a program.

There are at least three possible interrelated mechanisms contributing to the high degree of observed congruence. First, patients and staff simply learn about the characteristics of their treatment milieus, and perceptual congruence develops from a mutually shared reality of events. Value congruence must also develop to some extent through discussions of shared value orientations and through mutual attraction and similarity influences directed toward increasing congruence. Second, there is probably a strong tendency for patients and staff who share neither the perceptions of the treatment milieu nor the dominant value orientations to leave the program. Third, as actual treatment milieus change, expectations about ideal treatment milieus also change. This process tends to increase real–ideal congruence.

Thus the press toward program congruence or homogeneity is partly attributable to the following factors: initial self-selection, initial program selection, dropout and reselection by both individuals and programs, and actual changes occurring in individuals as they function within environments having particular dominant orientations. The degree of program congruence is important because both patient–staff and real–ideal congruence (at least for patients) is significantly related to patient morale, liking for staff, and hopefulness about treatment outcome. As a rule, interpersonal and group compatibility are positively related to similarity of perception, interpersonal attraction, and individual or group productivity criteria. These findings make it reasonable to consider selecting patients and staff for treatment programs on the basis of their background or value congruence with other individuals already in those programs. Work creating a variety of homogeneous or heterogeneous programs and studying their differential effects on various types of patients and staff may prove fruitful.

TOWARD A TAXONOMY OF SOCIAL ENVIRONMENTS

One of our most important findings is that the same three categories of environmental dimensions were identified in both hospital-based and community-based treatment programs. This facilitates the direct comparison of various types of treatment programs along commensurate dimensions. These three categories of dimensions are also useful in characterizing the social and organizational climates of a broad variety of groups and institutions.

Work in the Social Ecology Laboratory

Our central interest over the past few years has been the development of techniques by which psychosocial environments can be assessed. We have completed extensive work in seven institutional and group milieus (in addition to treatment environments), which are representative of three categories of environments: *"total" institutions* (correctional institutions and military training companies), *educational environments* (university student living groups and junior high and high school classrooms), and naturally occurring *community settings* (industrial or work milieus, social and task-oriented groups, and families). Table 14.1 summarizes the dimensions that are included in each of our nine Social Climate Scales.

Total Institutions

Our Correctional Institutions Environment Scale (CIES) assesses the social milieus of juvenile and adult correctional institutions (Moos, 1968; 1974a). We derived a final form of the CIES from data gathered from residents and staff in extensive national samples of more than 100 juvenile and 50 adult correctional units. The perceived climate dimensions of correctional institutions are very similar to those characterizing treatment environments. The majority of the correctional units we studied were for juvenile offenders, and it should be noted that juvenile units have a much more treatment-oriented milieu than do adult units, which are mainly custodial. The CIES has nine subscale dimensions. The Involvement, Support, and Expressiveness subscales assess Relationship dimensions; the Autonomy, Practical Orientation, and Personal Problem Orientation subscales assess Personal Development or Treatment Program dimensions; the Order and Organization, Program Clarity, and Staff Control subscales assess System Maintenance dimensions.

Thus the only difference in the perceived climate dimensions of treatment and correctional environments is that correctional institutions do not have an anger and aggression dimension. There was an anger and aggression subscale in an earlier form of the CIES. Designed to measure the extent to which residents are allowed and encouraged to argue with other residents and with staff, to become openly angry, and to display other aggressive behavior, this subscale was eliminated because of low item–subscale correlations and because most of the items had relatively extreme item splits and/or did not differentiate among correctional units. The tolerance in correctional milieus for the open expression of anger and aggression, even in verbal form, is rather low. This is in marked contrast to psychiatric treatment units, in which such expressions very seldom emphasize the open expression of anger and aggression as a "vector of development." The general similarity of the dimensions independently derived on the WAS, on the COPES, and on the CIES may allow investigators to compare directly the social milieus of treatment environments with those of correctional environments.

We have completed much additional work utilizing the CIES in research that substantially replicates and extends our earlier work on treatment environments. For example, one study revealed that juvenile correctional units characterized by greater emphasis on the Relationship dimensions of Involvement and Expressiveness and the Treatment Program dimensions of Autonomy and Personal Problem Orientation had residents who were more likely to like the staff and to feel that they were able to test their abilities and to increase their self-confidence. The residents on these units also tended to interact more with the staff (Moos, 1970).

Other research on the CIES includes the use of the scale in program comparisons and evaluations (e.g., Jesness et al., 1972), investigations of the relationships between perceived social climate and structural and organizational dimensions reported for correctional programs, studies of the correlates of individuals' perception and value discrepancies from the norms in their correctional units, and cross-cultural research systematically comparing open and closed prisons in the United Kingdom.

Our Military Company Environment Inventory (MCEI) assesses the social climates of military training companies as perceived by officers and enlisted men (Moos, 1973a). Our approach in developing the MCEI was similar to that used in the construction of the previous scales. The initial version of the MCEI was given to 13 training companies, and the Instrument was revised on the basis of a factor analysis conducted on a random sample of subjects taken from these companies. The factor analysis yielded 7 subscales, and the final version of the MCEI consists of 84 items (i.e., 12 items on each subscale).

As Table 14.1 indicates, the subscales also cluster in our three general categories. Whereas a dimension of Involvement significantly differentiates among the companies, it was not possible to identify a dimension made up of spontaneity or expressiveness items, even though these items were included in the initial item pool. However, the military environment has two distinctly different "support" dimensions—Peer Cohesion and Officer Support. It is difficult to find psychiatric or correctional programs in which

TABLE 14.1 SIMILARITIES OF SOCIAL CLIMATE DIMENSIONS ACROSS ENVIRONMENTS

Environment	Dimensions		
	Relationship	Personal Development	System Maintenance and System Change
Treatment environments (WAS and COPES)	Involvement Support Spontaneity	Autonomy Practical Orientation Personal Problem Orientation Anger and Aggression	Order and Organization Clarity Control
Total institutions Correctional institutions	Involvement Support Expressiveness	Autonomy Practical Orientation Personal Problem Orientation	Order and Organization Clarity Control
Military companies	Involvement Peer Cohesion Officer Support	Personal Status	Order Clarity Officer Control
Educational environments University student living groups	Involvement Emotional Support	Independence Traditional Social Orientation Competition Academic Achievement Intellectuality	Order and Organization Student Influence Innovation

Setting			
Junior high and high school classrooms	Involvement Affiliation Teacher Support	Task Orientation Competition	Order and Organization Rule Clarity Teacher Control Innovation
Community settings Social, task-oriented, and therapeutic groups	Cohesiveness Leader Support Spontaneity	Independence Task Orientation Self-Discovery Ander and Aggression	Order and Organization Leader Control Innovation
Work milieus	Involvement Peer Cohesion Staff Support	Task Orientation Competition	Work Pressure Clarity Control Innovation Physical Comfort
Families	Cohesion Expressiveness Conflict	Independence Achievement Orientation Intellectual–Cultural Orientation Recreational Orientation Moral–Religious Emphasis	Organization Control

support from peers is low and support from staff is high, or vice versa. In these environments, therefore, peer support and staff support merge into one Support dimension. In the more hierarchically arranged military environment, the enlisted men spend a great deal of time together and a dimension of Peer Cohesion which is quite separate from the dimension of Officer Support is thus identified.

It was only possible to identify one differentiating Personal Development dimension in the military environment. Items relevant to a practical task orientation were included in the initial item pool, and they characterized military companies adequately; however, they did not generally differentiate among them. Our Personal Status dimension is essentially an autonomy or independence dimension; it reveals how individual differences among enlisted men are recognized and respected and measures the emphasis on encouraging enlisted men to assume responsibility in the company. Finally, the System Maintenance dimensions independently identified in the military environment (i.e., Order, Clarity, and Officer [Staff] Control) are identical to those occurring in psychiatric and correctional environments.

We have conducted other research with the MCEI in collaboration with Harris Clemes. The MCEI has been utilized in 32 training companies, and company environment has been associated with the degree of negative affect of the men in the company. The results indicated that men are most anxious in companies with low Personal Status and high Officer Control. Men complain of more depression in companies that have low Peer Support and high Officer Control. Men feel most hostile in companies low in Involvement, Officer Support, and Clarity, and high in Officer Control. Thus men tend to feel most angry and hostile when they perceive that their officers do not listen to them, pay attention to them, or support them. Finally, Peer Cohesion was the only MCEI scale associated with company performance as measured by firing scores, physical training scores, and graded test scores. High Peer Cohesion was positively associated with high test scores and high total company performance.

Educational Environments

The University Residence Environment Scale (URES) assesses the social climates of university student living groups such as dormitories, fraternities, and sororities. The basic rationale and description of the development of the scale is detailed by Moos and Gerst (1974). The final

URES was derived from a random sample of data collected from 74 student living groups. Each of the 10 subscales has high internal consistency and test–retest reliability; moreover, the URES profile shows high stability over time.

The 10 dimensions identified in the URES are as follows.

1.   Involvement assesses the degree of commitment to the house and the amount of social interaction and feeling of friendship in the living group.

2.   Emotional Support assesses the extent of manifest concern for others in the house, efforts to aid one another with academic and personal problems, and the emphasis on open and honest communication.

3.   Independence assesses the diversity of thoughts and actions by students and the emphasis on acting in different ways without rigid regard for social sanction.

4.   Traditional Social Orientation assesses the stress on dating, going to parties, and other "traditional" heterosexual interactions.

5.   Competition assesses the degree to which a wide variety of activities (dating, grades, etc.) are cast into a competitive framework.

6.   Academic Achievement assesses the prominence of classroom accomplishments and concerns in the house.

7.   Intellectuality assesses the emphasis on cultural, artistic, and other scholarly activities in the house, as distinguished from purely academic emphasis on grades, studying, and so on.

8.   Order and Organization assesses the degree of formal structure or organization (e.g., rules, schedules, following established procedures) in the house and its neatness and orderliness.

9.   Student Influence assesses the extent to which student residents (not staff) control the running of the house; this dimension involves rule formulation and enforcement, the use of money, the selection of staff, and food and rooming policies.

10.   Innovation assesses both the organization's and the individual's spontaneity of behaviors and ideas and the number and variety of new and varied activities in the house.

Some of these dimensions differ from those identified previously, but again they seem to fall into the basic three categories of dimensions (see Table 14.1). University student residences are characterized along the two Relationship dimensions of Involvement and Emotional Support, the

System Maintenance dimension of Order and Organization, and two System Change dimensions labeled Student Influence and Innovation. Therefore, at least in terms of the number of identifiable climate dimensions, university student residences are more strongly oriented toward system change than toward system maintenance. This statement probably would not surprise many university student housing office administrators.

The Personal Development dimensions identified in university living groups are quite different from those identified in psychiatric or correctional environments because university students are interested in changing along quite different vectors of development. The URES has a dimension of Independence, as do the other scales. However, the additional Personal Development dimensions reflecting personal growth (Independence, Traditional Social Orientation, and possibly Competition) and intellectual growth (Academic Achievement and Intellectuality) are specifically appropriate to university living groups. These Personal Development dimensions identify the major directions in which university housing programs attempt to engender student development.

We have also developed a Classroom Environment Scale (CES) for evaluating the social climates of junior high and high school classrooms (Moos and Trickett, 1974). The CES has been utilized in more than 300 classrooms sampled from general and vocational high schools located in communities on the east and the west coasts. The CES, too, was derived using methods similar to those chosen for the development of our other Social Climate Scales. The nine subscales on the final form of the CES are as follows.

1.   Involvement measures the extent to which students pay attention to and show interest in the activities of the classroom.

2.   Affiliation measures the extent to which students work with and come to know one another within the classroom.

3.   Teacher Support measures the amount of help, concern, and friendship the teacher directs toward the students.

4.   Task Orientation measures the extent to which the activities of the class are centered around the accomplishment of specific academic objectives.

5.   Competition measures the amount of emphasis placed on student competition for grades and recognition.

6.   Order and Organization measures the emphasis on students' behaving in an orderly and polite manner and on the overall organization of assignments and classroom activities.

7.   Rule Clarity measures the degree to which rules for conduct in the classroom are explicitly stated and clearly understood.

8.   Teacher Control measures the degree to which student conduct in the classroom is delimited by the strict enforcement of rules.

9.   Innovation measures the extent to which students contribute in planning classroom activities and the amount of unusual and varying activities and assignments planned by the teacher.

Thus the Relationship dimensions found in junior high and high school classrooms are similar to those noted in other environments (e.g., Involvement, Affiliation, and Teacher Support). The System Maintenance dimensions of Order and Organization, Rule Clarity, and Teacher Control, as well as the System Change dimension of Innovation are also quite similar to those found in other environments, particularly university student residences. The two Personal Development dimensions differentiating among classrooms—Task Orientation and Competition—are also similar to two of the dimensions observed in university living groups (see Table 14.1). As might be expected, the results indicate that junior high and high school classrooms are less varied, than college living groups in their major goals for personal development.

Community Settings

Our final three Social Climate Scales relate to naturally occurring community settings. The Group Environment Scale (GES) assesses the social climates of various types of small groups, including therapeutically oriented groups, task-oriented groups, and social groups (Moos and Humphrey, 1973). The GES has been given to approximately 30 groups; roughly half have been therapy groups and the rest have been either social or task-oriented groups. The dimensions on the GES (see "Community Settings" in Table 14.1) are very similar to those previously identified in other settings. The final version of the GES has 90 items, which fall into 10 subscale dimensions. Cohesiveness, Leader Support, and Spontaneity are Relationship dimensions. Independence, Task Orientation, Self-Discovery, and Anger and Aggression are Personal Development dimensions. Order and Organization, Leader Control, and Innovation are System Maintenance and System Change dimensions. The subscales have high internal consistencies, and each significantly discriminates among different types of groups.

The Work Environment Scale (WES) is one of our two newly developed scales. Although not yet extensively utilized, the WES has been administered in a wide variety of work environments and completed by individuals of very diverse occupations (e.g., secretaries, fork-lift operators, research assistants, stock brokers, firemen, janitors, administrators, and recreational park workers) (Insel and Moos, 1972). The preliminary dimensions of organizational climate identified in work environments are relatively similar to those found in other environments, except for two additional System Maintenance dimensions (see Table 14.1). The Relationship dimensions on the WES are Involvement, Peer Cohesion, and Staff Support. Thus the work environment is similar to the military company environment in the sense that we can identify two separate support dimensions. The Personal Development dimensions of Autonomy and Task Orientation noted in work environments are by now familiar, as are the System Maintenance dimensions of Clarity and Control and the System Change dimension of Innovation. However, two additional System Maintenance dimensions were identified—Work Pressure and Physical Comfort. The Work Pressure dimension appears to be specifically and solely relevant to work environments, whereas the Physical Comfort dimension would probably have been identified in other environments, had we initially selected relevant items. Research on the differential correlates of these subscales is currently underway.

Our last Social Climate Scale is the Family Environment Scale (FES). Our final version of the FES has 10 subscale dimensions, which fall into the three categories of dimensions (Moos, 1973b). We do not yet know whether these dimensions will adequately characterize families, although our initial data on approximately 200 families looks quite promising. The initial subscales are as follows:

1.   Cohesion measures the extent to which family members are concerned with and committed to the family; it includes items designed to reflect enthusiasm, support and constructive activity.

2.   Expressiveness measures the extent to which family members are allowed and encouraged to act openly and to express their feelings directly.

3.   Conflict assesses the extent to which open expression of anger and aggression and generally conflictual interactions are characteristic of the family.

These three subscales assess Relationship dimensions.

4.   Independence assesses the extent to which family members are

encouraged to be self-sufficient and to make their own decisions; it includes items related to personal development and growth.

5.   Achievement Orientation assesses the emphasis on achievement, getting ahead in life, setting high goals, and so on.

6.   Intellectual–Cultural Orientation assesses the emphasis on intellectual and cultural activities, such as going to lectures, plays, and concerts; reading books; playing musical instruments; and engaging in artistic or craft activities.

7.   Active Recreational Orientation assesses the extent to which family members are encouraged to have hobbies, to be involved in a variety of activities outside work or school, and to have diverse interests.

8.   Moral–Religious Emphasis assesses the extent to which the family emphasizes and discusses ethical and religious issues and values.

These five subscales assess Personal Development dimensions.

9.   Organization measures the emphasis in the family on such variables as neatness, structuring family activities, financial planning, and punctuality.

10.   Control assesses the extent to which the family functions by relatively strict "rules and regulations" or procedures.

These two subscales assess System Maintenance dimensions.

Thus the three basic categories of dimensions identified in treatment environments also can characterize correctional units; military training companies; university student living groups; junior high and high school classrooms; therapeutic, social, and task-oriented groups; work environments, and families. With relatively few exceptions, the Relationship and the System Maintenance and System Change dimensions are similar across all the environments studied.

The Personal Development dimensions, on the other hand, vary a good deal across environments depending on the vectors along which a given environment attempts to direct the people functioning within it. In treatment environments, therefore, we use the designation Treatment Program dimensions to refer to our framework for assessing the directions in which the program attempts to change patients. In educational environments these dimensions are related to more traditional educational goals. In family milieus they are related to traditional concerns with the environments of developing children and adolescents.

It is quite important to be able to identify similar dimensions along which very different environments can be characterized, since this furnishes a means whereby, in principle, these environments can be directly compared, especially in terms of the Relationship and System Maintenance and System Change dimensions. This comparability may eventually help us to learn why an individual does very well in one environment but quite poorly in another.

In summary, only two important additions must be made to our original formulation to make it relevant to a broad range of environments. First, some milieus vary along a dimension that can be labeled Innovation—the extent to which variety, change, and new approaches are emphasized. A search had been made for a dimension of this type in treatment environments; unfortunately, however, the initial selection of items was not adequate to permit such a dimension to emerge. Since this dimension identifies the emphasis on system change, it belongs in the third category of dimensions—hence the expanded label, System Maintenance and System Change.

Second, the middle category of Treatment Program or Personal Development dimensions varies depending on the basic thrust or raison d'etre of the environment being studied. Environments orient the individuals functioning within them toward different "vectors of development." These different vectors of development essentially become the dimensions in our Personal Development category.

Comparing the social environments of a hospital-based or community-based treatment program with the social environment of a work milieu may illustrate the potential utility of the concepts just defined. Although on the surface these environments are rather remote from each other, they have a good deal in common. The relevant Relationship dimensions on the WAS and the COPES are Involvement, Support, and Spontaneity. The Relationship dimensions on the WES are Involvement, Staff Support, and Peer Cohesion. Involvement in a treatment program refers to the degree of activity and energy displayed by patients in the day-to-day functioning of the program. Involvement in a work milieu refers to the workers' concern with and commitment to their jobs. Support in a treatment program indicates the extent to which patients are encouraged to be helpful and supportive toward other patients and how supportive staff are toward patients. Staff support in a work milieu designates the extent to which management is supportive of workers and encourages workers to support one another. The subscales of Involvement and Support are roughly equivalent in both settings; however, a Peer Cohesion dimension quite separate from staff support emerges in the work milieu. In treatment programs Staff Support and Peer Support become one dimension, since they are highly related. Yet in a work setting they are relatively independent, reflecting the existence of two more or less separate subcultures—workers and supervisors. Furthermore, the dimension of Spontaneity, which is identified in treatment or therapeutic environments, does not appear as a separate dimension in work milieus.

In the Personal Development category, both treatment programs and work milieus have two dimensions in common—Autonomy and Practical or Task Orientation. Autonomy in a treatment program involves the independence and self-sufficiency encouraged in patients on such matters as making their own decisions. In a work milieu these issues are similar in that they are related to personal growth and independence (e.g., can employees use their own initiatives? are employees encouraged to learn more than one job?). Practical Orientation in a treatment program assesses the extent to which the patient's environment orients him toward preparing himself for release from the hospital. Such factors as training for new jobs and setting and working toward concrete goals are considered. In a work milieu, the component of Task Orientation measures the emphasis an environment places on good planning and efficiency and encouraging workers to "get the job done."

In terms of System Maintenance dimensions, both treatment programs and work milieus have dimensions of Clarity and Control. Clarity serves to ascertain how accurately patients and workers are aware of what to expect in their daily routines and how explicitly rules and policies are communicated. Control refers to the extent to which staff or supervisors use restrictive measures to keep patients or workers within necessary limits.

The foregoing example should convey the similarity of the threads in the fabrics of remotely related environments. The importance of this analysis appears more clearly if we imagine a patient who is discharged from a treatment program and gains employment in a particular work milieu. We are currently engaged in research and clinical work to determine whether diagnostic workups and predictions of behavior from one setting to another might benefit from this approach (Insel and Moos, 1974).

Other Indices of Perceived Climate

Since the nine Social Climate Scales just discussed were developed in our Social Ecology Laboratory, we were anxious to determine the adequacy of the three categories of dimensions in accounting for the organizational climate dimensions identified in other standard perceived climate scales. The results of eight investigators were utilized, as summarized in Table 14.2, which lists the subscales for several other scales. The overall conceptualization holds equally well for scales developed by other investigators and for our own. For example, the College and University Environment Scale (Pace, 1969) has five subscales:

1.   Community describes a friendly, cohesive, group-oriented campus and is clearly a Relationship dimension.
2.   Awareness describes an emphasis on personal, poetic, and political meaning and on self-understanding and reflectiveness; it is a Personal Development dimension.
3.   Scholarship, which describes an environment characterized by intellectuality, scholastic discipline, and academic achievement, is also a Personal Development dimension.
4.   Propriety describes a polite, considerate, mannerly, proper, and conventional environment in which group standards of decorum are important. Insofar as this dimension emphasizes order and organization and clarity within the environment, it belongs in the System Maintenance category.
5.   Practicality describes an environment characterized by organization, enterprise, material benefits, and social activities. Insofar as orderly supervision in the administration and in class work is its central aspect, this dimension also belongs in the System Maintenance category.

The second test reviewed—the Institutional Functioning Inventory (Peterson et al., 1970)—also provides dimensions for representing a college or university in terms of a number of characteristics judged to be of importance in American higher education. There are 11 dimensions, which appear in Table 14.2 separated into their appropriate categories. Institutional Esprit is certainly a Relationship dimension, whereas Freedom (lack of restraint on academic or personal life), Democratic Governance (extent of opportunity for participation in decision making), Self-Study and Planning (emphasis on continuous long-range planning for the total institution), Concern for Innovation (commitment to experimentation with new ideas for educational practice), and Human Diversity (heterogeneity of faculty and student body in background and attitudes) are quite clearly System Maintenance and System Change dimensions. The emphasis of these dimensions is mainly on system change, which tends to be more strongly prevalent in most university environments than is system maintenance. The other five dimensions, which belong in the Personal Development category, are as follows: Intellectual–Esthetic Extracurriculum (availability of activities and opportunities for intellectual and esthetic stimulation outside the classroom), Concern for Improvement of Society, Concern for Undergraduate Learning, Concern for Advancing Knowledge, and Meeting Local Needs (emphasis on providing educational and cultural opportunities for adults in the surrounding area). Table 14.2 also lists the subscale titles for two other organizational climate scales relevant to educational environments—the Learning Environment Inventory (Walberg, 1969) and the Organizational Climate Description Questionnaire (Halpin and Croft, 1963). The dimensions identified in these two scales clearly fall into our three major categories.

Table 14.2 also gives the subscales emerging from two questionnaires constructed for industrial environments—the Agency Climate Questionnaire (Schneider and Bartlett, 1970) and the Climate Questionnaire (Litwin and Stringer, 1968). The similarity between the dimensions identified in these scales and our own conceptualization is striking. For example, the ACQ has dimensions labeled as follows: (1) Managerial Support (managers take an active interest in agents as individuals), (2) Managerial Structure (managers require that agents strictly adhere to budgets), and (3) Agent Independence (agents receive an accurate picture of job potential when they are contacted, etc.). Some of the Litwin and Stringer dimensions are defined as follows: (1) Warmth (the feeling of general good fellowship that prevails in the work group atmosphere), (2) Support (the perceived helpfulness of the managers and other employees in the group), (3) Identity (the feeling that the employee belongs to the company and is a valuable member of the working team), (4) Responsibility (the feeling of being one's own boss and not having to double check all one's decisions, (5) Risk (the sense of riskiness and challenge in the job and in the organization), and (6) Structure (the feeling that the employees have about the constraints of the group, of rules, of regulations, etc.). The dimensions on these two scales developed for industrial organizations are very similar to those we have identified in very different environments.

Another example is provided by an assessment of the dimensions of group process conducted by Fairweather et al. (1969) in a comparison of a ward-based program and a community-based psychiatric treatment program. Fairweather et al. found three basic types of dimensions

TABLE 14.2 DIMENSIONS OF ORGANIZATIONAL CLIMATE SCALES

	Dimensions		
Instrument	Relationship	Personal Development	System Maintenance and System Change
College and University Environment Scale	Community	Awareness Scholarship	Practicality Propriety
Institutional Functioning Inventory	Institutional Esprit	Intellectual–Esthetic Extracurriculum Concern for Improvement of Society Concern for Undergraduate learning Concern for Advancing knowledge Meeting Local Needs	Freedom Democratic Governance Self-Study and Planning Concern for Innovation Human Diversity
Learning Environment Inventory	Intimacy Friction Cliquishness Apathy Favoritism	Difficulty Speed	Formality Goal Direction Democratic Disorganization Environment Diversity

Instrument			
Organizational Climate Description Questionnaire	Esprit Intimacy Consideration Disengagement	Thrust Hindrance	Production Emphasis Aloofness
Agency Climate Questionnaire	Managerial Support Intraagency Conflict New Employee Concern	Agent Independence	Managerial Structure
Climate Questionnaire	Warmth Support Conflict Identity	Responsibility Risk Standards Reward	Structure
Dimensions of Group Processes	Group Cohesiveness	Group Performance	Leadership and Role Delineation
Organizational Climate Index	Closeness Group Life	Intellectual Climate Personal Dignity Achievement Standards	Orderliness Impulse Control (Constraint)

characterizing group processes and labeled these dimensions (1) group cohesiveness (cohesiveness, morale, attraction to group, satisfaction with leader, etc.), (2) group performance (performance, reward, problem input, information input, etc.), and (3) leadership and role delineation (leadership, role clarity, etc.). These three types of dimensions are essentially identical to those derived by us.

In results that are based on both educational and industrial environments Stern (1970, pp. 68–70) has named six major types of dimensions based on extensive research with the Organizational Climate Index (OCI). The first two factor dimensions—Closeness and Group Life—appear to us to be Relationship dimensions. Three of Stern's dimensions seem to reflect Personal Development (as distinct from the basic types of relating that occur in the environment); these are called Intellectual Climate, Personal Dignity, and Achievement Standards. Stern's last two factors—Orderliness and Impulse Control or Constraint—are System Maintenance factors. Thus Stern's conceptualization is similar to our own, although Stern does not make a distinction between Relationship dimensions and Personal Development dimensions. He also does not include System Change dimensions in his category of Control or System Maintenance press.

This independent formulation, which is based on replicated factor analytic results, strongly supports the notion that only a limited number of relatively commensurate dimensions can characterize a broad diversity of social settings. The conceptual advantage of distinguishing between Relationship and Personal Development dimensions is that Relationship dimensions are extremely similar across environments, whereas Personal Development dimensions vary according to the overall purposes and goals of specific institutions. In addition, it seems important to include System Change dimensions because a substantial body of literature indicates that different milieus are differentially innovative and change oriented.

Stern summarizes the results of his second-order factor analyses as follows: "The first of the second-order factors describes a variety of press for facilitating growth and self-enhancement; the other reflects organizational stability and bureaucratic self-maintenance. These tend to confirm the hypothesized distinction drawn earlier between *anabolic* and *catabolic* press" (1970, p. 68). In general, our Relationship and Personal Development dimensions are similar to what Stern calls developmental or anabolic press, and our System Maintenance dimensions resemble what he calls control or catabolic press.

It may be more useful to think of developmental and control press without necessarily linking them to anabolic or catabolic (i.e., self-enhancing or self-destructive) effects. A press can be anabolic or catabolic, or it can have anabolic and catabolic effects simultaneously, depending on the circumstances under which it is utilized and the characteristics of the individuals subjected to it. If an emphasis on autonomy, which is most often clearly developmental and anabolic, is "applied" to the wrong patient or at the wrong time, it may have a catabolic effect. Current knowledge of the differential effects of social environment is not sufficient to sustain heavily value-laden general distinctions such as anabolic versus catabolic.

This distinction, moreover, was not completely substantiated in our work. Although Staff Control was to some extent catabolic, Order and Organization and Program Clarity were largely—but not totally—anabolic. The main effects of the emphasis on Anger and Aggression, which had been regarded by psychiatric staff as a Personal Development Press, were catabolic. Future research must assess the effects of more relationship-oriented, "benevolent" control on individuals in institutions. The evidence on the growth-inhibiting effects of System Maintenance dimensions is as yet unclear, particularly in institutions other than universities.

We have provided a framework within which further research on the effects of human environments can be planned. For example, relevant work in individual and group psychotherapy has focused almost exclusively on what we would call Relationship dimensions (e.g., empathy, warmth, and genuineness). Much of the previous work in group therapy has stressed cohesiveness, a dimension that is analogous to the concept of the "relationship" in individual therapy. Precious little work in either individual or group psychotherapy has been concerned with the measurement or the effects of what we call the Personal Development and System Maintenance dimensions.

Thus three major categories of dimensions are relatively adequate to describe the social environments of a variety of institutions and social groups. Further work is required in this area, and it is possible that additional dimensions will be identified; but the implications for the direct comparison of widely varying social milieus are nonetheless important. The concepts formulated will help investigators to construct additional perceived or organizational climate scales for other environments. At the minimum, we can conclude from this work that dimensions of Relationship, Personal Development, and System Maintenance and System Change must all be assessed if an adequate and reasonably complete picture of an environment is to emerge.

OVERALL IMPLICATIONS AND APPLICATIONS

We provide here an overall perspective on the salient dimensions of the physical and social environment and on the dimensions that influence the development and maintenance of (a) effective adaptation and coping behavior and (b) "social breakdown reactions," including medical and psychiatric symptomatology. The approach supplies some beginning conceptual and theoretical underpinning for community psychology and the community mental health movement. It suggests guidelines for more thorough and complete descriptions of individual clinical cases and overall treatment milieus. It has important implications for facilitating and evaluating social change, particularly in small group living settings. In our work in social ecology, we expand the traditional framework of human ecology to include issues of direct concern to the social and behavioral sciences (i.e., the identification of environmental variables that have impacts on the maintenance of effective and ineffective behaviors).

Our basic conceptualizations of human environments provide a general framework that is applicable to clinical situations, particularly in community-oriented consultation. We are increasingly asked to diagnose and change social settings, in addition to working separately with the individuals in those settings. Sensitivity to a broad range of environmental variables and their probable effects on individuals will help identify the causes of environmental "trouble spots" (e.g., high dropout, high turnover, high sickness or accident rates) and to suggest changes in them. Measures of environments aid in systematically comparing two or more milieus and are essential in evaluating the actual success of programs and social change attempts. Treatment outcome cannot be known specifically without assessing the characteristics of individuals; nor can the outcome of social systems change attempts be ascertained without assessing the characteristics of milieus. As discussed in Chapters 4 and 11, regular feedback about the environmental characteristics of an ongoing social system permits individuals participating in the system to plan, design, effect, and evaluate changes in it.

Eventually, the systematic use of information about relevant treatment and community environments of patients will yield far richer and more meaningful clinical case descriptions. The original Meyerian system included data about biological, psychological, and sociological (i.e., life situation) characteristics for each patient. However, there has never been any way of systematically describing the environments in which people function. Current case descriptions usually contain only general comments about life stress events (e.g., death of a family member, job changes, retirement, major physical illnesses). These descriptions should include at least as much detailed information about a patient's environment as data on his personality and behavior. A specific example is the attempt to determine what properties of the community environments contribute to the drinking problems of certain patients. The frequency with which individual patients encounter "alcoholic stimuli" (e.g., number of bottles of liquor visible in the house, number of social functions attended at which large quantities of alcohol are consumed, whether the spouse of the patient drinks heavily, whether the patient has a number of close friends who drink heavily) is at least as important in predicting drinking behavior as individual background or personality characteristics.

In this connection it should be noted that each of the six major ways in which environments have been characterized has been shown to have a central impact in the determination of various individual and group behaviors. Aggressive and violent behaviors are good examples; for example, Wolfgang (1958) reported homicidal activities peak in the hot summer months. Griffitt (1970) found that interpersonal attraction responses were significantly more negative under a "hot " condition (over 90°) than under a "normal" condition (about 68°). Different types of behavior settings also differentially elicit aggressive or hostile behavior. Gump et al. (1957) observed children in a camp setting and found that assertive, blocking, and attacking behaviors were much higher during swimming, whereas helping reactions are higher during arts and crafts. Raush et al. (1959) found that changes in hostility in hyperaggressive children were setting-specific; for example, one child showed a marked reduction in hostile responses toward adults in a structured group setting, whereas another showed such changes mainly during meal times.

Many organizational structure dimensions have been related to the frequency of aggressive behavior, most notably indices of space and population density (crowding). For example, Swift (1964) concluded that conflicts between children are more numerous when play space is restricted. Other studies have revealed correlations between high population density areas and high crime rates for juveniles and adults (Schmid, 1960). In terms of the personal and behavioral characteristics of the inhabitants of the milieu, perhaps the most relevant example is that of the "interpersonal reflex" (Leary, 1957) or "behavioral reciprocity." Aggression begets aggression, and the proportion of hostile actions that are "sent" by an individual often parallels the proportion he "receives." For example, Purcell and Brady (1964) found that the interpersonal response of affection was preceded by the interpersonal stimulus of affection 80% of the time and by the interpersonal stimulus of aggression 0% of the time. According to the results of Couch (1970), knowledge of the immediately preceding interpersonal stimulus is a better predictor of interpersonal hostility than a combination of personality need and ego defense variables. These findings should give significant pause to anyone who attempts to make predictions from personality needs alone.

There have been many demonstrations of social climate and reinforcement effects on aggression, particularly in groups and families. Lewin et al. (1939) found that the same group may change markedly (from apathy to aggression, or vice versa) when it acquired a new leadership atmosphere under a different chief. Milgram (1964) has shown that subjects who are not usually aggressive can be made to behave very aggressively under experimenter and group pressure encouragement. Thus the evidence indicates that ecological variables, behavior settings, dimensions of organizational structure, behavioral characteristics of milieu inhabitants, social and organizational climates and reinforcement variables have important impacts on various indices of aggressive and violent behavior.

Similar analyses can be carried out, and similar conclusions probably would hold for most other clinically relevant behaviors. This analysis in no way minimizes the importance of individual dispositions, since it is clinically obvious that some individuals are more prone to express certain behaviors (including aggressive and violent behaviors) than others. In addition, individual dispositions may have their effects in interaction with environmental conditions. On the other hand, the significance of this work on the development of taxonomies of environmental variables can hardly be overemphasized, especially in its implications for behavior prediction and behavior change. Knowledge of the probable behavioral and attitudinal effects of different environmental arrangements is at least as central an issue for understanding behavior as is knowledge about traditional personality theory and psychotherapy.

As we pointed out earlier, the categorization of environmental dimensions into six broad types may or may not have general utility. The categories are overlapping, and certain variables can as easily be placed into one category as another. Nevertheless, our framework serves to identify some initial directions for an overall organization of this field. Our example of aggression and violence illustrates the potential clinical relevance of a coherent set of concepts regarding environmental and stimulus variables. That is, this framework is of central relevance, not only for aggression but for the entire range of behaviors with which mental health professionals must deal.

In the broadest perspective, environmental and stimulus variables appear to reduce and shape the potential variability in human behavior. In this sense our six major types of dimensions are interrelated. The geographical and meteorological environment contributes to the form of the environment of architecture and physical design, which has demonstrable effects on the types of behavior settings. Behavior settings, in turn, constrain the potential range of organizational structure, methods of institutional functioning, and the personal and behavioral characteristics of individuals who choose to inhabit the behavior settings. Next the behavior settings, organizational structures, and sets of milieu inhabitants themselves give rise to different psychosocial characteristics and organizational climates. Finally, any of the foregoing types of variables may affect the reinforcements that are likely to occur in a specific setting. Decisions about specific valued reinforcements may then, in a feedback loop, affect the resulting geographical and architectural environment. Any of these levels of environmental variables may be influenced by any other level, although some levels (e.g., personal characteristics of milieu inhabitants and organizational climates) may be more closely related than others (e.g., geographical variables and organizational structure).

As we pointed out in Chapter 11, the six types of environmental dimensions also provide guidelines for compiling program descriptions. Each method of environmental description gives a different perspective on a treatment program, and the use of all six should enhance the accuracy and completeness of program descriptions. The dimensions are clearly useful for constructing complete descriptions of other social environments (e.g., university living groups and junior high and high school classrooms). A more detailed knowledge of the components of social systems should improve the matching of individuals with environmental settings that meet their needs, hence facilitate personal growth.

It is well established that social milieus have important physiological and "health-related" effects (Cobb et al., 1963; Mason, 1968). A systematic conceptualization of environments makes it possible to test more differentiated hypotheses about the effects of specific environmental dimensions on given physiological indices (Kiritz and Moos, 1973). The potential importance of this area is indicated by Caffrey's observation (1969) that the incidence of coronaries varies both among environments and among individuals, as well as the finding by Klerman et al. (1969) that the same psychopharmacological agent may have different therapeutic effects in different treatment settings. Genetic and developmental studies also require more differentiated information about environmental characteristics. The observation that home environments of individuals with certain chromosomal abnormalities are or are not "disharmonic" (e.g., Nielsen, 1970) simply does not prove anything and is no longer sufficient.

Even though it is not yet clear how levels of environmental description will eventually relate to one another, we realize that all are directly relevant to the central tasks of the behavioral sciences. Psychologists and behavioral scientists are being asked to help design physical and social systems capable of maximizing the probabilities of human growth and facilitating effective functioning and excellence. We need information about the common task requirements for effective functioning in different milieus. We know that different environments may facilitate different preparatory activities for coping in new environments, thus that cultural and social groups obtain differential preparation for environmental transitions. We need to identify the behaviors related to survival, learning, and adaptation in different social systems, as well as the environmental factors related to the ability to withstand stress effectively.

Since we know that disorders of human functioning are at least partly rooted in social systems, research toward effective modification of institutions to promote constructive handling of life stresses must have high priority. Bergin (1966) has suggested that we actively study the naturally occurring therapeutic conditions in society. Anastasi (1967) has added the important point that environments must not be ordered along a simple favorable–unfavorable continuum because, for example, an environment favoring the development of independence and self-reliance may differ significantly from one favoring the development of social conformity or abstract thinking. We cannot obtain definitive information on any of these areas without learning more about the dimensions of social and physical environments and about the types of initiatives, adaptive behaviors, and preparatory and coping mechanisms that are likely to be successful in each.

Our central tasks of understanding, predicting, and changing behavior compel us to learn more about environmental dimensions and to formulate valid concepts about them. The optimal arrangement of environments is probably the most powerful behavior modification technique we currently have available. Social and behavioral scientists are now asked to consult on the probable behavioral and attitudinal effects of environmental changes, precisely because human beings can now control and change their environments. Each institution in our society is attempting to set up conditions for the maximization of certain types of behaviors and/or certain directions of development. Families, hospitals, prisons, business organizations, secondary schools, universities, communes, and various other groups arrange selected environmental conditions that, presumably, maximize certain effects. There is of course the greatest disagreement about the effects that should be maximized and about which conditions maximize them. In this sense it can be cogently argued that our most important task is the systematic description and classification of environments and their differential costs and benefits to adaptation.

The field of social ecology, although currently somewhat vague and undifferentiated, presents a developing multidisciplinary focus around which clinical psychologists and psychiatrists, with their detailed knowledge of human adaptation and coping skills, can fruitfully interact with other social science professionals who are primarily concerned with formulating and constructing new environments. The potential for radically altering day-to-day clinical practice over the next decade or two is much greater than we now realize.

REFERENCES

Anastasi, A. Psychology, psychologists, and psychological testing. *American Psychologist,* **22**:297–306, 1967.

Bergin, A. Some implications of psychotherapy research for therapeutic practice. *Journal of Abnormal Psychology,* **71**:235–246, 1966.

Caffrey, B. Behavior patterns and personality characteristics related to prevalence of coronary heart disease in American monks. *Journal of Chronic Diseases,* **22**: 93–103, 1969.

Cobb, S., French, J., Kahn, R., & Mann, F. An environmental approach to mental health. *Annals of the New York Academy of Sciences,* **107**:596–606, 1963.

Couch, A. The psychological determinants of interpersonal behavior. In Gergen, K. & Marlowe, D. (Eds). *Personality and social behavior,* Addison-Wesley, Reading, Mass., 1970.

Fairweather, G., Sanders, D., Cressler, D., & Maynard, H. *Community life for the mentally ill,* Aldine, Chicago, 1969.

Griffitt, W. Environmental effects on interpersonal affective behavior: Ambient effective temperature and attraction. *Journal of Personality and Social Psychology*, **15**: 240–244, 1970.

Gump, P., Schoggen, P., & Redl, F. The camp milieu and its immediate effects. *Journal of Social Issues*, **13** : 40–46, 1957.

Halpin, A. & Croft, D. *The organizational climate of schools*. Midwest Administration Center, University of Chicago, Chicago, 1963.

Insel, P. & Moos, R. The Work Environment Scale. Social Ecology Laboratory, Department of Psychiatry, Stanford University, Palo Alto, Calif., 1972.

Insel, P. and Moos, R. Psychological environments: Expanding the scope of human ecology. *American Psychologist*, in press, 1974.

Jesness, C., DeResi, W., McCormick, P., & Wedge, R. *The Youth Center research project*. American Justice Institute and California Youth Authority, Sacramento, Calif., 1972.

Kiritz, S. & Moos, R. Physiological effects of social environments. *Psychosomatic Medicine*, in press, 1973.

Klerman, G., Goldberg, S. & Davis, D. Relationship between the hospital milieu and the response to phenothiazines in the treatment of schizophrenics, Paper presented at Semaine Interdisciplinaire des Neuroleptiques, Liege, Belgium, May 11–16, 1969.

Leary, T. *Interpersonal diagnosis of personality*. Ronald Press, New York, 1957.

Lewin, K., Lippitt, R., & White, R. Patterns of aggressive behavior in experimentally created "social climates." *Journal of Social Psychology*, **10**: 271–299, 1939.

Litwin, G., & Stringer, R. Motivation and organizational climate. Division of Research, Harvard Business School, Cambridge, Mass., 1968.

Mason, J. A review of psychoendocrine research on the pituitary-adrenal cortical system. *Psychosomatic Medicine*, **30**:576–607, 1968.

Milgram, S. Group pressure and action against a person. *Journal of Abnormal and Social Psychology*, **69**: 137–143, 1964.

Moos, R. The assessment of the social climates of correctional institutions. *Journal of Research in Crime and Delinquency*, **5**: 174–188, 1968.

Moos, R. Differential effects of social climates of correctional institutions. *Journal of Crime and Delinquency*, **7**: 71–82, 1970.

Moos, R. *Military Company Environment Inventory Manual*. Social Ecology Laboratory, Department of Psychiatry, Stanford University, Palo Alto, Calif., 1973a.

Moos, R. *Family Environment Scale Preliminary Manual*. Social Ecology Laboratory, Department of Psychiatry, Stanford University, Palo Alto, Calif., 1973b.

Moos, R. *Correctional Institutions Environment Scale Manual*. Consulting Psychologists Press, Palo Alto, Calif., 1974.

Moos, R. and Gerst, M. University Residence Environment Scale Manual. Consulting Psychologists Press, Palo Alto, Calif., 1974.

Moos, R. & Humphrey, B. *Group Environment Scale Technical Report*. Social Ecology Laboratory, Department of Psychiatry, Stanford University, Palo Alto, Calif., 1973.

Moos, R. and Trickett, E. Classroom Environment Scale Manual. Consulting Psychologists Press, Palo Alto, Calif., 1974.

Nielsen, J. Criminality among patients with Kleinfelter's Syndrome and XYY Syndrome. *British Journal of Psychiatry*, **117**: 365–369, 1970.

Pace, R. *College and University Environment Scale, Technical manual*, 2nd ed. Educational Testing Service, Princeton, N.J., 1969.

Peterson, R., Centra, J., Hartnett, R., & Linn, R. *Institutional Functioning Inventory, Preliminary technical manual*, Educational Testing Service, Princeton, N.J., 1970.

Purcell, K. & Brady, D. *Assessment of interpersonal behavior in natural settings*. Final Progress Report, Childrens' Asthma Research Institute and Hospital, Denver, Colorado, 1964.

Schneider, B. & Bartlett, C. Individual differences and organizational climate. II. Measurement of organizational climate by the multi-trait, multi-rater matrix. *Personnel Psychology*, **23**: 493–512, 1970.

Raush, H., Dittman, A., & Taylor, T. Person, setting, and change in social interaction. *Human Relations*, **12**: 361–378, 1959.

Schmid, C. Urban crime areas. *American Sociological Review*, **25**: 527, 542, 655–678, 1960.

Stern, G. *People in context: Measuring person environment congruence in education and industry*. Wiley, New York, 1970.

Swift, J. W. Effects of early group experience: The nursery school and day nursery. In Hoffman, M. & Hoffman, L. (Eds.). *Child development research*, Vol. 1, Russell Sage Foundation, New York, 1964.

Walberg, H. Social environment as a mediator of classroom learning. *Journal of Educational Psychology*, **60**: 443–448, 1969.

Wolfgang, M. *Patterns in criminal homicide*. University of Pennsylvania Press, Philadelphia, 1958.

REFERENCES   390

WARD ATMOSPHERE SCALE
SCORING KEY

Below is the scoring key for the subscales of the different forms of the Ward Atmosphere Scale. The Real Ward, Ideal Ward, and Expectation forms are directly parallel, and all items are scored in the same direction on all three forms. The 40 items included in the Short Form are marked with an asterisk. An item listed as "true" (T) is scored 1 point if marked "true" by the individual taking the scale, and an item listed as "false" (F) is scored 1 point if marked "false." The total subscale score is simply the number of items answered in the scored direction.

The Ward Atmosphere Scale and Manual have been published and are available for interested users (Moos, 1974a). Users should note that some changes have been made in the WAS, as presented in this Manual, to facilitate its general utility. *(a)* One item (No. 93, unscored) was added to make the WAS an even 100 items. *(b)* Two items were dropped from the Involvement subscale in order to reduce it to 10 items. These two items (96 and 97) remain in the WAS, but are not scored on the regular 10 subscales. Item 96 is scored on The Dropout Scale and item 97 is scored on The Community Tenure Scale. *(c)* The items were reordered both to facilitate hand-scoring and to make the first 40 items the Short Form (Form S) items. *(d)* Form C, used to describe the current or "Real" ward, is called Form R in the Manual.

Involvement

Real, Ideal, and Expectation Form Item Number	Scoring Direction	
1*	T	Patients put a lot of energy into what they do around here.
11*	T	This is a lively ward.
21*	T	The patients are proud of this ward.
31*	F	There is very little group spirit on this ward.
41	F	Nobody ever volunteers around here.
51	T	Patients are pretty busy all of the time.
61	F	The ward has very few social activities.
71	F	Very few things around here ever get people excited.
81	T	Discussions are pretty interesting on this ward.
91	T	Patients often do things together on the weekends.

Support

Real, Ideal, and Expectation Form Item Number	Scoring Direction	
2*	F	Doctors have very little time to encourage patients.
12*	T	The staff know what the patients want.
22*	T	Staff are interested in following up patients once they leave the hospital.
32*	F	Nurses have very little time to encourage patients.
42	F	Doctors spend more time with some patients than with others.
52	T	The healthier patients on this ward help take care of the less healthy ones.
62	F	Patients rarely help each other.
72	T	The ward staff help new patients get acquainted on the ward.
82	F	Doctors sometimes don't show up for their appointments.
92	T	Staff go out of their way to help patients.

Spontaneity

Real, Ideal, and Expectation Form Item Number	Scoring Direction	
3*	F	Patients tend to hide their feelings from one another.
13*	T	Patients say anything they want to the doctors.
23*	F	It is hard to tell how patients are feeling on this ward.
33*	F	Patients are careful about what they say when staff are around.
43	T	Patients set up their own activities without being prodded by the staff.
53	F	When patients disagree with each other, they keep it to themselves.
63	T	It's o.k. to act crazy around here.
73	F	Patients tend to hide their feelings from the staff.
83	T	Patients are encouraged to show their feelings.
93	(Filler item)	The ward always stays just about the same.

Autonomy

Real, Ideal, and Expectation Form Item Number	Scoring Direction	
4*	T	The staff act on patient suggestions.
14*	F	Very few patients have any responsibility on the ward.
24*	T	Patients are expected to take leadership on the ward.
34*	T	Patients here are encouraged to be independent.
44	T	Patients can leave the ward whenever they want to.
54	T	Patients can wear what they want.
64	F	There is no patient government on this ward.
74	T	Patients can leave the ward without saying where they are going.
84	F	Staff rarely give in to patient pressure.
94	F	The staff discourage criticism.

Practical Orientation

Real, Ideal, and Expectation Form Item Number	Scoring Direction	
5*	T	New treatment approaches are often tried on this ward.
15*	F	There is very little emphasis on making patients more practical.
25*	T	Patients are encouraged to plan for the future.
35*	F	There is very little emphasis on what patients will be doing after they leave.
45	F	There is very little emphasis on making plans for getting out of the hospital.
55	T	This ward emphasizes training for new kinds of jobs.
65	F	Most patients are more concerned with the past than with the future.
75	T	Patients are encouraged to learn new ways of doing things.
85	F	Staff care more about how patients feel than about their practical problems.
95	T	Patients must make plans before leaving the hospital.

Personal Problem Orientation

Real, Ideal, and Expectation Form Item Number	Scoring Direction	
6*	F	Patients hardly ever discuss their sexual lives.
16*	T	Patients tell each other about their personal problems.
26*	T	Personal problems are openly talked about.
36*	T	Patients are expected to share their personal problems with each other.
46	F	Patients talk very little about their pasts.
56	F	Patients are rarely asked personal questions by the staff.
66	T	Staff are mainly interested in learning about patients' feelings.
76	F	The patients rarely talk about their personal problems with other patients.
86	T	Staff strongly encourage patients to talk about their pasts.
96	(Filler item)	It's hard to get a group together for card games or other activities.

Anger and Aggression

Real, Ideal, and Expectation Form Item Number	Scoring Direction	
7*	T	Patients often gripe.
17*	T	Patients often criticize or joke about the ward staff.
27*	F	Patients on this ward rarely argue.
37*	T	Staff sometimes argue with each other.
47	T	Patients sometimes play practical jokes on each other.
57	F	It's hard to get people to argue around here.
67	F	Staff never start arguments in group meetings.
77	T	On this ward staff think it is a healthy thing to argue.
87	F	Patients here rarely become angry.
97	(Filler item)	A lot of patients just seem to be passing time on the ward.

Order and Organization

Real, Ideal, and Expectation Form Item Number	Scoring Direction	
8*	T	Patients' activities are carefully planned.
18*	T	This is a very well organized ward.
28*	T	The staff make sure that the ward is always neat.
38*	F	The ward sometimes gets very messy.
48	T	Most patients follow a regular schedule each day.
58	F	Many patients look messy.
68	F	Things are sometimes very disorganized around here.
78	T	The staff set an example for neatness and orderliness.
88	T	Patients are rarely kept waiting when they have appointments with the staff.
98	F	The day room is often messy.

Program Clarity

Real, Ideal, and Expectation Form Item Number	Scoring Direction	
9*	T	The patients know when doctors will be on the ward.
19*	F	Doctors don't explain what treatment is about to patients.
29*	T	If a patient's medicine is changed, a nurse or doctor always tells him why.
39*	T	Ward rules are clearly understood by the patients.
49	F	Patients never know when a doctor will ask to see them.
59	T	On this ward everyone knows who's in charge.
69	T	If a patient breaks a rule, he knows what will happen to him.
79	F	People are always changing their minds here.
89	F	Patients never know when they will be transferred from this ward.
99	T	Staff tell patients when they are getting better.

Staff Control

Real, Ideal, and Expectation Form Item Number	Scoring Direction	
10*	F	The staff very rarely punish patients by restricting them.
20*	F	Patients may interrupt a doctor when he is talking.
30*	T	Patients who break the ward rules are punished for it.
40*	T	If a patient argues with another patient, he will get into trouble with the staff.
50	F	Staff don't order the patients around.
60	T	Once a schedule is arranged for a patient, the patient must follow it.
70	F	Patients can call nursing staff by their first name.
80	T	Patients will be transferred from this ward if they don't obey the rules.
90	T	It's not safe for patients to discuss their personal problems around here.
100	T	It's a good idea to let the doctor know that he is boss.

Appendix B

COMMUNITY-ORIENTED PROGRAMS ENVIRONMENT SCALE SCORING KEY

Below is the scoring key for the subscales of the different forms of the Community-Oriented Programs Environment Scale. The Real program, Ideal program, and Expectation forms are directly parallel, and all items are scored in the same direction on all three forms. The 40 items included in the Short Form are marked with an asterisk. An item listed as "true" (T) is scored 1 point is marked "true" by the individual taking the scale, and an item listed as "false" (F) is scored 1 point is marked "false." The total subscale score is simply the number of items answered in the scored direction.

The Community-Oriented Programs Environment Scale and Manual have been published and are available for interested users (Moos, 1974b). Users should note that some changes have been made in the COPES, as presented in this Manual, to facilitate its general utility. *(a)* Two items were dropped from the Involvement subscale to reduce COPES to an even 100 items. *(b)* The items were reordered both to facilitate hand-scoring and to make the first 40 items the Short Form (Form S) items. *(c)* Form C, used to describe the current or "Real" program, is called Form R in the Manual.

Involvement

Real, Ideal, and Expectation Form Item Number	Scoring Direction	
1*	T	Members put a lot of energy into what they do around here.
11*	T	This is a lively place.
21*	T	The members are proud of this program.
31*	F	There is very little group spirit in this program.
41	F	Very few members ever volunteer around here.
51	F	A lot of members just seem to be passing time here.
61	F	This program has very few social activities.
71	T	Members are pretty busy all of the time.
81	T	Discussions are very interesting here.
91	T	Members often do things together on weekends.

Support

Real, Ideal, and Expectation Form Item Number	Scoring Direction	
2*	T	The healthier members here help take care of the less healthy ones.
12*	F	Staff have relatively little time to encourage members.
22*	F	Members seldom help each other.
32*	T	Staff are very interested in following up members once they leave the program.
42	T	Staff always compliment a member who does something well.
52	T	The staff know what the members want.
62	F	Staff sometimes don't show up for their appointments with members.
72	F	There is relatively little sharing among the members.
82	T	Members are given a great deal of individual attention here.
92	T	The staff go out of their way to help new members get acquainted here.

Spontaneity

Real, Ideal, and Expectation Form Item Number	Scoring Direction	
3*	F	Members tend to hide their feelings from one another.
13*	T	Members say anything they want to the staff.
23*	F	It is hard to tell how members are feeling here.
33*	F	Members are careful about what they say when staff are around.
43	T	Members are strongly encouraged to express themselves freely here.
53	T	Members spontaneously set up their own activities here.
63	F	When members disagree with each other, they keep it to themselves.
73	T	Members can generally do whatever they feel like here.
83	F	Members tend to hide their feelings from the staff.
93	T	Members are strongly encouraged to express their feelings.

Autonomy

Real, Ideal, and Expectation Form Item Number	Scoring Direction	
4*	F	There is no membership government in this program.
14*	T	Members can leave here anytime without saying where they are going.
24*	T	Members are expected to take leadership here.
34*	F	The staff tend to discourage criticism from members.
44	T	Members can leave the program whenever they want to.
54	T	Members can wear whatever they want.
64	T	The staff almost always act on members' suggestions.
74	F	Very few members have any responsibility for the program here.
84	T	Members here are very strongly encouraged to be independent.
94	F	Staff rarely give in to pressure from members.

Practical Orientation

Real, Ideal, and Expectation Form Item Number	Scoring Direction	
5*	T	This program emphasizes training for new kinds of jobs.
15*	F	There is relatively little emphasis on teaching members solutions to practical problems.
25*	T	Members are expected to make detailed specific plans for the future.
35*	F	There is relatively little discussion about exactly what members will be doing after they leave the program.
45	F	There is relatively little emphasis on making specific plans for leaving this program.
55	F	Most members are more concerned with the past than with the future.
65	T	Members here are expected to demonstrate continued concrete progress toward their goals.
75	T	Members are taught specific new skills in this program.
85	F	Staff care more about how members feel than about their practical problems.
95	T	Members must make detailed plans before leaving the program.

Personal Problem Orientation

Real, Ideal, and Expectation Form Item Number	Scoring Direction	
6*	F	Members hardly ever discuss their sexual lives.
16*	T	Personal problems are openly talked about.
26*	F	Members are rarely asked personal questions by the staff.
36*	T	Members are expected to share their personal problems with each other.
46	F	Members talk relatively little about their past.
56	T	Members tell each other about their intimate personal problems.
66	T	Staff are mainly interested in learning about members' feelings.
76	F	The members rarely talk with each other about their personal problems.
86	F	Members are rarely encouraged to discuss their personal problems here.
96	T	Staff strongly encourage members to talk about their past.

Anger and Aggression

Real, Ideal, and Expectation Form Item Number	Scoring Direction	
7*	F	It's hard to get people to argue around here.
17*	T	Members often criticize or joke about the staff.
27*	F	Members here rarely argue.
37*	T	Staff sometimes argue openly with each other.
47	T	Members sometimes play practical jokes on each other.
57	T	Staff encourage members to express their anger openly here.
67	F	Staff here never start arguments.
77	T	Members often gripe.
87	T	Staff here think it is a healthy thing to argue.
97	F	Members here rarely become angry.

Order and Organization

Real, Ideal, and Expectation Form Item Number	Scoring Direction	
8*	T	Members' activities are carefully planned.
18*	T	This is a very well organized program.
28*	T	The staff make sure that this place is always neat.
38*	F	This place usually looks a little messy.
48	T	Members here follow a regular schedule every day.
58	F	Some members look messy.
68	F	Things are sometimes very disorganized around here.
78	F	The dayroom or living room is often untidy.
88	T	Members are rarely kept waiting when they have appointments with staff.
98	T	The staff strongly encourage members to be neat and orderly here.

Clarity

Real, Ideal, and Expectation Form Item Number	Scoring Direction	
9*	T	If a member breaks a rule, he knows what the consequences will be.
19*	T	If a member's program is changed, staff always tell him why.
29*	F	Staff rarely give members a detailed explanation of what the program is about.
39*	T	The program rules are clearly understood by the members.
49	F	Members never know when staff will ask to see them.
59	T	The members always know when the staff will be around.
69	T	Everyone knows who's in charge here.
79	F	People are always changing their minds here.
89	F	Members never quite know when they will be considered ready to leave the program.
99	F	There are often changes in the rules here.

Staff Control

Real, Ideal, and Expectation Form Item Number	Scoring Direction	
10*	T	Once a schedule is arranged for a member, the member must follow it.
20*	F	The staff very rarely punish members by taking away their privileges.
30*	T	Members who break the rules are punished for it.
40*	T	If a member fights with another member, he will get into real trouble with the staff.
50	F	Staff don't order the members around.
60	T	It is important to carefully follow the program rules here.
70	F	Members can call staff by their first names.
80	F	Members may interrupt staff when they are talking.
90	T	Members will be transferred or discharged from this program if they don't obey the rules.
100	T	The staff make and enforce all the rules here.

REFERENCES

Moos, R.   *Ward Atmosphere Scale Manual,* Palo Alto: Consulting Psychologists Press, 1974a.

Moos, R.   *Community-Oriented Programs Environment Scale Manual,* Palo Alto, Consulting Psychologists Press, 1974b.

Author Index

Subject Index